Teaching and Learning in a Concept-Based Nursing Curriculum

A How-To Best Practice Approach

Donna D. Ignatavicius, MS, RN, CNE, ANEF
President
DI Associates, Inc.

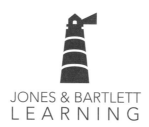

JONES & BARTLETT
L E A R N I N G

World Headquarters
Jones & Bartlett Learning
5 Wall Street
Burlington, MA 01803
978-443-5000
info@jblearning.com
www.jblearning.com

Jones & Bartlett Learning books and products are available through most bookstores and online booksellers. To contact Jones & Bartlett Learning directly, call 800-832-0034, fax 978-443-8000, or visit our website, www.jblearning.com.

Production Credits
VP, Executive Publisher: David D. Cella
Executive Editor: Amanda Martin
Acquisitions Editor: Rebecca Stephenson
Editorial Assistant: Christina Freitas
Senior Vendor Manager: Sara Kelly
Senior Marketing Manager: Jennifer Scherzay
Product Fulfillment Manager: Wendy Kilborn
Composition and Project Management: S4Carlisle
 Publishing Services
Cover Design: Kristin E. Parker
Rights & Media Specialist: Robert Boder
Media Development Editor: Shannon Sheehan
Cover Image (Title Page, Part Opener, Chapter Opener):
 ©aleksandarvelasevic/DigitalVision Vectors/Getty
Printing and Binding: Edwards Brothers Malloy
Cover Printing: Edwards Brothers Malloy

Library of Congress Cataloging-in-Publication Data
Names: Ignatavicius, Donna D., author.
Title: Teaching and learning in a concept-based nursing curriculum : a how-to
 best practice approach / by Donna Ignatavicius.
Description: First edition. | Burlington, Massachusetts : Jones & Bartlett
 Learning, [2018] | Includes bibliographical references and index.
Identifiers: LCCN 2017021577 | ISBN 9781284127362 (pbk. : alk. paper)
Subjects: | MESH: Education, Nursing--methods | Curriculum | Teaching |
 Nursing Evaluation Research--methods
Classification: LCC RT73 | NLM WY 18 | DDC 610.73071/1--dc23 LC record available at https://lccn.loc.gov/2017021577

6048

Printed in the United States of America
21 20 19 18 17   10 9 8 7 6 5 4 3 2 1

Contents

Preface ix

Contributors xi

Reviewers xii

Acknowledgments xiii

PART I **Introduction to the Concept-Based Curriculum and Conceptual Learning in Nursing Education**   **1**

Chapter 1 Essential Elements of an Effective Nursing Curriculum 3

Introduction to Curriculum 3

Faculty Role in Nursing Curriculum
Development and Revision 4

Role of Nursing Program Accreditation. . . . 6

Components of an Effective Nursing
Curriculum. 6

    Mission and Philosophy 8

    Organizing Curriculum
    Framework 8

    Program Outcomes 10

    Curriculum Models. 12

    Plan of Study and Degree Plan. 13

    Course Development 18

Curriculum Approval
Process 20

Chapter Key Points 20

Chapter References and Selected
Bibliography 21

Chapter 2 Traditional Learning Versus Conceptual Learning 23

Introduction to Teaching and Learning. . . . 23

How Learning Occurs. 25

Characteristics of Traditional Teaching
and Learning 25

Characteristics of a Concept-Based
Curriculum and Conceptual
Teaching/Learning. 26

    Key Building Blocks of the
    Concept-Based Curriculum
    Structure 26

    Meaningful Learning and
    Constructivism 27

    Benefits of the Conceptual
    Learning Approach 28

Chapter Key Points 33

Chapter References and Selected
Bibliography 34

Chapter 3 Developing a Nursing Concept-Based Curriculum: A 12-Step Approach 37

Introduction to the Nursing Concept-
Based Curriculum 37

    Concept-Based Curriculum for
    Prelicensure U.S. Registered
    Nursing Programs 38

Concept-Based Curriculum for
Prelicensure Canadian Registered
Nursing Programs 38

Concept-Based Curriculum for
Prelicensure Practical/Vocational
Nursing Programs 39

Preplanning for Transition from a
Traditional to a Concept-Based
Nursing Curriculum 39

The 12-Step Approach to Concept-Based
Curriculum Development 41

Step 1: Review and Revise the
Nursing Department and
School of Nursing Mission
and Philosophy 42

Step 2: Develop the Organizing
Curriculum Framework 42

Step 3: Establish Program
Outcomes 43

Step 4: Determine the Plan of
Study or Degree Plan 43

Step 5: Select and Define Nursing
Curriculum Concepts 46

Step 6: Select Exemplars for Each
Concept 48

Step 7: Write Course Descriptions
and Student Learning
Outcomes 50

Step 8: Determine Where Each
Concept Will Be Introduced 51

Step 9: Develop a Concept
Presentation for Each
Curriculum Concept 52

Step 10: Determine Where Each
Exemplar Will Be Placed in the
Curriculum .54

Step 11: Develop Each Course
Syllabus and Lesson Plan/
Study Guide 54

Step 12: Select Appropriate
Clinical Experiences and
Activities That Are Conceptually
Focused 55

Chapter Key Points 55

Chapter References and Selected
Bibliography 56

PART II Teaching and Learning in a Concept-Based Nursing Curriculum   57

Chapter 4 Developing Student Learning Outcomes for Conceptual Learning 59

Introduction to Developing Student
Learning Outcomes for Conceptual
Learning 59

Developing Course Student Learning
Outcomes 60

Developing Conceptual Content
Student Learning Outcomes by
Learning Domain 61

Cognitive Domain 61

Psychomotor Domain 63

Affective Domain 65

Measuring Achievement of
Course SLOs 66

Measuring Achievement of
Conceptual Content Student
Learning Outcomes by Learning
Domain 67

Cognitive Domain 68

Psychomotor Domain 69

Affective Domain 70

Chapter Key Points 71

Chapter References and Selected
Bibliography 71

Chapter 5 Teaching and Learning in the Concept-Based Classroom 73

Introduction to Teaching and
Learning in the Concept-Based
Classroom 73

Characteristics of Today's Learners 74

Learning Preferences 75

Thinking Styles 75
Developmental Stage 76
Demographic Characteristics 77
The Role of Collaborative Learning 78
The Flipped Versus Scrambled
Classroom 79
Fostering Clinical Imagination 80
Relationship of Student Learning
Outcomes to Conceptual Learning 81
Selected Strategies and Activities
to Promote Active Conceptual
Learning 81
Pair Discussions 82
Case Studies 83
Graphic Organizers 85
Test Item Checks 86
Send a Problem 87
Collaborative Testing 87
Storytelling. 87
Video Clips and Sounds 90
Gaming 91
Social Media 92
Chapter Key Points 92
Chapter References and Selected
Bibliography 93

Chapter 6 Clinical Teaching and Learning in a Concept-Based Nursing Curriculum 95

Introduction to Clinical Teaching and
Learning in a Concept-Based
Curriculum. 95
The Traditional Model of Clinical
Teaching. 96
Clinical Learning in the Concept-Based
Curriculum. 97
Preparing for Concept-Based Clinical
Experiences. 98
Role of the Clinical Coordinator 99
Role of the Academic-Practice
Liaison 99
Role of the Educational Resource
Unit 100
Mentoring the Clinical Nurse
Educator 100

Connecting Conceptual Clinical
Learning with Classroom, Laboratory,
and Simulation Learning 106
Selecting and Managing a
Concept-Based Curriculum
Clinical Learning Environment 107
Conceptual Clinical Learning Activities
and Assignments 108
Interprofessional Activities
and Assignments 109
Safety-Focused Activities and
Assignments 110
60-Second Assignment. 112
Quality Improvement
Assignments 112
Concept Mapping. 112
Socratic Questioning 114
Peer-to-Peer Interaction 115
Reflections 115
Organizing Conceptual Clinical
Learning Activities and Assignments . 115
Chapter Key Points 122
Chapter References and Selected
Bibliography 123

Chapter 7 Teaching in the Concept-Based Online Learning Environment 125

Introduction to Online Learning 125
Types of Online Learning 126
Methods Used in Designing Online
Learning 126
Netiquette and Communication 127
Online Presence 129
Social Presence. 131
Cognitive Presence. 132
Teaching Presence 132
Learning Management Systems 132
Using Learning Management
System Tools for Classroom
Preparation. 133
Ensuring Course Consistency
Within the LMS 136
Designing and Structuring the
Course 137

Fostering Conceptual Thinking in
Interactive Discussion Forums........137

Delineating the Role of Nurse
Educators in Online Course
Development.......................140

Chapter Key Points 145

Chapter References and Selected
Bibliography 145

Chapter 8 Using Concept Mapping for Conceptual Learning 147

Introduction to Concept Mapping 147

Assimilation Theory as a Basis for
Concept Mapping 148

Terminology Associated with
Developing Concept Maps 149

Use of Concept Mapping in the Concept-
Based Nursing Curriculum 150

Using Concept Maps in a
Prelicensure Nursing Program ..151

Using Concept Maps in a
Graduate Nursing Program 153

How to Develop a Meaningful Concept
Map 154

The Step-by-Step Approach
to Concept Map Development.......156

Step 1: Determine the Main
Concept or Focus Question.....157

Step 2: Clarify or Define Concepts
and Sub-Concepts..............157

Step 3: Create a Parking Lot for
Sub-Concepts 157

Step 4: Organize and Prioritize the
Information 158

Step 5: Arrange the Sub-Concepts
Around the Central Focus or
Concept........................158

Step 6: Draw Lines Using Arrows
to Connect Sub-Concepts 159

Step 7: Label the Lines with Linking
Words That Show Concept
Relationships...................159

Step 8: Add Pictures and Color for
Visual Appeal and Clarity 159

Step 9: Make a Key and Include
References 161

Step 10: Revise the Concept
Map as Needed................161

Faculty and Student Development......161

Learning Tool or Graded
Assignment: Evaluating
a Concept Map.................163

Adding Concept Maps to a
Portfolio........................163

Chapter Key Points 164

Chapter References and Selected
Bibliography 164

Chapter 9 Using Case Studies Effectively in a Concept-Based Curriculum 167

Introduction to Case Studies...........167

The Nursing Process and Critical
Thinking..............................168

Clinical Reasoning and Clinical
Judgment 169

Translating Nursing Knowledge into
Practice..............................171

Effective Use of Case Studies for
Conceptual Learning and Clinical
Reasoning 172

Single Case Studies, Exercises,
and Challenges................172

Unfolding and Continuing Case
Studies 175

Chapter Key Points 180

Chapter References and Selected
Bibliography 181

PART III Evaluation in a Nursing Concept-Based Curriculum 183

Chapter 10 Evaluating Learning in the Concept-Based Curriculum Classroom 185

Introduction to Evaluation of
Conceptual Learning in the Concept-
Based Curriculum Classroom.........186

Validity and Reliability
Considerations 187

Learning Domain
  Considerations 187
Other Considerations for
  Developing Evaluation
  Methods 187
Examinations and Quizzes 188
  Cognitive Test Anxiety. 188
  NCLEX®-Style Tests 189
  Commercial Standardized
    Testing 205
  Quizzes 206
Papers and Projects. 206
Chapter Key Points 207
Chapter References and Selected
  Bibliography 209

**Chapter 11 Evaluating Learning
             in the Concept-Based
             Curriculum Clinical
             Setting 211**
Introduction to Evaluation of Learning
  in the Concept-Based Curriculum
  Clinical Setting. 212
Validity and Reliability Considerations. . .212
Direct Care Activities. 213
  Formative Evaluation of Direct Care
    Activities in the Community-
    Based Clinical Setting. 213
  Summative Evaluation of
    Direct Care Activities
    in the Community-Based
    Clinical Setting 216
Standardized Patient Methodology 222
Clinical Simulation. 223
Objective Structured Clinical
  Evaluation 224
Focused Learning Activities. 224
  Reflection Papers. 225
  Clinical Paper Assignments 227
  Data Mining Assignments 228
  Compare and Contrast
    Assignments 231
  Graphic Organizers. 231

Chapter Key Points 231
Chapter References and Selected
  Bibliography. 232

**Chapter 12 Determining
             Systematic Methods for
             Concept-Based
             Curriculum Program
             Evaluation 233**
Introduction to Program Evaluation. 234
Commonly Used Program Evaluation
  Models 234
The Systematic Plan for Program
  Evaluation 235
  Program Outcomes 236
  Curricular Outcomes 238
  Faculty Outcomes. 242
Evaluating Concept-Based Curriculum
  Outcomes 243
Chapter Key Points 245
Chapter References and Selected
  Bibliography 246

**Appendix A Lesson Plan/Student
             Study Guide. 247**
**Appendix B Concept Presentation:
             Mobility 249**
**Appendix C Concept Presentation:
             Clinical Judgment. 251**
**Appendix D Example of Lesson
             Plan for Concept
             Introduction: Gas
             Exchange 253**
**Appendix E Lesson Plan/Student
             Study Guide for
             Exemplar 255**
Glossary 257
Index 263

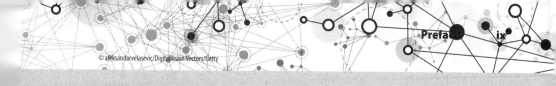

Preface

The modern-day concept-based curriculum (CBC) has been adopted by many prelicensure nursing programs in the United States and Canada in the past decade; however, few resources exist to assist faculty and administrators in developing, implementing, and evaluating this type of curriculum. Graduate students in nursing education tracks or postmasters' certificates in nursing education continue to have minimal instruction about the rapid movement from traditional teaching to conceptual learning.

This book meets the needs of both groups. For prelicensure nursing faculty, administrators, and curriculum committees, it provides practical tools and strategies to help develop and operationalize an effective and successful CBC. Where appropriate, application for conceptual learning in graduate programs is also included. In graduate nursing education programs, the book should be required for curriculum courses to assist students for preparation as novice nurse educators.

▶ What's Inside

This book presents a reader-friendly, accessible, "how-to" approach to each topic and is divided into three major parts, with a total of 12 chapters. Part I consists of three chapters (Chapters 1 to 3) that present an introduction to CBC and conceptual learning. Chapter 1 begins with a review of the essential elements of an academic curriculum. Chapter 2 compares traditional teaching with conceptual learning. Chapter 3 presents the author's 12-step approach to developing a CBC in nursing, including tips on faculty buy-in and how to get started.

Part II consists of six chapters (Chapters 4 to 9) that focus on teaching and learning in a CBC. Numerous tips, tools, and strategies are described with examples that are currently used in many nursing programs. Conceptual learning in the classroom, online, clinical, and laboratory settings is addressed.

Finally, Part III consists of three chapters (Chapters 10 to 12) that discuss assessment and evaluation in a nursing CBC in detail. Chapters 10 and 11 target assessment of student learning. Chapter 12 focuses on systematic program evaluation.

▶ Pedagogical Features

Given the book's two-pronged target audience, the major pedagogical features include:

- Chapter Learning Outcomes at the beginning of each chapter
- Chapter Key Points at the end of each chapter
- Boxed features throughout each chapter that highlight the most important content or expand on content
- Multiple examples of specific teaching/ learning and evaluation tools within applicable chapters

- Five appendices (A to E) at the end of the text that present teaching and learning tools for a CBC
- Glossary of bolded text terms with definitions in alphabetical order at the end of the text
- Comprehensive and current Chapter References and Selected Bibliography at the end of each chapter that provide the evidence for the content

All of these features help emphasize the most important information while making the content accessible to the reader.

I hope that you enjoy this book as an effective tool in your practice as a novice or "seasoned" nurse educator, dean, or director.

Donna D. Ignatavicius, MS, RN, CNE, ANEF

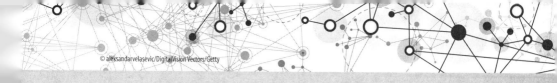

Contributors

Deanne A. Blach, MSN, RN
President
DB Productions of NW AR, Inc.
Green Forest, Arkansas

Nicole M. Heimgartner, MSN, RN, COI
Subject Matter Expert
Elsevier
Louisville, Kentucky

Kristin E. Oneail, MSN, RN
Clinical Nurse Liaison
United Health Care
Walbridge, Ohio

Cherie Rebar, PhD, MBA, RN, COI
Professor of Nursing
Wittenberg University
Springfield, Ohio

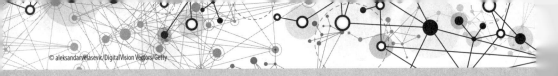

Reviewers

Dot Baker, RN, MS(N), PHCNS-BC, EdD
Professor
Wilmington University
Georgetown, Delaware

Laurie Bladen, PhD, RN, MBA
Assistant Professor
Clarion University of Pennsylvania
Clarion, Pennsylvania

Pamela S. Covault, MSN, RN, CNE
Director of Nursing
Neosho County Community College
Chanute, Kansas

Marie A. Cueman, PhD, RN
Associate Professor
Felician University
Rutherford, New Jersey

Sharon Kitchie, PhD, RN
Adjunct Instructor
Keuka College
Keuka Park, New York

Dolores Minchhoff, DNP, CRNP
Assistant Professor
Pennsylvania College of Health
  Sciences
Lancaster, Pennsylvania

Anita K. Reed, MSN, RN
Department Chair Community Health
  Practice
St. Elizabeth School of Nursing
Lafayette, Indiana

Kristen D. Zulkosky, PhD, RN, CNE
Assistant Professor
Pennsylvania College of Health
  Sciences
Lancaster, Pennsylvania

Acknowledgments

I would like to thank Christina Freitas, Editorial Assistant and Rebecca Stephenson, Acquisitions Editor at Jones & Bartlett Learning for their guidance and support. I would also like to thank my contributors for their knowledge and expertise, and Lee Henderson, editor extraordinaire, for mentoring me for many years in writing skills and for sharing his creativity in developing the flow chart on How to Determine If a Test Item Is at the Applying or Higher Level.

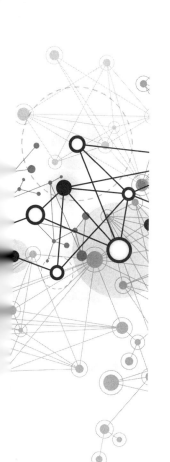

PART I

INTRODUCTION TO THE CONCEPT-BASED CURRICULUM AND CONCEPTUAL LEARNING IN NURSING EDUCATION

CHAPTER 1   Essential Elements of an Effective
            Nursing Curriculum 3

CHAPTER 2   Traditional Learning Versus
            Conceptual Learning 23

CHAPTER 3   Developing a Nursing Concept-Based
            Curriculum: A 12-Step Approach 37

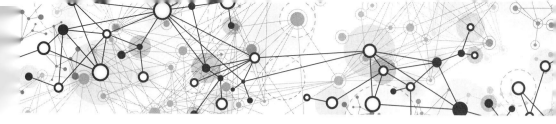

CHAPTER 1

Essential Elements of an Effective Nursing Curriculum

Donna Ignatavicius

CHAPTER LEARNING OUTCOMES

After studying this chapter, the reader will be better able to:

1. Define the term *curriculum*.
2. Explain the role of faculty in curriculum development or revision.
3. Describe the key components of an effective nursing curriculum.
4. Differentiate how curriculum for generalist and advanced practice educational programs are organized.
5. Identify the three stages of the backward design approach for curriculum development or revision.
6. Compare three common types of curricular models.
7. Explain the process for developing a nursing course, including the course syllabus.
8. Describe the typical process for formal curriculum approval.

▶ Introduction to Curriculum

Broadly defined, **curriculum** is the formal and informal structure and process in which a learner gains the knowledge, skills, attitudes, and abilities to meet established educational outcomes. *Formal* curriculum is outlined in the educational institution's catalog, student handbook, and faculty handbook. The *informal* curriculum includes learning opportunities that are not necessarily planned. These opportunities provide "teachable moments" for the educator and enriches the student's learning.

An educational program's curriculum also has a structure and a process. *Structure* indicates how the curriculum is organized; it includes the essential elements for an effective curriculum (whether new or revised) and is reviewed in this chapter. Sometimes referred to as instruction, *process* is how the curriculum is operationalized and delivered; it incorporates adult learning theories and models that are briefly discussed in Chapter 2.

Concept-based nursing curricula are used most often in prelicensure programs, which is the primary focus of this book. However, considerations for graduate nursing curricula are also addressed where appropriate. Selected differences for Canadian nursing programs are included throughout this book.

▶ Faculty Role in Nursing Curriculum Development and Revision

According to the National League for Nursing's (NLN's) Standards of Practice for the academic nurse educator, nursing faculty are responsible for developing and revising their program's curriculum (NLN, 2012) (**BOX 1-1**). The educational institution's role description for full-time faculty should include a statement that indicates that curriculum design and revision is a required part of the role (Keating, 2015). Some faculty may express concern that curriculum development or revision is time-consuming. Novice faculty may feel they are not qualified to help make curricular changes. Others, especially faculty who have been teaching in a program for many years, may not want to make changes and think that the existing curriculum is adequately serving the needs of both faculty and students.

According to Billings and Halstead (2016), curricular revision is inevitable. Changes in society, community influences, and educational research drive the need for the dynamic process of curriculum revision. In 2010, a major study of nursing

---

BOX 1-1 Examples of Academic Nurse Educator Standards of Practice for Curriculum Design and Revision

NLN Competency IV: Participate in Curriculum Design and Evaluation of Program Outcomes

- Demonstrates knowledge of curriculum development, including identifying program outcomes, developing competency statements, writing learning objectives, and selecting appropriate learning activities and evaluation strategies.
- Bases curriculum design and implementation decisions on sound educational principles, theory, and research.
- Revises the curriculum based on assessment of program outcomes, learner needs, and societal and healthcare trends.
- Collaborates with external constituencies throughout the process of curriculum revision.

Modified from the National League for Nursing (NLN). (2012). The scope of practice for academic nurse educators, 2012 revision. New York: NLN. Copyright © Wolters Kluwer. Reprinted with permission.

education in the United States by the Carnegie Foundation for the Advancement of Teaching called for a radical transformation in nursing education to better prepare future nurses with the knowledge and skills to provide the safest care possible (Benner, Stephen, Leonard, & Day, 2010). In response to the call for this change, nurse educators must revise their curricula and design instructional strategies to achieve the graduate competencies that reflect this goal (Emory, 2014).

Curricular revision usually begins with full faculty discussion about the need for change, but the support of the educational institution's administration and nursing program administrator is vital. External stakeholders, such as employers and alumni, and current students also should be part of the curriculum development or revision process from the beginning. These constituencies can provide valuable information about the competencies that the new graduates need to be successful. In addition, they can provide insight on changes or new trends in the healthcare community.

Most nursing programs have a curriculum committee made up of a sub-group of full-time faculty who are responsible for curriculum revision. If the program has a small number of faculty, the curriculum committee may function as a "committee of the whole," meaning that all faculty are members of the curriculum committee. That decision is made by the nursing faculty. The nursing curriculum committee also may represent faculty across types of programs, such as associate degree (AD) and baccalaureate (BSN) degree programs, or committees may be dedicated to each type of program. Usually, graduate and undergraduate programs have their own separate curriculum committees, but again, this depends on the number of total faculty. Nursing faculty in smaller colleges and universities often cross-teach; that is, they teach at both the undergraduate and graduate levels. In this case, the school may have only one nursing curriculum committee that serves all program levels.

Many nursing faculty, especially in the United States, have not received formal education in curriculum, instruction, and evaluation. For most programs, full-time faculty need a minimum of a master's in nursing degree, but not necessarily focused on nursing education. Although many new faculty are clinical experts, they are not educational experts. The nurse administrator can be very helpful in facilitating the curriculum change by providing resources, such as research articles on curricular trends, or hiring a nationally known outside expert in nursing curriculum. The role of the consultant should be to help guide and facilitate the faculty's curricular work. He or she should also provide information about national trends in nursing education and curriculum development. However, the consultant should *not* revise the program's curriculum because curriculum development is the responsibility of nursing faculty.

Another source of information to help guide faculty in the curriculum revision process is new graduate and/or employer survey data. Survey data are usually collected at the time of graduation and/or within 6 to 12 months after graduation. These data are analyzed, aggregated, and trended by graduating cohort, program option, and physical location (unless online). The survey findings can then help drive the faculty's decisions about the need for curriculum change.

Prelicensure practical nursing and registered nursing programs are regulated by state boards of nursing (in the United States) or provincial regulatory nursing bodies (in Canada). These organizations provide myriad regulations that influence how nursing curricula are developed. Adherence to these laws is not optional. For example, in California, the number of contact hours allocated for theory must be equal to that for clinical contact hours in a prelicensure registered nursing program.

▶ Role of Nursing Program Accreditation

Most nursing programs at all levels seek to obtain additional recognition by a national nursing education accreditation body. This voluntary process demonstrates whether the nursing program meets national standards of excellence in addition to the regulations of their own state or province. Nursing accreditation provides opportunities for graduates to have more choices for employment and continued education.

Currently there are the following three nursing education accreditation organizations in the United States:

- National League for Nursing Commission for Nursing Education Accreditation (NLN CNEA) (www.nln.org/accreditation-services)
- Commission of Collegiate Nursing Education (CCNE) (www.aacn.nche.edu /ccne-accreditation)
- Accreditation Commission for Education in Nursing (ACEN) (www.acenursing.org)

Nursing education accreditation standards do not mandate the use of any one curricular model or instructional process. However, all three accrediting bodies require that nursing curricula incorporate national and state standards and guidelines (e.g., Quality and Safety Education for Nurses [QSEN] competencies, NLN Competencies, and *Essentials*). The standards also reflect the need for faculty to utilize best practices in nursing education and teaching/learning. **BOX 1-2** provides examples of curricular criteria needed for initial or ongoing nursing program accreditation in the United States.

▶ Components of an Effective Nursing Curriculum

The components of an effective nursing curriculum typically include:

- Mission/Philosophy
- Organizing Curricular Framework
- Program Outcomes
- Curricular Model
- Plan of Study/Degree Plan
- Course Development
- Program Assessment Plan (discussed in Chapter 12)

Whether faculty are developing a new curriculum or revising a current one, all of these components need to be created or reviewed.

BOX 1-2 Example of Curriculum Standard with Criteria for Accreditation Commission for Education in Nursing Accreditation

Standard V: Culture of Learning and Diversity—Curriculum and Evaluation Processes

Faculty design program curricula to create a culture of learning that fosters the human flourishing of diverse learners through professional and personal growth, and supports the achievement of expected student learning outcomes. Professional nursing standards and other professional standards appropriate to the program type are foundational curricular elements and are clearly integrated throughout the curriculum. Teaching, learning, and evaluation processes take into consideration the diverse learning needs of students and are designed to support student achievement of learning outcomes. Distance learning programs are held to the same curricular, teaching/learning, and evaluation standards as campus-based programs. The program's culture of learning and diversity related to the implementation of curriculum and teaching/learning/evaluation processes is evident through the creation of a positive learning environment and achievement of the following associated quality indicators.

V-A. The curriculum is designed to foster achievement of clearly delineated student learning outcomes that are specific to the program mission and type (i.e., practical/vocational, diploma, associate, bachelor's, master's, postmaster's, and clinical doctorate) and aligned with expected curricular program outcomes.

V-B. The curriculum incorporates professional nursing standards and other professional standards and guidelines, associated with practical nursing/vocational nursing and RN licensure, advanced practice registered nurses certification, and/or other graduate level practice competencies aligned with practical/vocational, diploma, associate, bachelor's, master's, postmaster's certificate, and clinical doctorate types.

V-C. The program's curriculum is sequenced, designed, and implemented to progressively support student achievement of learning outcomes and the acquisition of competencies appropriate for the intended practice role.

V-D. The curriculum is up-to date, dynamic, evidence-based, and reflects current societal and health care trends and issues, research findings, and contemporary educational practices.

V-E. The curriculum provides students with experiential learning that supports evidence-based practice, intra- and interprofessional collaborative practice, student achievement of clinical competence, and as appropriate to the program's mission and expected curricular outcomes, expertise in a specific role or specialty.

V-F. The curriculum provides experiential learning that enhances student ability to demonstrate leadership, clinical reasoning, reflect thoughtfully, provide culturally responsive care to diverse populations, and integrate concepts, including, but not limited to context and environment of care delivery, knowledge and science, personal and professional development, quality and safety, patient-centered care, and teamwork into their practice.

Modified from National League for Nursing Commission for Nursing Education Accreditation. Accreditation Standards for Nursing Education Programs. Approved Feburary 2016. Retrieved from www.nln.org/accreditation-services/standards-for-accreditation. Permission to reproduce granted by the NLN Commission for Nursing Education Accreditation.

Mission and Philosophy

Some schools have either a mission or philosophy, and others have both. Simply stated, a university, college, or school's **mission** is a broad statement about the institution's goal or purpose. For example, a community college's mission might be: "To provide qualified graduates who meet the needs of the community in providing service and excellence in the workforce." A nursing department or college of nursing's mission should be consistent and in alignment with that of its educational institution.

A **philosophy** flows from the mission and is generally described as a set of beliefs and their related concepts (Keating, 2015). A nursing program or department or college of nursing's philosophy typically includes faculty's beliefs about professional nursing, adult learning, and the role(s) of nursing graduates. A nursing department or college of nursing's philosophy should also be consistent with that of its educational institution.

A nursing department or college of nursing's mission and/or philosophy drives curriculum development and revision. For example, if the faculty believes that professional nurses use current evidence for making clinical judgments, the curriculum should include a focus on the knowledge and skills associated with evidence-based practice. If the faculty believe adult learning and thinking is the primary focus of the program, processes to ensure learning and thinking need to be planned (see Chapter 2 for detail on teaching and learning).

Organizing Curriculum Framework

An **organizing curriculum framework**, also referred to as an *organizational framework* and formerly called the *conceptual framework,* identifies the major underpinnings, themes, or core concepts that organize a program's curriculum. In earlier years, accrediting organizations and boards of nursing required the identification of "threads" that were depicted in a conceptual framework, but there is currently no requirement by most regulatory or accrediting bodies to create this graphic representation. A few programs continue to use a diagram to show the relationship of core concepts or themes that are emphasized in the curriculum.

A few programs also continue to use the metaparadigm of person, environment, health, and nursing as an organizing approach. However, this approach is outdated and seldom used (Keating, 2015). In addition, a single nursing theory is no longer appropriate for nursing education and is not required by U.S. state boards of nursing or accrediting agencies. Some programs include caring theory, which is broad and aligns with professional nursing practice.

Prelicensure and registered nursing to BSN programs prepare students for entry into practice as *nurse generalists.* The Institute of Medicine's (IOM's) *Future of Nursing* report renewed interest in entry-level (generic) master's degree programs in nursing (Keating, 2015). After completing nurse generalist courses at the baccalaureate level, the student completes the graduate courses for advanced practice. Staff nurses prepared at this level can better meet the needs of the population they work with and manage the demands of a changing healthcare system. Organizing frameworks for graduate programs vary based on whether the program prepares the student for generalist or advanced practice.

Organizing Frameworks for Nurse Generalist Programs

Core curricular concepts in an organizing framework are sometimes referred to as core curricular organizers, metaconcepts, or themes. These concepts need to be consistent with state or provincial and national standards or guidelines. For example, the organizers for an AD in nursing program might include concepts consistent with the QSEN's competencies (www.qsen.org) and the National League for Nursing's Differentiated Graduate Competencies for Graduates of Associate Degree Programs (www.nln.org). An example of an AD in nursing program's core themes are listed in **BOX 1-3**.

The framework for U.S. BSN programs also must align with the AACN's *The Essentials of Baccalaureate Education for Professional Nursing Practice* (referred to most commonly as the *BSN Essentials*) (www.aacn.nche.edu). Additionally, many BSN programs have adopted the 10 Massachusetts Future of Nursing core competencies, which include the QSEN competencies plus communication, leadership, professionalism, and systems-based practice (Sroczynski, Gravlin, Route, Hoffart, & Creelman, 2011). Each core professional nursing concept should be defined to ensure that faculty and students use these terms consistently.

In Canada, over 100 entry-level competencies for new registered nurse (RN) graduates are divided into five categories (http://www.nurses.ab.ca/content/dam/carna/pdfs/DocumentList/Standards/RN_EntryPracticeCompetencies_May2013.pdf):

- Professional responsibilities and accountability
- Knowledge-based practice
- Ethical practice
- Service to the public
- Self-regulation

All nursing program curricula are designed to meet these competencies, but each program may determine its plan of study and curricular model.

Organizing Frameworks for Advanced Nursing Practice Programs

In the United States, advanced practice registered nurses (APRNs) have typically been prepared clinically at the master's level as a certified nurse midwife (CNM), certified

---

BOX 1-3 Examples of an Associate Degree in Nursing Program's Core Organizing Themes

- Patient-Centered Care
- Safety and Quality
- Informatics and Technology
- Nursing Judgment and Evidence-Based Practice
- Teamwork and Interprofessional Collaboration
- Nursing Professionalism

nurse practitioner (CNP), nurse anesthetist (CRNA), or clinical nurse specialist (CNS). APRNs are required to hold both an RN and APRN license. The AACN set a goal that master's programs for the APRN be phased out and replaced with the doctor of nursing practice (DNP). Students preparing for functional roles, such as nurse educators, clinical nurse leaders (CNLs), case managers, and nurse administrators, typically receive the master's of nursing degree.

In the United States, the expectations for designing a graduate curriculum include the following requirements:

- Alignment with either AACN's *The Essentials of Master's Education in Nursing* or *The Essentials of Doctoral Education for Advanced Nursing Practice* (www.aacn .nche.edu), depending on role
- Congruence with the *Consensus Report for APRN Practice*, published by the National Council of State Boards of Nursing (Cahill, Alexander, & Gross, 2014)
- Congruence with nationally established competencies for APRN roles

Program Outcomes

This textbook supports the backward design approach to strengthen nursing program curricula. **Backward design (BD)** is a pedagogical approach that has been used in secondary education for some time. More recently, BD has been applied in higher education health professions education (Emory, 2014). Simply described, BD is a three-stage process that includes the following:

1. Developing desired student learning outcomes and program outcomes
2. Determining evaluation strategies
3. Determining course content, student expectations, and teaching/learning strategies

The first stage of BD is the development of desired or expected student learning outcomes and program outcomes. **Student learning outcomes (SLOs)** can be defined as the desired expectations regarding knowledge, skills, and attitudes that students are expected to achieve during an educational program. SLOs organize the curriculum and guide student learning and evaluation. They can be categorized into three levels:

- End-of-program SLOs (one of two types of program outcomes)
- Course SLOs
- Unit, modular, or weekly SLOs

This section describes end-of-program student learning outcomes. The other two levels of SLOs are briefly discussed later in this chapter under *Course Development* and in more detail in Chapter 4.

Two types of program outcomes are usually developed for a nursing program as part of curriculum development or revision. The first type delineates the end-of-program graduate competencies or student learning outcomes (also known as program learning outcomes [PLOs]) and usually begin with: "At the end of the _____ program, the graduate will be able to. . . ." Each type of program must have its own new graduate outcomes written as competency statements while incorporating the program's core organizing concepts. In some states, all programs use the same standardized PLOs (e.g., Alabama, Kansas, Wyoming).

It is important to note that if a program offers more than one option to achieve the degree or certificate, the PLOs must be the same for all options. For instance, the BSN PLOs in **BOX 1-4** would apply for generic BSN graduates, LPN/LVN-to-BSN graduates, and RN-to-BSN graduates preparing for the same degree. Box 1-4 presents an example of the PLOs for a BSN program; **BOX 1-5** delineates those for an MSN program preparing students for the functional roles of nurse educator and administrator.

When developing PLOs, the faculty need to plan how to measure whether the new graduate has achieved these competencies as part of the program systematic evaluation plan. Determining evaluation strategies is the second stage of the BD approach to curriculum development. For example, the PLOs for the BSN

BOX 1-4 Examples of Program Learning Outcomes for a Bachelor of Science in Nursing Program

By the end of the BSN program, the graduate will be able to:

- Apply knowledge from liberal arts and sciences as a foundation for the generalist nursing role.
- Provide safe, evidence-based nursing care for patients and families in a variety of health inpatient and community care settings.
- Collaborate with the interprofessional healthcare team using informatics and technology to facilitate communication and improve care.
- Utilize leadership and management of care principles within the legal and ethical framework of the generalist nursing role.
- Demonstrate global awareness, social justice, and advocacy for diverse individuals and groups to promote health and prevent illness.
- Participate in quality improvement initiatives to promote optimal clinical outcomes for diverse patients and families.

BOX 1-5 Examples of Program Learning Outcomes for an Master of Science in Nursing Program

Upon successful completion of the MSN program, the graduate will be able to:

- Demonstrate professional scholarship, leadership, and global awareness to advance professional and personal development.
- Contribute to nursing science through systematic inquiry and dissemination of research findings.
- Synthesize concepts from nursing and appropriate related disciplines as a foundation for advanced nursing roles.
- Evaluate the design of healthcare systems to determine their effectiveness in providing and improving quality care.
- Integrate informatics and technology in advanced nursing roles to achieve positive outcomes.
- Advocate for nursing and healthcare policy to meet the needs of a diverse society in a changing healthcare environment.

program in Box 1-4 might be measured using one or more of the following sample assessments:

- Performance on a standardized comprehensive examination that predicts NCLEX® performance (for pre-RN licensure BSN options)
- Portfolio containing graded assignments that demonstrate PLO achievement
- End-of-program clinical performance examination (CPE)

Data for the second type of program outcomes indicate program success and are also a part of the program's evaluation plan. The faculty predetermine desired levels of achievement for graduate performance and compare those expected levels with actual levels of achievement. For example, "The first-time pass rate for graduates taking the NCLEX-PN® will be at least 80%."

Curriculum Models

After faculty determine the program's end-of-program SLOs and the indicators for program success, they need to select a curricular model to ensure outcome achievement. Over the past 15 years, many experts in nursing education have called for a change in prelicensure nursing curricula due to content saturation, which fosters superficial learning and memorization rather than deep learning and understanding (Benner, 2012; Forbes & Hickey, 2009; Giddens & Brady, 2007; Ironside, 2004). This section briefly describes three major curricular models—traditional, concept-based, competency-based. The most successful nursing programs often combine several models.

The traditional block model that focuses on medical diagnoses does not promote critical thinking and nursing judgment such that students learn to "think like a nurse." The newer concept-based and competency-based models decrease content saturation and focus on the knowledge and skills needed for safe, quality nursing practice.

Traditional Curriculum Model

In the traditional block model, courses are centered around care of various populations, such as community health, adult health, maternal and child health, and mental and behavioral health. As new clinical standards and knowledge become available, faculty add them to the already content-laden curriculum, creating an "additive curriculum" problem. Students and faculty alike become overwhelmed with the amount of content to teach and learn. Students compartmentalize knowledge and are not usually able to transfer learning from one context to another.

Nursing faculty are assigned to courses in a traditional model depending on their clinical expertise. As a result, these clinical experts tend to teach content in more detail than is needed for a prelicensure nursing program to prepare a beginning nurse generalist. Surprisingly, in view of the increasing number of Baby Boomers turning 65 years of age, many nursing programs have no separate course or focus on care of older adults in their curricula. In many programs, the number of credits allocated for specialty courses is higher or the same as those allocated for adult health and gerontology content. This imbalance becomes an issue when compared to the NCLEX® test plan that emphasizes adult health. Additionally, new nursing graduates are more likely employed in settings for adult care, especially for older adults.

Concept-Based Curriculum Model

Concept-based curriculum (CBC) models are based on brain research that demonstrates how people learn. Many primary and secondary educational schools have been using concept-based curricula for 10 to 15 years in the United States (Erickson, 2002, 2008), but higher education has been slower to adopt this approach. In a CBC approach, specific concepts are identified as the focus of the curriculum. *Concepts* are classifications/categories of information (knowledge) that can be ideas or mental images. A **concept-based curriculum**, then, is designed by organizing specific content around identified program concepts (Giddens, Caputi, & Rodgers, 2015). Chapter 3 describes a 12-step process to developing a CBC in nursing education.

The CBC approach in nursing is gaining national and international popularity because of the following:

- Is student-centered (what the students need) rather than teacher-centered (what the educator wants or likes to teach)
- Requires student engagement in thinking and learning
- Enables students to transfer learning from one context to another
- Decreases the amount of content in the curriculum
- Helps develop nursing judgment so students can "think like a nurse" (Tanner, 2006)
- Focuses on conceptual learning (discussed in Chapter 2)

Competency-Based Curriculum Model

Competencies are the knowledge, skills, and attitudes (KSAs) that make up a person's job or role. They are context-specific and show demonstration of abilities, behaviors, and skills in a variety of situations. A competency-based curricular model outlines expected competencies that guide student behaviors and indicate how they are measured. While delineated expected outcomes are essential to guide curriculum development, the KSAs also must be identified. Therefore, most nursing programs using the CBC model include a combination of concepts, conceptual learning, and competencies to plan the most effective curriculum.

> **Remember This . . .**
>
> - Concepts are classifications or categories of knowledge that can be ideas or mental images.
> - Competencies are the knowledge, skills, and attitudes (KSAs) that make up a person's job or role. They are context-specific and show demonstration of abilities, behaviors, and skills in a variety of situations.

Plan of Study and Degree Plan

The PLOs guide the faculty in deciding on the knowledge, skills, attitudes, and abilities that students need as part of the nursing curriculum. Not all nursing programs offer a college degree upon graduation. Some schools, such as career or technical programs, award a certificate or diploma rather than a college degree. Examples of programs that do not typically offer a degree include practical nursing/vocational nursing (PN/VN) programs and diploma programs in nursing. Some diploma programs preparing for registered nursing practice offer both a diploma and a degree if they have degree-granting approval.

A **plan of study** (also referred to as a program of study) outlines the sequence of courses needed for a student to graduate from a program. If an institution awards a degree, the plan of study may be referred to as the **degree plan**. The length of a nursing program varies depending on type of nursing program and whether the program is traditional, accelerated, completion, or part time.

Most nursing programs require that a certain number of general education courses be taken in the liberal arts and sciences before admission or taken concurrently with nursing courses, depending on the program. The liberal arts and science courses serve as the foundation for nursing knowledge and practice. Students taking these required courses before acceptance into the nursing program are often referred to as *prenursing students*, although their admission into the nursing courses is not guaranteed.

A nursing program's plan of study is typically divided into a set of prenursing and nursing courses. For example, a BSN program may be structured as a 2 + 2 curriculum (2 years of lower division general education [prenursing] courses plus 2 years of upper division nursing courses) or a 1 + 3 curriculum (1 year of prenursing courses and 3 years of nursing courses mixed with general education courses). Other programs, such as those participating in the Wyoming statewide curriculum called ReNew, use a 1 + 2 + 1 design. In this structure, students take the first year of their general education courses and then complete their AD in nursing requirements during the next 2 years. The last year (2 semesters) allows students to achieve their BSN degree.

Considerations for Course Decisions

In view of healthcare advances and current trends in nursing practice, faculty are faced with determining which competencies they want their graduates to meet. Knowledge in areas such as informatics and technology, multicultural care, genetics and genomics, and quality improvement must be considered by faculty as they design nursing curricula in preparation for both the generalist and advanced practice roles. Increased emphasis on interprofessional education and collaboration, transition management and care coordination, ethics, and social justice in health care today also affect which concepts are included into the curriculum. Faculty need to stay current in health care changes and trends to be prepared to develop a contemporary curriculum that best meets the needs of today's nursing graduates.

Another consideration for course decisions is whether to separate courses by specialty, such as in a block curriculum, or plan courses that focus on care of individuals, families, and communities across the lifespan. This integrated approach reduces content duplication and fragmentation and is therefore easier for students to learn. It is often used as part of a CBC, but is not limited to that application. For example, courses in an integrated curriculum may be numbered like Nursing Concepts I, II, III, and IV or specify a general type of health problem, such as Health Promotion for Patients with Chronic Health Problems.

Support courses for a traditional BSN nursing program should include the first three courses below (referred to as the Basic 3Ps), Evidence-Based Practice, and one or more of the remaining course examples, as follows:

- Pathophysiology
- Pharmacology
- Physical/Health Assessment

- Evidence-Based Practice
- Informatics in Health Care
- Law and Ethics in Health Care
- Leadership and Management of Care
- Cultural and Global Awareness
- Current Issues and Trends in Nursing and Health Care

These support courses are strategically placed in the plan of study to assist the students in deeper understanding of program content.

Generalist Nursing Program Length

Including the general education courses, a *traditional* generic PN/VN program is typically between 1 and 2 years in length for a total of 36 to 45 semester credits. A traditional generic diploma or AD in nursing program preparing the RN is between 2 and 3 years in length and typically varies between 60 and 72 semester credits. A traditional generic baccalaureate program is 4 years, or approximately 120 semester credits. Proprietary institutions, career schools, and some public colleges may use quarter credits rather than semester credits at a 2:3 ratio. For example, a 120-semester credit program equals 180 quarter credits. Courses offered in the quarter system are typically 10 to 11 weeks rather than 15 to 16 weeks. However, some proprietary systems offer courses of 5 to 8 weeks each for the entire program.

Some BNS programs offer *accelerated* or second-degree options for students who have previously achieved college degrees. For example, one of the fastest growing program types is the accelerated BSN (ABSN) program option (Billings & Halstead, 2016). Students accepted into this type of program are required to have at least a baccalaureate degree in another field, often with a math and science background. After qualified students complete any remaining required courses (often anatomy and physiology and microbiology), they are admitted to the nursing program to complete the nursing courses in 12 to 16 months.

Other nursing programs require that students attend courses year-round. These programs are also categorized as accelerated because a student can graduate within a shorter amount of time than when courses are not offered during the summer. For example, some BSN programs in Canada and the United States are 3 years rather than 4 because students attend classes for 12 months for three semesters each year. (Canada's entry into registered nursing practice is at the BSN level.) ABSN programs are very intense and require dedicated students.

Many proprietary programs in the United States that offer the AD in nursing degree also conduct classes year-round. Students can often graduate in about 1½ years and are eligible to take their NCLEX-RN®.

Completion programs provide students with advanced standing to complete a first or higher degree. For example, an LPN/LVN may be admitted into an AD nursing program's LPN/LVN-to-RN option. The student must complete any required general education courses, take a transition to professional nursing course, and meet all of the qualifications for program admission. RN-to-BSN completion programs have grown tremendously as a result of the *Future of Nursing* initiative to have 80% of all RNs in the United States educated at the BSN level to better enable collaboration with other healthcare professionals. Most of these programs are offered in an online format (see Chapter 7).

Part-time nursing program options allow working students to complete the program over a longer period than what is expected for full-time students. This option is not as common today because program outcomes have not typically been as positive when students choose to complete a program on a part-time basis. In these programs, students tend to work full-time and have family commitments preventing them from spending adequate time on learning and studying.

Advanced Practice Nursing Program Length

Graduate nursing programs vary widely in length depending on whether the awarded degree is a masters or doctoral degree and for which role the student is being prepared. For example, the CRNA student is required to take additional sciences classes and pharmacology to ensure competence in anesthesia administration. In addition, many graduate students take graduate courses on a part-time basis. The minimum number of semester credits for a master's degree in nursing is usually 30 to 36.

Nursing Program Course Sequence

To plan the nursing program's plan of study or degree plan, the faculty must consider a number of factors (**BOX 1-6**), including how to offer the program (e.g., full time, part time, accelerated) and which program options should be planned. Of critical importance is the need to ensure that foundational courses needed for more difficult advanced courses are placed early in the program to provide prerequisite knowledge and skills. For example, a pathophysiology course is usually taught before a pharmacology course because it is easier for the students to learn pharmacology content if they understand why drugs are given and for which health problems they are used. **TABLE 1-1** presents a typical traditional degree plan for an AD nursing program.

Another consideration for course content sequencing is whether students can transfer into the program from another educational institution, with or without advanced standing. For example, many students chose to take their prelicensure general education courses in a community college before applying to a BSN nursing program because they are generally less expensive than those offered in a 4-year school.

BOX 1-6 Common Factors to Consider When Developing a Nursing Program Plan of Study or Degree Plan

- Board of nursing or provincial regulatory requirements
- State or provincial higher education requirements
- Institution and nursing accreditation standards
- Professional nursing standards and competencies
- Requirements for institutional graduation (core courses)
- Institutional policies
- Length of program and program options (also called tracks) (e.g., part time, accelerated, completion)
- Number, qualifications, and expertise of full-time and part-time faculty
- Physical space and resources
- Learning resources (including technology for alternative delivery formats)
- Opportunities for interprofessional education
- Fiscal resources
- Nature of students (e.g., traditional vs. nontraditional learners)
- Level of students (e.g., generalist vs. advanced practice role preparation)

TABLE 1-1 Example of a Typical Traditional Associate Degree in Nursing Program Plan of Study or Degree Plan

Type of Course	Credits for Each Course
General Education Credits (23 credits total)	
English I	3
Algebra II (or other math)	3
Anatomy (with laboratory)	4
Physiology (with laboratory)	4
General Psychology	3
Developmental Psychology	3
Humanities	3
Nursing Credits (42 credits total)	
Semester 1 (all 16-week courses)	
Foundations of Nursing Practice	8 (5T, 3C)
Introduction to Pharmacology	3 (3T, 0C)
Semester 2	
Adult Health I Nursing Practice (10 weeks)	6 (4T, 2C)
Mental Health Nursing Practice (5 weeks)	3 (2T, 1C)
Introduction to Gerontology (5 weeks)	2 (2T, 0C)
Semester 3 (all courses 8 weeks)	
Adult Health II Nursing Practice	5 (3T, 2C)
Maternal Child Health Nursing Practice	6 (4T, 2C)
Semester 4	
Adult Health III Nursing Practice (10 weeks)	6 (4T, 2C)
Concept Synthesis/Capstone (5 weeks)	3 (1T, 2C)
Program Total Credits	65

T = Theory; C = clinical/laboratory.

Course Development

After the faculty decide on a plan of study or degree plan, each course must be developed and formatted for the course syllabus. The course syllabus is a *legal document* among the nursing program, faculty, and students. Therefore, any changes to the syllabus must go through a formal approval process, described later in this chapter. At a minimum, components of a course syllabus should consist of the following:

- Course title and number
- Number of total course credits (with breakdown of theory/clinical credits if applicable)
- Prerequisite and/or corequisite course requirements
- Course description (should match the school catalog description)
- Course student learning outcomes (may be called objectives or competencies)
- Student learning assessment methods
- Required and recommended textbooks and other learning resources

Additionally, there may be an attached course calendar, topical outline, and/or lesson plans or study guides for students.

> **Remember This . . .**
>
> - The course syllabus is a legal document among the nursing program, faculty, and students. Therefore, any changes to the syllabus must go through a formal approval process.

The first step in developing course syllabi is to determine how many credits each course should be, the title of the course, and any division among theory (didactic), clinical, and laboratory credits. For example, a beginning nursing course with a clinical component may be a total of 7 credits with 4 credits of theory and 3 credits of laboratory/clinical experience. Or, the two components may be split into two courses: one theory and one clinical. The advantage of one total course is that there is one course syllabus with one course description and one set of course student learning outcomes. The disadvantage of this approach is that a student must pass all of the components of the course. If she or he fails the course, the larger number of credits for the course can lower the student's grade point average significantly. For that reason, some programs have smaller credit courses and split the theory (didactic) and clinical courses. However, if a student passes the clinical course and fails the companion theory course, he or she does not need to or be required to retake the successfully achieved course.

Writing the Course Description

The next task is to write the course description in one or two sentences to briefly provide an overview of the course. Course descriptions should be different for each course in the curriculum. If more than one degree option or track is offered, they all should have the same syllabus for a course offered in all tracks. For example, if the Evidence-Based Practice course is 3 credits and offered in a generic BSN and RN-to-BSN completion program in the same college, the syllabus for the two options should be the same, especially the course description—for example, classroom versus

> **BOX 1-7** Example of a Typical Course Description for the Adult Health I Nursing Course in a Bachelor of Science in Nursing Program
>
> Built on the Foundations of Nursing course, this course focuses on safe, evidence-based nursing care of the adult patient with common acute and chronic health problems. Students will have the opportunity to apply professional nursing skills in caring for one or two patients using simulation and community clinical agencies.

online instruction. **BOX 1-7** shows an example of a course description for Concepts in Adult Health I in a BSN program as part of a course syllabus.

Based on the course description and in alignment with the end-of-program outcomes for new graduates, the course SLOs should be thoughtfully written using one verb as the first word in each outcome to describe the expected student behavior. The faculty need to consider how student achievement of each outcome can be measured.

Determining Course Content and How It Is Evaluated

The third stage of BD for curriculum is determining course content, student expectations (through SLO and competency statements), and teaching/learning strategies. Faculty determine which concepts or topics will be included in each course based on current nursing practice. Topic changes and associated SLOs at this level do not require formal curriculum approval and can be changed when needed as part of the faculty's academic freedom. However, a change in one course may affect other courses. Communication among faculty is essential to ensure a well-designed curriculum that is current and aligned.

Course topics should be consistent with the course description and course SLOs. The course topics should not be selected based on a single textbook or other resource. Rather, the faculty should design the course, select essential content needed to meet learning outcomes, and then decide on the "best fit" learning resources, including the textbook, if appropriate. A course should *not* include every topic in the selected textbook.

> **Remember This . . .**
>
> - The course topics should not be selected based on a single textbook or other resource. Rather the faculty should design the course and then decide on the "best fit" learning resources, including the textbook, if appropriate.

Faculty typically design a course calendar based on weekly or unit/modular content. After determining the topics, a lesson plan or study guide can help delineate the specific topical SLOs, topical outline, teaching/learning strategies, assignments, and assessment methods. The lesson plan also may designate the associated course SLOs for each unit or topic. Appendix A provides an example of a lesson plan in a traditional curriculum. As the lesson plan illustrates, the unit SLOs guide the delivery of instruction (where the topic is taught; e.g., online or classroom), learning activities (how it is learned), and how it is evaluated. Evaluation includes formative versus summative evaluation and is discussed in detail later in this textbook.

The overall course evaluation criteria are outlined in the syllabus to show how the course grade is obtained. For example, for a face-to-face course (classroom) in a Basic Pharmacology course of a BSN program, the evaluative methods to determine the grade might be:

Unit tests (4)	300 points (75 points each)
Final comprehensive examination	100 points
Health teaching project	50 points
Quizzes/homework	50 points
TOTAL possible for course	500 points

▶ Curriculum Approval Process

Before major curricular revision can be implemented, the curriculum goes through a formal curriculum approval process. Although each state, province, and region has its own regulations or procedures, the basic process typically includes the following sequence of approvals:

- Approval by the nursing curriculum committee
- Approval by full nursing faculty
- Approval by the college, school, or university curriculum committee, senate, and/or administration
- Approval by the state or provincial regulatory higher education and nursing education body
- Approval by the nursing accrediting organization (if the program is nursing accredited)

This process is often time-consuming and must be built into a timeline prior to curriculum implementation. During the approval process, faculty and school advisors need to alert prenursing students in a timely manner that a new curriculum is being considered and how it will likely affect them. Ideally, the students should be notified of major changes a year prior to implementation of the curriculum. Most nursing accreditation bodies require a minimum of 4 months' notice and substantive change report before a new curriculum is implemented.

▶ Chapter Key Points

- Curriculum is the formal and informal structure and process in which a learner gains the knowledge, skills, attitudes, and abilities to meet established educational outcomes.
- Faculty have the primary role in developing and revising nursing curriculum; curriculum development should be part of the nursing faculty's role description (see Box 1-1).
- The key components of an effective nursing curriculum include the Mission or Philosophy, Organizing Curriculum Framework, Program Outcomes, Curriculum Model, Plan of Study or Degree Plan, and Course Development.

- Nurse generalist curricula are usually organized based on the QSEN competencies, Nurse of the Future competencies, BSN Essentials, and/or the NLN Differentiated New Graduate Competencies.
- Advanced nursing practice curricula are organized based on the MSN/Doctorate Program Essentials, APRN standards of practice, and/or the National Council of State Boards of Nursing Consensus Report.
- Backward design is an approach to curriculum development or revision.
- The most common curricular models are traditional, concept-based, and competency-based. In a traditional model, courses are planned according to populations and nursing specialty; the curriculum focuses on medical diagnoses.
- In a concept-based curriculum, nursing concepts are often taught across the lifespan to develop deep learning and nursing judgment. They are context-specific and show demonstration of abilities, behaviors, and skills in a variety of situations.
- Course development involves creating a course syllabus and the lesson plan/study guide. The syllabus is a legal document that includes the course title; credit allotment; course description; prerequisite and corequisite courses, if any; course student learning outcomes (SLOs); required textbooks; and course evaluative methods.
- Each course needs a lesson plan and calendar of topics, unit/weekly SLOs, teaching/learning strategies, assignments, and assessments of student learning.
- A new curriculum or curriculum revision requires a formal approval process by the nursing program or department faculty, college or school curriculum or faculty approval, state or provincial nursing regulatory approval, and nursing accrediting body approval, if applicable.

▶ Chapter References and Selected Bibliography

Benner, P. (2012). Educating nurses: A call for radical transformation: How far have we come? *Journal of Nursing Education, 51*(4), 183–184.

Benner, P., Stephen, M., Leonard, V., & Day, L. (2010). *Educating nurses: A call for radical transformation.* San Francisco, CA: Jossey-Bass.

Billings, D. M., & Halstead, J. A. (2016). *Teaching in nursing: A guide for faculty* (5th ed.). St. Louis, MO: Elsevier.

Cahill, M., Alexander, M., & Gross, L. (2014). The 2014 NCSBN report on APRN regulation. *Journal of Nursing Regulation, 4*(3), 3–12.

Emory, J. (2014). Understanding backward design to strengthen curricular models. *Nurse Educator, 39*(3), 122–125.

*Erickson, L. (2002). *Concept-based curriculum and instruction.* Thousand Oaks, CA: Corwin Press.

Erickson, L. (2008). *Stirring the head, heart, and soul: Redefining curriculum, instruction, and concept-based learning.* Thousand Oaks, CA: Corwin Press.

Forbes, M. O., & Hickey, M. T. (2009). Curriculum reform in baccalaureate nursing education: Review of the literature. *International Journal of Nursing Education Scholarship, 6*(1), 1–16.

Giddens, J. F., & Brady, D. (2007). Rescuing nursing education from content saturation: The case for a concept-based curriculum. *Journal of Nursing Education, 46*(2), 65–69.

Giddens, J. F., Caputi, L., & Rodgers, B. (2015). *Mastering concept-based teaching: A guide for nursing educators.* St. Louis, MO: Mosby.

*Ironside, P. M. (2004). "Covering content" and teaching thinking: Deconstructing the additive curriculum. *Journal of Nursing Education, 43*(1), 5–12.

Keating, S. B. (2015). *Curriculum development and evaluation in nursing.* New York, NY: Springer Publishing.

McDonald, M. (2014). *The nurse educator's guide to assessing learning outcomes* (3rd ed.). Burlington, MA: Jones & Bartlett Learning.

National League for Nursing (NLN). (2012). *The scope of practice for academic nurse educators* (2012 revision). New York, NY: NLN.

Sroczynski, M., Gravlin, G., Route, P. S., Hoffart, N., & Creelman, P. (2011). Creativity and connections: The Future of Nursing Education and Practice: The Massachusetts initiative. *Journal of Professional Nursing, 27*(6), e64–e70.

*Tanner, C. A. (2006). Thinking like a nurse: A research model of clinical judgement in nursing. *Journal of Nursing Education, 45*(6), 204–211.

*Indicates classic reference.

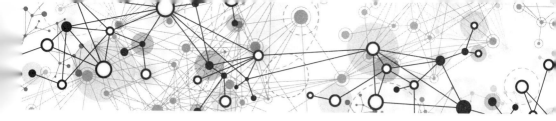

CHAPTER 2

Traditional Learning Versus Conceptual Learning

Donna Ignatavicius

CHAPTER LEARNING OUTCOMES

After studying this chapter, the reader will be better able to:

1. Explain the role of teaching and learning in higher education.
2. Differentiate the three major learning domains.
3. Briefly describe how learning occurs in the brain based on recent research.
4. Compare the characteristics of traditional and conceptual teaching and learning.
5. List the key building blocks of a concept-based curriculum (CBC) structure.
6. Explain the need to align a CBC with the NCLEX® test plan and/or the appropriate *Essentials* documents.
7. Identify five major benefits of concept-based teaching and conceptual learning.

▶ Introduction to Teaching and Learning

For many years, the mission of most colleges and universities has been *teaching, research, and service. Teaching*, though, is what the educator does through instructional methods and is therefore "teacher-centered." *Learning* is what students do and is therefore student-centered. Learning should be the core mission of higher education to ensure that students can apply the knowledge, skills, and attitudes (KSAs) needed to prepare for careers or jobs. This textbook focuses on facilitating learning as the primary focus of the nurse educator with an introduction in this chapter.

Since 1997, O'Banion and others have called for an education revolution in which *learning* (rather than teaching) is the primary goal of higher education. The Learning College environment emphasizes the role of the faculty as facilitators of student learning. The key principles of a Learning College are summarized in **BOX 2-1**.

Learning occurs in one or more of three domains and can be applied to nursing education—*cognitive* (using and applying knowledge), *psychomotor* (performing skills as part of total care), and *affective* (appreciating and developing professional attitudes). Each domain has one or more taxonomies (classification systems) that help show growth and progression in a variety of learning environments. For example, Anderson and Krathwohl revised Bloom's 1956 cognitive taxonomy in 2001 (Anderson, et al., 2001) (**TABLE 2-1**). Anderson and Krathwohl changed the noun terminology of Bloom to verbs that more specifically identify the cognitive processing that occurs in the brain. These researchers also placed creating (synthesis) at a higher thinking level than evaluating. To promote thinking and learning, faculty need to plan activities that help students apply knowledge in simulated and actual clinical practice experiences.

BOX 2-1   O'Banion's Key Principles of a Learning College

- Creates a substantive change in student learning.
- Engages learners as full partners in learning with learners taking responsibility for their choices.
- Offers many options for meaningful student learning.
- Promotes collaborative learning.
- Succeeds when student learning can be documented.

Reproduced with permission from O'Banion, T. & Wilson, C. (2010). Focus on learning: A learning college reader. Phoenix: League for Innovation in the College Community.

TABLE 2-1   Anderson and Krathwohl's Taxonomy to Update Bloom's Cognitive Taxonomy

Bloom's Terminology (Nouns)	Anderson and Krathwohl's Taxonomy (Verbs)
Knowledge	Remembering
Comprehension	Understanding
Application	Applying
Analysis	Analyzing
Synthesis	Evaluating
Evaluation	Creating

▶ How Learning Occurs

Many definitions and descriptions of learning exist in the literature; however, the science of learning is based on neurobiology research, which demonstrates that meaningful learning produces connections between information and allows students to apply knowledge in a variety of contexts. Kumaran et al. (2009) found that new neuronal connections were created or expanded in the brain during each meaningful learning experience, resulting in long-term **deep learning**. Strong neuronal connections are essential for good judgment and decision-making, particularly in new situations.

Giddens, Caputi, and Rodgers (2015) summarized the brain's function into three major categories: sensing, integrating, and responding. All three of these categories of brain function are essential to learning. *Sensing* refers to data input by the brain through the senses—auditory, visual, olfactory, and touch—which is coordinated by the thalamus. *Integrating* refers to how the brain processes the data and makes sense of it, including making connections to previous knowledge (by the frontal lobe of the cerebral cortex). *Responding* refers to what the brain does with the integration of data (by the frontal, parietal, and/or temporal lobes of the cerebral cortex and basal ganglia).

One of the most common definitions of learning states that learning results in a *change* in behavior as a result of gaining knowledge and experience (Ambrose, Bridges, Dipietro, Lovett, & Norman, 2010). For example, when a student learns how to perform a sterile procedure, he or she observes the demonstrated behavior (either face-to-face or video), hears the instructor's explanation, reads the procedure in the print or digital skills book, and practices the procedure, thereby using multiple senses (*sensing*). Then the student's brain processes this knowledge/skill and connects it to other knowledge—for example, gloving, handwashing, and principles of sterile technique learned earlier (*integrating*). The student's response is a *change* in behavior if the procedure is performed correctly (*responding*). With experience, that performance improves with more efficiency. If the student cannot perform sterile technique, deep learning has not occurred. Although the student's precise knowledge acquisition cannot be measured, the application of the knowledge can be assessed, as illustrated in this example.

▶ Characteristics of Traditional Teaching and Learning

Historically, most nursing education programs were based on the Tyler curricular model, which was designed in the 1940s (Getha-Eby et al., 2014). This traditional model was used to provide state and national standards for nursing education program approval and accreditation, and resulted in a list of curricular content topics to be "covered" in each program.

Over time curricular content has expanded to include more current topics and issues relevant to nursing and health care. However, faculty are often hesitant to delete topics that have been in their curriculum since inception. For example, Maslow's Hierarchy of Needs has been included in prelicensure nursing curricula since the 1960s. Yet Maslow's pyramid may not assist students or nurses today in prioritizing patient care. This practice of retaining old content while adding new content has led to the *additive* curriculum, resulting in content saturation. As a result, a number of nursing education experts and researchers have called for *desaturation* of the nursing curriculum for the past 15 years (Diekelmann, 2002; Giddens & Brady, 2007; Ironside, 2004).

Traditional pedagogies use a lecture-style format often accompanied by numerous PowerPoint slides. This *teaching* approach helps faculty "cover" large amounts of course content in a certain timeframe. However, it promotes rote memorization, inaccurate connections, and short-term **superficial learning** in which knowledge is fragmented, disorganized, and compartmentalized in the student's mind. In this model, students are passive learners who often cannot cognitively process large amounts of information. As a result, learners cannot connect new knowledge to previous learning and cannot transfer learning to new contexts, thus limiting thinking and decision-making.

Lecture-style presentations have been identified by nursing education researchers as a contributing factor to the difficulty of new nursing graduates in providing safe and effective patient care (Benner, 2012; Benner, Stephen, Leonard, & Day, 2010). Yet, nursing education has been slow to embrace the transition from teaching to learning.

One reason for the reluctance to accept this paradigm shift is that many nursing faculty have not been formally educated, mentored, and/or developed in their role as academic nurse educators. Therefore, they tend to teach students as they were taught during their own prelicensure educational program and do not recognize the need to change. Other faculty may be resistant to change either because they do not want to invest the time and energy to learning a newer approach or because they do not see the change as a benefit to students or faculty. Additional discussion about faculty "buy-in" is discussed in the next chapter of this textbook.

▶ Characteristics of a Concept-Based Curriculum and Conceptual Teaching/Learning

As mentioned in Chapter 1, an educational curriculum has a structure and a process. For this textbook, the *structure* is the concept-based curriculum (CBC) model; the *process* is concept-based or conceptual teaching and learning.

Key Building Blocks of the Concept-Based Curriculum Structure

The two major building blocks of the CBC structure are concepts and exemplars. **Concepts** are classifications/categories of information (knowledge) that can be ideas or mental images. They are not objects or things and can be flexible and dynamic. In nursing education, they are used to organize curricular content into a CBC. Although used most often in prelicensure nursing education, the CBC may be used in RN-to-BSN or MSN programs and in advanced practice programs.

Using a CBC model is not new to nursing education. In fact, in the 1970s and 1980s, grand theories and conceptual models, such as those developed by Orem, Roy, King, and Rogers, were used as a basis for nursing curricula. Specific theory-related terminology was integrated into the nursing program for faculty and student use. For example, Sister Roy's stress and adaptation model emphasized the importance for the nurse to identify the patient's internal and external stressors as a basis for nursing interventions. Dorothea Orem's self-care theory advocated the need for nurses to promote patient self-management and care. Although today's nursing programs do not typically select a single nursing theory upon which to base their curricula, the concepts of self-care and stress management are very important in the provision of whole-person or whole-family care.

Dr. Jean Giddens began the current trend in CBC for nursing programs in 2004 at the University of New Mexico's BSN program. She and her team of nurse educator colleagues developed the first new-generation CBC that identified concepts in several areas: Health and Illness concepts, Health Care Recipient concepts, and Professional Nursing and Health Care concepts (Giddens, 2017). Examples of concepts in each of these categories are listed in Chapter 3. Most CBC nursing programs use some or all of these concepts. Other programs have added concepts or modified some of the language of the Giddens' list.

Exemplars are specific content topics that relate to and represent identified concepts. For the Health and Illness concepts, the exemplars tend to be health problems experienced by patients, clients, and residents. Exemplars for health and illness/wellness concepts may be disease processes such as chronic heart failure (concept of perfusion) and osteoarthritis (concept of mobility). For professional nursing and health care concepts, the exemplars are often "softer" topics, such as ethics, scope of nursing practice, and social justice. Chapter 3 provides additional commonly used exemplars by concept and describes the CBC process in more detail.

Meaningful Learning and Constructivism

Concept-based teaching is an innovative approach that ensures meaningful learning to help students apply patterns of knowing across a variety of contexts. Students are able to organize content, create connections, develop critical thinking, and make decisions that keep patients safe and provide quality care through conceptual learning (Erickson, 2007). In other words, they are able to effectively use the three brain functions associated with deep learning: sensing, integrating, and responding to change their behavior.

> ### Remember This . . .
>
> *Concept-based teaching is an innovative approach that ensures meaningful learning to help students apply patterns of knowing across a variety of contexts.*

The tenets of meaningful learning are based on an older philosophy called *constructivism* as advocated by a number of learning theorists, including David Ausubel (1963). **Constructivism** is similar to Malcolm Knowles' classic adult learning theory (1984) which posits that 1) new knowledge is best understood if it can be connected to previous knowledge or experiences and 2) previous knowledge and experiences influence the understanding and interpretation of new knowledge. Understanding requires synthesis into a learner's existing network of knowledge rather than merely adding to the collection of knowledge. The best way to assess this process is to determine how the learner uses that knowledge.

Meaningful learning enables transfer of KSAs to real-world situations (Novak, 2010). It creates deep understanding which students then can transfer to real-world problem solving and decision making using judgment and critical thinking. Deep understanding and transfer of knowledge patterns are vital in nursing practice. Nurses often encounter new situations in which they must readily recall, connect, and apply essential knowledge to promote patient safety (Getha-Eby et al., 2014).

Benefits of the Conceptual Learning Approach

Unlike traditional pedagogies in which students are passive, disengaged learners, **conceptual learning** is student-centered and requires active engagement (**TABLE 2-2**). Students are full partners in the learning process, and learning is the responsibility of the students. These characteristics are similar to the key principles outlined by O'Banion for the Learning College (see Box 2-1).

Primary benefits of the conceptual learning approach for nursing education programs include the following:

- Decreased content saturation
- Increased focus on nursing practice, not on medical diagnosis
- Opportunities for collaborative learning
- Increased thinking and nursing judgment
- Student engagement in the learning process

Decreased Content Saturation

In a conceptual learning environment, content is carefully and purposefully selected for inclusion in the curriculum. This content prepares the nursing student for real-world practice and focuses on keeping patients and their families safe. Therefore, a CBC helps desaturate the curriculum (Giddens & Brady, 2007).

One of the challenges in revising or developing any curriculum is achieving faculty consensus on which content to include. One guide that can assist prelicensure nursing faculty is either the NCLEX-RN® or NCLEX-PN® test plan (see www.ncsbn.org). Nursing faculty who teach in prelicensure programs may be reluctant to delete existing medical diagnosis curriculum content for fear that the content will be tested on the NCLEX®. However, the current licensure test plans are not organized by medical diagnosis, but rather by integrated processes and client needs categories. Nursing faculty need to consider the NCLEX® as a guide when selecting concepts and exemplars for their CBC. **TABLE 2-3** provides examples of Giddens' concepts as they compare to selected NCLEX® topics.

TABLE 2-2 Comparison of Traditional and Conceptual Teaching and Learning	
Traditional Teaching and Learning	**Conceptual Teaching and Learning**
Is teacher-centered	Is student-centered
Is content-driven	Is process-driven
Promotes rote memorization and surface/superficial learning	Promotes deep learning
Uses passive learning	Uses active learning
Focuses on large amount of content using lecture format	Focuses on smaller amount of content to allow cognitive processing

TABLE 2-3 Comparison of Selected NCLEX® Topics with Giddens' Concepts	
NCLEX® Concept	**Giddens' Concept**
Collaboration	Collaboration
Safety	Safety
Continuity of care	Care coordination
Management concepts	Leadership
Quality improvement	Healthcare quality
Ethical practice	Ethics
Health promotion/Disease prevention	Health promotion, patient education
Therapeutic communication	Communication
Coping mechanisms	Coping
Stress management	Stress
Aging process, newborn	Development
Family dynamics	Family dynamics
Cultural awareness	Culture
Elimination	Elimination
Mobility/Immobility	Mobility
Nutrition and hydration	Nutrition
F & E imbalances	F & E balance
Rest and sleep	Sleep
Nonpharmacological comfort interventions/ Pharmacological pain management	Pain
Ante/Intra/Postpartum care	Reproduction
Substance abuse disorder	Addiction

BOX 2-2 Suggested Concepts for Selected *BSN Essentials*

Essential VI. Interprofessional Communication and Collaboration for Improving Patient Outcomes

- Communication
- Collaboration
- Advocacy
- Safety
- Scopes of practice
- Caring
- Group dynamics

Essential VIII. Professionalism and Professional Values

- Communication
- Informed consent
- Ethics
- Culture
- Accountability
- Professional identity
- Advocacy

Other national guidelines for faculty to consider include the *Essentials* documents for each type of nursing program. For both prelicensure BSN and RN-to-BSN programs, the American Association of Colleges of Nursing's (AACN's) *The Essentials of Baccalaureate Education for Professional Nursing Practice* (referred to most commonly as the *BSN Essentials*) can be a valuable resource for determining the most important concepts to include in a BSN curriculum. **BOX 2-2** illustrates the relationship of selected *BSN Essentials* with concepts that might be included in a BSN curriculum.

Few graduate nursing program curricula formally acknowledge that they are concept-based or emphasize conceptual learning. However, the nature of *The Essentials of Master's Education in Nursing* and *The Essentials of Doctoral Education for Advanced Nursing Practice* lend themselves to identifying key concepts and teaching conceptually. For example, *Essential VI* for master's education is Health Policy and Advocacy. Related concepts for this topic include the following:

- Healthcare delivery system
- Ethics
- Globalization
- Health disparities
- Healthcare economics
- Political activism

Students in graduate programs that lead to advanced clinical practice must also learn primary diagnosis, pharmacology, and best practices in patient care.

Increased Focus on Nursing Practice

Another very important benefit to using the conceptual approach is the increased focus on nursing practice rather than an emphasis on medical diagnoses. As part of prerequisite general education courses in a *traditional* curriculum, professional nursing students take anatomy and physiology. These courses are usually organized by body system, and the student frames the content through that lens.

After completing all or most of these science courses, the student is accepted into the nursing sequence portion of the program. The first major nursing course typically introduces the student to the role of the nurse, nursing process, communication, and nursing care to meet basic human needs, such as comfort and nutrition. This course tends to be organized by concepts, even in a traditional model, because students must have basic knowledge and skills that serve as the foundation for the remainder of the curriculum. Students no longer organize content by body system and begin learning using a conceptual approach. They may also take corequisite health assessment and pharmacology courses.

After successfully completing these first course(s), students then take courses organized by medical diagnosis associated with body system and divided into "specialty" areas. The students are required to again change their framework for learning. The focus of specialty content tends to emphasize pathophysiology, medical diagnosis, and treatment, with less attention to the role of the nursing in providing safe, quality care.

By contrast to the previous description of a traditional nursing curriculum, a *conceptual* approach throughout all nursing courses places emphasis on nursing care in a collaborative and changing health care system. Students can transfer knowledge and patterns of learning about nursing practice across the curriculum.

Opportunities for Collaborative Learning

In a conceptual curriculum, students are provided with opportunities for collaborative learning in pairs or larger groups (**FIGURE 2-1**). Peer learning is effective and promotes teamwork, which prepares diverse students for nursing practice in the workplace. Students who are **English Language Learners (ELLs)** (also referred to as students who have English as a Second Language [ESL]) can benefit from working in groups as they refine their use of English, the most difficult language to learn. Examples of pair and group activities that are appropriate in a CBC classroom or clinical setting are described in Chapter 5 of this textbook.

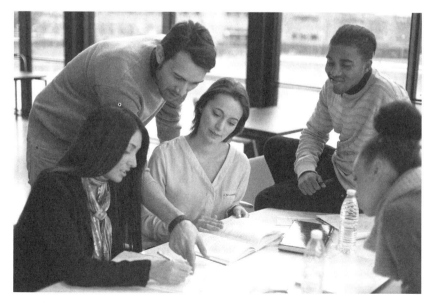

FIGURE 2-1 Nursing students in a classroom working on a case study in collaborative groups
© jacoblund/iStock/Getty

BOX 2-3 Interprofessional Education Collaborative Competencies

- *Values/Ethics for Interprofessional Practice:* Work with individuals of other professions to maintain a climate of mutual respect and shared values.
- *Role-Responsibilities:* Use the knowledge of one's own role and those of other professions to appropriately assess and address the healthcare needs of the patients and to promote and advance the health of populations.
- *Interprofessional Communication:* Communicate with patients, families, communities, and other professionals in health and other fields in a responsive and responsible manner that supports a team approach to the maintenance of health and the prevention and treatment of disease.
- *Teams and Teamwork:* Apply relationship-building values and the principles of team dynamics to perform effectively in different team roles to plan, deliver, and evaluate patient-/population-centered care and population health programs and policies that are safe, timely, efficient, effective, and equitable.

Modified from Interprofessional Education Collaborative (IPEC). (2016). Core competencies for interprofessional collaborative practice: 2016 update. Washington, DC: Interprofessional Education Collaborative. Reprinted with permission.

Another opportunity for collaboration is interprofessional education. **Interprofessional education (IPE)** allows students from two or more health professions to learn together during the same learning activity or in the same setting and promotes team building. Teamwork is included in the Interprofessional Education Collaborative (IPEC) initiative competencies (IPEC, 2016) (**BOX 2-3**). Examples of IPE activities are included elsewhere in this textbook.

Increased Thinking and Nursing Judgment

Learning conceptually increases student thinking (Erickson, 2007). Thinking conceptually helps nursing students learn to "think like nurses." In her meta-analysis study, Tanner (2006) found that nurses in practice increase thinking and clinical judgment skills as they become more confident and competent as practitioners. The nurse brings his or her knowledge and experience, ethical comportment, and knowledge of the patient to provide appropriate and timely clinical judgments. Tanner's model of clinical judgment includes the following elements:

- Noticing (which triggers additional data collection)
- Interpreting (based on data)
- Responding (if needed, and based on the interpretation of data)
- Reflecting (determining is the situation is resolved and what is learned)

In Canada, these elements and considerations are part of *relational practice*. Relational nursing practice also includes consideration of the healthcare system (Doane & Varcoe, 2015).

A study by Ashley and Stamp (2014) showed that novice nursing students developed clinical judgment and reasoning skills in a high-fidelity simulated laboratory experience. The scenario for the sophomores focused on a patient with hypoglycemia; the scenario for the juniors focused on a patient with chest pain. After this learning activity, the researchers interviewed the 104 sophomore and junior level nursing students. Although differences in the levels of clinical judgment were noted between the two subgroups, the following five themes emerged from content analysis of the data:

- Thinking like a nurse
- Importance of nursing assessment
- Looking for answers to resolve the patient's problem
- Need for communication using SBAR (situation, background, assessment, recommendation)
- Magical or reflective thinking

The biggest differences between the analysis of sophomore and junior data included that the juniors were more systematic in their thinking and decision making.

Student Engagement in the Learning Process

A successful conceptual approach requires responsibility for learning and active student engagement in the learning process (Erickson, 2007; Getha-Eby et al., 2014). In a traditional curriculum, deep learning is not common and students forget memorized information. As a result, nursing faculty review normal anatomy and physiology, human development, pathophysiology, and other content that students should know. Students realize that they do not need to be responsible or accountable for learning because many faculty "spoon feed" students. "Spoon feeding" the content to students does not result in deep learning. Students again memorize the reviewed content for the short term and become passive learners.

In a CBC, faculty are obligated to engage students in each educational setting through active and innovative learning strategies. Recent trends in creating a flipped or scrambled classroom are based on this student accountability for learning. The educator must outline student expectations for before class, during class, and after class to facilitate that learning. The same principle applies for learning that occurs online, in a laboratory, or in a community clinical agency or unit.

> ### Remember This . . .
>
> *A successful conceptual approach requires responsibility for learning and active student engagement in the learning process. Recent trends in creating a flipped or scrambled classroom are based on this student accountability for learning.*

▶ Chapter Key Points

- *Teaching* is what the educator does through instructional methods and is therefore teacher-centered. *Learning* is what students do and is therefore student-centered.
- Advances in neurobiology (brain) research demonstrate that meaningful deep learning produces connections between information and allows students to apply knowledge in a variety of contexts.
- The *teaching* approach helps faculty "cover" large amounts of course content in a certain timeframe, but promotes rote memorization, inaccurate cognitive connections, and short-term superficial learning.
- The key building blocks of a CBC are concepts and exemplars.

- For both prelicensure BSN and RN-to-BSN programs, the American Association of Colleges of Nursing's (AACN's) *The Essentials of Baccalaureate Education for Professional Nursing Practice* (referred to most commonly as the *BSN Essentials)* can be a valuable resource for determining the most important concepts to include in a BSN curriculum.
- The nature of *The Essentials of Master's Education in Nursing* and *The Essentials of Doctoral Education for Advanced Nursing Practice* lend themselves to identifying key concepts and teaching conceptually.
- Meaningful learning creates deep understanding, which students then can transfer to real-world problem solving and decision making using judgment and critical thinking.
- Primary benefits of the conceptual learning approach for nursing education programs include decreased content saturation, increased focus on nursing practice, opportunities for collaborative learning, increased thinking and nursing judgment, and student engagement in the learning process.

▶ Chapter References and Selected Bibliography

Ambrose, S., Bridges, M. W., Dipietro, M., Lovett, M. C., & Norman, M. K. (2010). *How learning works.* San Francisco: Jossey-Bass.

American Association of Colleges of Nursing. (2008). *The Essentials of Baccalaureate Education for Professional Nursing Practice.* Retrieved November, 2016 from www.aacn.nche.edu/education-resources/BaccEssentials08.pdf.

American Association of Colleges of Nursing. (2011). *The essentials of master's education in nursing.* Retrieved November, 2016 from www.aacn.nche.edu/education-resources/MastersEssentials11.pdf.

*Anderson, L. W., Krathwohl, D. R., Airasian, P. W., Cruikshank, K. A., Mayer, P. E., Pintrich, P. R. . . . Wittrock, M. C. (2001). *A taxonomy for learning, teaching and assessing: A revision of Bloom's taxonomy of educational objectives.* San Francisco: Jossey-Bass.

Ashley, J., & Stamp, K. (2014). Learning to thinking like a nurse: The development of clinical judgment in nursing students. *Journal of Nursing Education, 53*(9), 519–525.

*Ausubel, D. P. (1963). *The psychology of meaningful verbal learning: An introduction to school learning.* New York, NY: Grune & Stratton.

Benner, P. (2012). Educating nurses: A call for radical transformation—how far have we come? *Journal of Nursing Education, 51*(4), 183–184.

Benner, P., Stephen, M., Leonard, V., & Day, L. (2010). *Educating nurses: A call for radical transformation.* San Francisco: Jossey-Bass.

*Diekelmann, N. (2002). "Too much content. . . ." Epistemologies' grasp and nursing education. *Journal of Nursing Education, 41*(11), 469–470.

Doane, G. H., & Varcoe, C. (2015). *How to nurse: Relational inquiry with individuals and families in changing health and health care contexts.* Philadelphia, PA: Wolters Kluwer.

*Erickson, L. (2002). *Concept-based curriculum and instruction.* Thousand Oaks, CA: Corwin Press.

Erickson, L. (2007). *Concept-based curriculum and instruction in the thinking classroom.* Thousand Oaks, CA: Corwin Press.

Erickson, L. (2008). *Stirring the head, heart, and soul: Redefining curriculum, instruction, and concept-based learning.* Thousand Oaks, CA: Corwin Press.

Getha-Eby, T. J., Beery, T., Xu, Y., & O'Brien, B. A. (2014). Meaningful learning: Theoretical Support for concept-based teaching. *Journal of Nursing Education, 53*(9), 494–500.

Giddens, J. F. (2017). *Concepts for nursing practice* (2nd ed.). St. Louis, MO: Elsevier.

Giddens, J. F., & Brady, D. P. (2007). Rescuing nursing education from content saturations: The case for a concept-based curriculum. *Journal of Nursing Education, 46*(2), 65–69.

Giddens, J. F., Caputi, L., & Rodgers, B. (2015). *Mastering concept-based teaching: A guide for nursing educators.* St. Louis, MO: Elsevier.

Interprofessional Education Collaborative (IPEC). (2016). Core competencies for interprofessional collaborative practice: 2016 update. Washington, D.C.: IPEC.

*Ironside, P. M. (2004). "Covering content" and teaching thinking: Deconstructing the additive curriculum. *Journal of Nursing Education, 43*(1), 5–12.

*Knowles, M. (1984). *Androgogy in action.* San Francisco, CA: Jossey-Bass.

Kumaran, D., Summerfield, J. J., Hassabis, D., & Maguire, E. A. (2009). Tracking the emergence of conceptual knowledge during human decision-making. *Neuron, 63*(6), 889–901.

Lasater, K., & Nielson, A. (2009). The influence of concept-based learning activities on students' clinical judgement development. *Journal of Nursing Education, 48*(8), 441–446.

Novak, J. D. (2010). *Learning, creating, and using knowledge: Concept maps as facilitative tools in schools and corporations.* Mahwah, NJ: Lawrence Erlbaum.

O'Banion, T., & Wilson, C. (2010). *Focus on learning: A learning college reader.* Phoenix, AZ: League for Innovation.

*Tanner, C. A. (2006). Thinking like a nurse: A research-based model of clinical judgment in nursing. *Journal of Nursing Education, 45*(6), 204–211.

---

*Indicates classic reference.

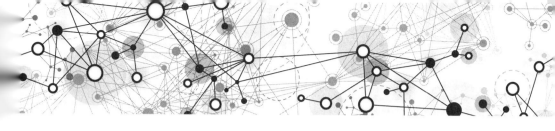

CHAPTER 3

Developing a Nursing Concept-Based Curriculum: A 12-Step Approach

Donna Ignatavicius

▶ Introduction to the Nursing Concept-Based Curriculum

A number of nursing programs in the United States and Canada have implemented or are developing concept-based curricula that best meet the needs of their students, faculty, and geographic region. Unfortunately, there is a paucity of literature on *how* to structure an effective concept-based curriculum (CBC). Following a general overview, this chapter outlines the author's 12-step approach to developing a CBC. This process is based on the literature and the author's years of experience in assisting with CBC development throughout the United States and Canada.

Concept-Based Curriculum for Prelicensure U.S. Registered Nursing Programs

During the 1980s and 1990s, several new nursing textbooks were published that were organized by pathophysiological concepts, such as obstruction, ischemia, and dyspnea. Faculty were not instructed or professionally developed in how to teach using these unique resources. The author of this CBC book used one of these texts in a large mid-Atlantic BSN program in the mid-1980s and found that students had difficulty understanding this conceptual approach. As a result, students performed poorly on their nursing licensure examination. Since that time, Lynn Erickson and her colleagues published multiple articles and books on developing a concept-based curriculum and inquiry-based learning in K through 12 education (Erickson, 2002, 2007; Erickson & Lanning, 2014).

In 2004, Dr. Jean Giddens and her colleagues at the University of New Mexico began the current concept-based nursing curricular movement based on the works of Erickson and the pathophysiological concept nursing textbook written by Carrieri-Kohlman, Lindsey, and West (2003). Although this more current CBC model and conceptual learning have been implemented in a number of nursing programs, no two curricula are exactly alike unless a state or province designs a common core curriculum that all of its programs use. Oregon and North Carolina were two of the earliest states to develop a statewide CBC. The Oregon model included universities and community college programs, but the North Carolina model included only state associate degree (AD) programs in community colleges.

Since these earlier statewide curricula were developed, other states have implemented their own unique plans. All prelicensure RN nursing programs in Wyoming and New Mexico, for example, have recently implemented a seamless curriculum that allows students to transition easily from the AD in nursing to graduation from a BSN program. Each program in Wyoming may select its own concepts and exemplars integrated into statewide-developed lifespan courses. By contrast, all New Mexico programs use a predetermined concept list selected by a state faculty consortium and based on data from a national survey of concepts published by Giddens (Giddens, Wright, & Gray, 2012). AD in nursing programs in Texas and Alabama also incorporate a preplanned concept list as they phase in their statewide CBC for multiple community colleges.

Concept-Based Curriculum for Prelicensure Canadian Registered Nursing Programs

A few nursing schools in Canada have developed or are developing a CBC for BSN programs. Examples include the University of Manitoba in Winnipeg, The British Columbia Institute of Technology in Burnaby, and Kwantlen Polytechnic University in Surrey. These program curricula are largely based on the Giddens' concepts, with additional concepts that are specific or unique to Canadian professional nursing practice (Doane & Varcoe, 2015). Examples of these concepts are found in **BOX 3-1**.

> **BOX 3-1** Examples of Professional Nursing and Health Care Concepts Unique to Canadian Professional Nursing Practice
>
> - Relational Inquiry
> - Cultural Safety
> - Global Citizenship
> - Followership
> - Accessibility
> - Social Justice
> - Health Care Context

Data from Doane, G. H., & Varcoe, C. (2015). *How to nurse: Relational inquiry with individuals and families in changing health and health care contexts*. Philadelphia: Wolters Kluwer Health.

Concept-Based Curriculum for Prelicensure Practical/Vocational Nursing Programs

The Minnesota statewide collaborative curriculum project led by Dr. Sue Field is an excellent example of using the CBC for practical nursing (PN) programs (Field et al., 2014). This PN curriculum may be taught using a conceptual model or traditional medical model. Role-specific competencies that demonstrate achievement of PN curricular student learning outcomes (SLOs) emphasize the Knowledge (K), Practice Know How (P), and Ethical Comportment (E) needed for each concept. These competencies represent the cognitive, psychomotor, and affective domains of learning and are aligned with the NCLEX-PN® test plan, Minnesota Scope of Practice for Practical Nursing, and revised standards published by the National Association of Practical Nursing Education and Service (NAPNES) (Field et al., 2014).

▶ Preplanning for Transition from a Traditional to a Concept-Based Nursing Curriculum

According to Erickson and Lanning (2014), preplanning work is needed to "set the stage" for a successful CBC. According to these K through 12 educational experts, the following three preliminary steps are required:

1. Examine the hidden impediments to change.
2. Assemble a learning team.
3. Shape a shared vision of concept-based instruction.

In nursing education, the most important preplanning considerations are similar to Erickson and Lanning's steps and include the need to 1) obtain faculty buy-in, 2) educate faculty before and throughout the process, and 3) form a curriculum faculty work group. These considerations are interrelated and require the use of change theory, administrative support, stakeholder input, faculty commitment, and adequate resources to attain the goal. Each step is briefly discussed later in this chapter.

Before any new curriculum can be developed, it is essential to identify all facilitators and any overt or hidden barriers to the process to obtain faculty buy-in.

BOX 3-2 Potential Reasons Why Nursing Faculty May Not Support Curriculum Revision or a Concept-Based Curriculum

- Currently have better-than-national first-time NCLEX® pass rates.
- Too much time needed to revise the curriculum.
- Need to recalculate faculty load; some faculty may lose their jobs if specialty content decreases.
- Too many new inexperienced faculty who do not have knowledge about curriculum development.
- Not enough knowledge about how to structure or teach a CBC.
- Clinical partners may not buy into the conceptual learning approach.

As mentioned in Chapter 1, some faculty are eager to make changes that can improve student learning and thinking. Others may be reluctant to change from a curricular model that they have used for many years to one that is very different. Some of the reasons that faculty cite for maintaining a traditional curriculum are listed in **BOX 3-2**.

Remember This . . .

Before any new curriculum can be developed, it is essential to identify all facilitators and barriers to the process to obtain faculty buy-in.

Faculty education about the CBC can be achieved through reading pertinent literature that describes the benefits and process of conceptual learning; attending local, regional, or national CBC conferences; and discussing the revision process with program faculty where the CBC is used. Understanding the nature of conceptual learning and how to develop a meaningful curriculum are crucial to successful planning and implementation.

When the current CBC movement began, professional development for faculty was lacking. Many nurse educators did not know how to teach conceptually, and there were very few resources to assist them. As a result, some programs experienced a temporary decrease in first-time NCLEX® pass rates. However, program outcomes rebounded fairly quickly as faculty and students became more comfortable with the conceptual approach. For example, the North Carolina AD in Nursing program 3-year average NCLEX-RN® pass rate from 2012 to 2014 was 88%; the national average for that same period was 82% (www.ncbon.com). Given these statistics and anecdotal reports of program outcomes throughout the United States, worry about low NCLEX® pass rates as a reason for avoiding curriculum revision is unwarranted.

Curriculum revision and development are time-consuming projects, but ultimately improve the quality of nursing education. As mentioned in Chapter 1, one of the major responsibilities and competencies of the academic nurse educator is curriculum revision. As a group, nursing faculty drives the curricular process, and thus must learn and consider best practices in curriculum development.

Another concern is the calculation of faculty load and possible loss of hours or positions as curricular content is reduced. In many BSN programs, faculty tend to teach the theory/didactic courses or the didactic portion of combined theory/clinical

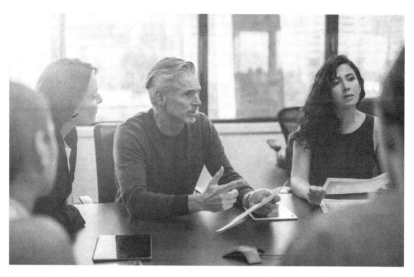

FIGURE 3-1 Faculty work group working to develop new nursing concept-based curriculum
© xavierarnau/E+/Getty

courses alone. In AD and PN/VN programs, faculty often team or turn teach. Each faculty member is usually required to have X amount of load hours depending on how many contact hours or credits are taught. In a new curricular model, faculty might need to be flexible and teach part or all of a course to meet full-time load requirements. However, a CBC should not result in loss of faculty positions.

Faculty and clinical staff education is essential for a successful curricular revision and implementation. Planning a conceptual approach requires a new way of thinking, organizing knowledge, and making sense of learning. Erickson (2007) describes learning in a traditional curriculum as two-dimensional, incorporating only factual content and process/skills. A CBC adds the third dimension of concepts that represent the big ideas or mental images that promote deep learning and understanding. Nursing programs need to have an ongoing dialogue with their stakeholders, including their advisory committee, alumni, and clinical partners, about the benefits of conceptual instruction and the need to obtain their input into curricular decisions.

The last preplanning step is to create a small work group of three to five faculty who are well respected, communicate effectively, and are knowledgeable about curriculum development and conceptual teaching and learning (**FIGURE 3-1**). The primary goal of this group is to shape a shared vision of CBC while keeping the entire faculty fully aware of their work. All faculty should have the opportunity to have input during each step of the curriculum development process.

▶ The 12-Step Approach to Concept-Based Curriculum Development

Chapter 1 describes the essential components of an effective curriculum. This section incorporates those components and provides details for developing a CBC using the author's 12-step process (**BOX 3-3**). Each step is described in the following section

BOX 3-3 Ignatavicius' 12-Step Approach to Concept-Based Curriculum Development

Step 1: Review and revise the Nursing Department/School of Nursing mission and philosophy.

Step 2: Develop the organizing curriculum framework.

Step 3: Establish program outcomes.

Step 4: Determine the plan of study or degree plan.

Step 5: Select and define nursing curriculum concepts.

Step 6: Select exemplars for each concept.

Step 7: Write course descriptions and student learning outcomes.

Step 8: Determine where each concept will be introduced.

Step 9: Develop a concept presentation for each curriculum concept.

Step 10: Determine where each exemplar will be placed in the curriculum.

Step 11: Develop each course syllabus and lesson plan/study guide.

Step 12: Select appropriate clinical experiences and activities that are conceptually focused.

and includes a brief discussion of student learning assessment when indicated. More detail on Assessment and Evaluation in a nursing CBC may be found in Part III of this book in Chapters 10, 11, and 12.

Step 1: Review and Revise the Nursing Department and School of Nursing Mission and Philosophy

The nursing philosophy for a program, department, or school should flow from its mission and be congruent with those of the institution (Keating, 2015). It typically includes a definition of nursing practice that aligns with national standards that guide nursing practice and nursing education. As part of the definition of nursing, many programs include the Quality and Safety Education for Nurses (QSEN) concepts and/or the Nurse of the Future competencies. Chapter 1 describes the components of a philosophy and mission statement.

Step 2: Develop the Organizing Curriculum Framework

From the mission/philosophy, the faculty can then select the core organizing concepts or themes upon which to build the curriculum. Recall from Chapter 2 that concepts are classifications/categories of information that can be big or broad ideas or mental images. Some programs use the entire list of curricular concepts as their organizing or organizational framework. Most programs select a subset of 6 to 10 professional nursing concepts that align with the mission/philosophy as their core curricular organizers. These organizing concepts reflect the underpinnings of the curriculum and what will be emphasized, such as safety, collaborative care, professionalism, and patient-centered care, based on the faculty's definition of nursing. Not all programs use an organizing framework because it may not be required by their state or province.

Step 3: Establish Program Outcomes

Most nursing programs using a CBC combine concepts with competencies. Competencies are the knowledge, skills, and attitudes that make up a person's role. They are context-specific and show demonstration of abilities and skills (behaviors) based on knowledge in a variety of situations. These behaviors demonstrate "thinking like a nurse."

In nursing education, SLOs are used to delineate competencies and help organize the curriculum. As mentioned in Chapter 1, they can be categorized into three levels:

- End-of-program SLOs (also called program learning outcomes [PLOs])
- Course SLOs
- Unit, modular, or weekly SLOs

At this point in curriculum development, the only SLOs that can be developed are those for the new graduate at the end of the nursing program, sometimes referred to as end-of-program outcomes or new graduate outcomes. These outcomes specify graduate competencies related to the core organizers. For example, if safety and patient-centered care are two of the core organizing concepts for a PN program, then an appropriate graduate outcome might be: "Provide *safe, patient-centered care* to individuals across the lifespan in a variety of community-based health care settings."

If a school, college, or university has more than one type of nursing program (e.g., generic AD and RN-to-BSN), each program must have its own list of new graduate outcomes. These outcomes should be leveled by program to show clear differences in graduate knowledge, skill, and attitude. Chapter 4 of this book discusses developing SLOs in detail.

Step 4: Determine the Plan of Study or Degree Plan

The **plan of study (POS)**, also referred to as the **program of study**, provides a list of courses by term in a sequence from program admission to graduation. If graduates receive a college degree upon program completion, the POS may be referred to as a **degree plan**. Faculty must decide on which courses and sequence of courses will enable the students to meet the end-of-program outcomes. Box 1-5 in Chapter 1 reviews factors that faculty must consider when developing the POS.

Faculty are also responsible for assigning the number of credits for each course and translating those credits to student contact hours within the approved total number of program credits or clock hours. For most nursing programs:

- 1 didactic/theory course credit = 1 contact hour per week (1:1) over a semester. For a 15-week semester, that means the student would have a total of 15 contact hours, or 1 contact hour/credit × 15 weeks. For a 2-credit course, the contact hours would be 1 contact hour/credit × 15 weeks × 2 credits = 30 contact hours, and so forth. If the course is taught over an 8-week term, the same number of contact hours must be included. For instance, a 2-credit didactic course with 30 contact hours over an 8-week period would require 3.75 hours a week of class (3.75 hours per week × 8 weeks = 30 contact hours).
- 1 laboratory/clinical course credit = 3 contact hours per week over a semester (3:1). For a 15-week semester, that means that the student would have a total of 45 contact hours for the semester (3 contact hours/credit × 15 weeks × 1 credit = 45 contact hours). Those hours could be distributed in any way that the nurse educator thinks would be the best for the student. In some colleges, laboratory and/or clinical courses are calculated at 2:1 rather than at 3:1.

If the program results in awarding a degree, part of the POS includes the prenursing general education or liberal arts and science courses required by the institution (Keating, 2015). For a generic or accelerated BSN degree, students are typically required to take most or all of their liberal arts and sciences prior to being admitted to the nursing program. This practice may vary depending on the school, state, province, or region.

In a CBC, courses are often developed using a lifespan approach rather than dividing the content in several courses based on population. For example, rather than teaching about caring for children and adolescents with diabetes mellitus (DM) in one course, teaching about caring for the pregnant woman with gestational diabetes in another course, and teaching chronic care of adults with diabetes in yet another course, a lifespan approach requires that students learn how to care for patients with diabetes across the lifespan in the same course. This approach prevents content duplication and promotes deep learning. However, keeping one or more population-based courses does not prevent the program from using a conceptual approach to teaching and learning.

Some nursing programs keep their maternal health/childbearing content in a separate course because the content is unique. Faculty members decide which POS they think would be best for students. Currently there is no evidence to support one POS versus another, but an increased focus on care for older adults should be a major goal of every nursing program, given the large Baby Boomer population moving into older adulthood.

Another way that courses may be delineated is by grouping concepts by category and developing courses around those categories. For example, consider these first nursing semester *concept-focused* courses for a BSN program:

Introduction to Health Concepts	4 credits
Professional Nursing I	3 credits
Nursing Practicum I	3 credits
Basic Pathophysiology	4 credits

The Introduction to Health Concepts course might be similar to the more traditional Foundations or Fundamentals of Nursing course, but taught conceptually. The focus of this didactic course would be on health concepts across the lifespan that serve as a foundation for the rest of the curriculum. Examples of these concepts are Nutrition, Elimination, and Oxygenation (or Gas Exchange). The Professional Nursing I course would include beginning concepts that are needed to develop professional behavior and identity, such as Clinical Judgment (Nursing Process), Communication, and Safety. The Nursing Practicum I course would allow students to apply concepts learned in the concurrent didactic courses in community clinical settings and/or simulation.

One of the advantages of a separate clinical course is the expectation for students to apply both Health and Professional Nursing concepts in the clinical setting. In most nursing programs, however, student failures tend to occur more often in didactic courses than clinical courses. In the previous semester course example, if a student passes Nursing Practicum I and Professional Nursing I, but fails Introduction to Health Concepts, the student needs only to retake the one failed course without any supporting clinical experience. From a legal perspective, students who successfully complete any course cannot be made to retake it. For this reason, many programs offer combined didactic/clinical courses that require the student to successfully complete both the theory and clinical requirements to pass the course.

Using a lifespan approach to integrate populations can be challenging when seeking approval from the state board of nursing. Some states require that theory and/or clinical topics and time be specified by population. For example, in California, the Board of Registered Nursing must be able to clearly see where pediatric, obstetric, older adult, adult, and mental health nursing care is being taught and practiced in the curriculum. Although this task can be challenging to "carve out," it can be done in an integrated, concept-focused plan of study. **BOX 3-4** provides an example of how this required information might be provided.

The last Professional Nursing course in a CBC is usually devoted to leadership and healthcare system concepts. In addition, the program may have a 1- or 2-credit

---

BOX 3-4 Sample Plan of Study for an Associate Degree Program in Nursing Using a Concept-Based Curriculum

Year 1
Nursing Semester 1
HC I: Introduction to Health Concepts Across the Lifespan   7 cr. (5T, 2C/L)
(NOTE: Introduction to Care of Older Adults included.)

Professional Nursing I   2 cr.
Pharmacology I   1 cr.
Total   *10 cr.*

Nursing Semester 2
HC II: Care of Individuals and Families with Common Health Conditions   7 cr. (4T, 3C)
(NOTE: Adult, mental health, pediatric, normal peripartum content included.)

Professional Nursing II   2 cr.
Pharmacology II   1 cr.
Total   *10 cr.*

Year 2
Nursing Semester 3
HC III: Care of Individuals and Families with Complex Health Problems   7 cr. (4T, 3C)
(NOTE: Adult, pediatric, mental health, high risk peripartum content included.)

Professional Nursing III   1 cr.
Pharmacology III   1 cr.
Total   *9 cr.*

Nursing Semester 4
First 8 weeks:
HC IV: Care of Individuals with Multisystem and Emergent Health Problems   3 cr. (2T, 1C)
(NOTE: Focus on adult health.)

Professional Nursing III   2 cr.
Second 8 weeks:
Concept Synthesis   1 cr.
Capstone Clinical Immersion   3 cr.
Total   *9 cr.*

HC = Health Concepts; cr. = credit; T = theory (either online or classroom); C = clinical experience; L = laboratory experience.

didactic Concept Synthesis course and a clinical Capstone course in which students can apply all program concepts while under the supervision of either a preceptor or clinical instructor (see Box 3-4).

Step 5: Select and Define Nursing Curriculum Concepts

Steps 4 and 5 are sometimes interchanged, depending on faculty preference. The author finds that it is usually better to at least plan the approach for the plan of study before determining concepts for the curriculum. However, there are times when it is more important for faculty to select concepts before naming and sequencing the courses.

Select Nursing Concepts

Selecting nursing concepts can be a challenge: Which concepts do we need? Should we use all of the Giddens' concepts or only part of them? Should we categorize the concepts similarly or differently than Giddens? How many concepts do we need for an effective curriculum? Unfortunately, there are no definitive answers to these questions. However, nursing programs typically begin with a review of the established and recently refined concept list published by Giddens in her revised book entitled *Concepts for Nursing Practice* (2nd ed.) in 2017.

Dr. Giddens divides the 58 concepts in her book into three major categories and 12 subcategories, or macroconcepts. According to Erickson (2007), **macroconcepts** provide disciplinary breadth; that is, they are broad and provide a way to link sub-concepts, sometimes called microconcepts (Giddens, Caputi, & Rodgers, 2015). **Microconcepts** are more specific and provide disciplinary depth for understanding and deep learning (Erickson, 2007).

The three major Giddens' categories are Health Care Recipient Concepts, Health and Illness Concepts, and Professional Nursing and Health Care Concepts. Examples of concepts in each major Giddens' category are listed in **TABLE 3-1**. Health Care

TABLE 3-1 Categories and Examples of Giddens' Concepts for Nursing Practice		
Health Care Recipient	**Health and Illness**	**Professional Nursing and Health Care**
Development	Reproduction	Professional Identity
Functional Ability	Clotting	Leadership
Family Dynamics	Nutrition	Safety
Culture	Coping	Ethics
Spirituality	Anxiety	Health Disparities
Self-Management	Addiction	Health Policy

Data from Giddens, J. F. (2017). *Concepts for nursing practice* (2nd ed.). St. Louis, MO: Elsevier.

Recipient Concepts include concepts that represent the unique characteristics of a patient, such as Development, and concepts that can influence a patient's health care decisions and preferences, such as Culture. Health and Illness Concepts are related to health promotion, such as Nutrition and Perfusion, or actual health problems, such as Pain and Addiction. Professional Nursing and Health Care Concepts represent nursing attributes and role and professional nursing competences. They also include issues in health care delivery and infrastructure (Giddens, 2017).

To illustrate Giddens use of macroconcepts and microconcepts, within the major category of Professional Nursing and Health Care Concepts, there are four sub-categories (or *macroconcepts)*. Six concepts are grouped under the *macroconcept* of Nursing Attributes and Roles within the major category. These concepts include the following (Giddens, 2017):

- Professional Identity
- Clinical Judgment
- Leadership
- Ethics
- Patient Education
- Health Promotion

Prelicensure nursing programs vary greatly in the number of concepts they chose. There is no evidence that shows how many concepts should be included for a successful and effective CBC. When developing its statewide nursing curriculum, the New Mexico Nursing Education Consortium used data obtained through a survey of a small group of nursing programs across the country to determine the most commonly used concepts to include (Giddens et al., 2012). Large-scale research is needed to determine which concepts are used by the most successful CBC programs to ensure best practices in curriculum development.

From the author's experience, most PN/VN and AD in nursing programs select 20 to 35 total concepts and divide them into Professional Nursing and Health/Illness (H/I) or Health Concept categories; this model is a "modified" CBC. In this model, Health Care Recipient concepts may not be "called out" as curricular concepts, but are integrated throughout each course. For example, Culture is typically introduced in the first nursing course, but then discussed across the curriculum in multiple contexts and courses.

BSN programs may use more than 35 concepts because they include a major emphasis on evidence-based practice, leadership, health policy, and healthcare quality. Some BSN programs use all 58 Giddens' concepts (a more "purist" CBC approach), whereas others either delete concepts from the published list or add more concepts to the list.

> **Remember This . . .**
>
> *Prelicensure nursing programs vary greatly in the number of concepts they chose. There is no evidence that shows how many concepts should be included for a successful and effective CBC.*

Interestingly, only 9 of 31 Giddens' H/I Concepts represent health problems; the remaining 22 concepts in this category are health promotion–oriented. For this reason, many programs, including the community college RN programs in Texas, use only the health promotion–oriented concepts and relabel some of the health problem concepts as exemplars. For example, Pain is a Giddens' H/I Concept, but it can be relabeled to Comfort with pain as the primary exemplar. Addiction can be an exemplar for the H/I Concept of Coping rather than its own concept label. Likewise, Psychosis can be an exemplar for Cognition rather than a concept. Many programs use only Health Concepts (removing the Illness portion) and label Illness Concepts as exemplars. The author found that students and faculty better grasp an understanding of concepts when they are more consistent within a major category. Nursing program faculty members decide which concepts to use and if and when concepts should be relabeled to facilitate both student and faculty understanding.

Define Nursing Concepts

Each selected concept, including the core organizing concepts, requires a definition. Nurse educators can use Giddens' definitions, edit those definitions, or create their own definitions using a variety of resources. The author advocates using Giddens' definitions when possible if they are clearly understood and fit for the nursing program. However, if faculty members do not agree with a concept's definition as published in Giddens, they should utilize multiple sources and create a new definition. Be sure that all definitions are clear and concise for students and that faculty members are comfortable with the language used.

Most concepts can be defined in one sentence. For example, the Giddens' definition of Elimination is "the excretion of waste products" (Giddens, 2017, p. 156). This definition is clear, concise, and easily understood by both students and faculty. However, the concept of Sexuality is more complex and, therefore, Giddens' definition is quite lengthy. A more concise definition is offered in a widely used medical-surgical nursing textbook: "Sexuality is a complex integration of physiologic, emotional, and social aspects of well-being related to intimacy, self-concept, and role relationships" (Ignatavicius, Workman, & Rebar, 2018, p. 27). This amalgamated definition was developed by the author based on a review of multiple definitions from a variety of well-respected resources.

Step 6: Select Exemplars for Each Concept

The most challenging and often most frustrating step in developing a CBC is the selection of exemplars due to lack of faculty consensus. As mentioned in Chapter 2, **exemplars** are specific content topics that relate to and represent identified concepts. These selected topics are then taught and learned through the lens of the concept they represent.

In prelicensure nursing education, some nurse educators think they have to "teach everything" in textbooks because the content might be on the NCLEX® examination. In fact, both the NCLEX-RN® and NCLEX-PN® are not focused on medical diagnoses. In most cases, the medical diagnosis is not included in test items (unless needed to answer the question) because nurses at a generalist level do not make the diagnosis. Rather the NCLEX® is a nursing-focused test that measures minimum safety to practice as a beginning licensed PN/VN or RN. Do not feel compelled to include all topics that are discussed in any textbook, even one that is considered a resource for programs using a CBC. The decision for exemplar selection belongs to faculty.

> **Remember This . . .**
>
> *Do not feel compelled to include all topics that are discussed in any textbook, even one that is considered a resource for programs using a CBC.*

One way to think about exemplars is to compare them to drug prototypes. In a Pharmacology course, whether a basic or advanced course, the educator cannot teach every drug and students cannot learn every drug. Therefore, the most sensible approach is to help students learn the major drug classifications and several drug prototypes (exemplars) in each classification. Other helpful ways of learning about drug therapy is to learn the nursing implications within the drug classification using common suffixes, such as the "-statins," "-olols," and "-prils."

Likewise, the nurse educator cannot teach every disease, illness, and professional nursing issue, and students cannot learn all of that content. Programs using this traditional curricular method suffer from content saturation, causing students to rely on memorization for superficial learning. The difficult question, then, is which exemplars does an effective CBC *need* to include?

The following can be used for determining exemplars for H/I or Health Concepts:

- Research national websites for common health problems, including www.cdc.gov and www.healthypeople.gov in the United States or www.publichealth.gc.ca in Canada.
- Research state and provincial websites to identify major public health issues and concerns.
- Research local and regional public health issues or common health problems.

TABLE 3-2 delineates examples of common exemplars organized by selected Health Concepts.

TABLE 3-2 Examples of Health Concepts with Common Exemplars for a Prelicensure Nursing Concept-Based Curriculum

Mobility	Mood and Affect	Immunity	Nutrition
Fractures	Depression	Infection*	Peptic ulcer disease/GERD
Parkinson's disease	Bipolar disorder	Rheumatoid arthritis	Cholecystitis
Spinal cord injury	Anxiety disorder	Lupus erythematosus	Obesity
Scoliosis		Multiple sclerosis	Failure to thrive
Osteoarthritis			

*This nursing program designated Giddens' concept of Infection as an exemplar for Immunity to maintain the health promotion focus of Health Concepts.
GERD = Gastroesophageal reflux disease.

To determine the most important exemplars for Professional Nursing and Health Care concepts, research established national and state or provincial standards, guidelines, and competencies published by well-respected nursing and interprofessional organizations, including regulatory agencies. If selecting Health Care Recipient concept exemplars, research the most common demographic data that describe the local, state, provincial, and/or national population. For example, programs in the southwestern United States would want to include Hispanic (especially Spanish and Mexican) and American Indian/Native American cultures as exemplars for the concept of Culture.

After all of these data are collected from a variety of sources, the curricular work group or faculty as a whole begin to determine which exemplars represent which concepts. Be sure to indicate the evidence for why each exemplar should be included. For example, preventing and managing chronic health failure and hypertension are included in the goals for Healthy People 2020. The group may want to use a brainstorming session to develop the first draft of the exemplars. For example, one might think that exemplars for the concept of Acid-Base Balance could include chronic kidney disease (CKD) and chronic obstructive pulmonary disease (COPD). However, COPD could be an exemplar for the concept of Gas Exchange (or Oxygenation), and CKD could be an exemplar for the concept of Elimination.

One way to make a decision about where a Health concept exemplar is *best* placed is to think about an entire population of people across the lifespan experiencing the health problem. For instance, not all patients with COPD have an acid-base imbalance, but *all* of them have a disease affecting gas exchange. Likewise, not all patients with CKD have an acid-base imbalance, but *all* of them have a disease that affects urinary elimination. Therefore, the best placement of COPD is under the concept of Gas Exchange and CKD is best placed as an exemplar under Elimination. Acid-Base Balance would be an interrelated concept for both exemplars, as discussed under Step 10.

Remember This . . .

One way to make a decision about where a Health concept exemplar is best placed is to think about an entire population of people across the lifespan experiencing the health problem.

For Professional Nursing and Health Care Concepts, select exemplars that focus on major issues and concerns in the profession and across the interprofessional collaborative care team in a variety of health care settings. **TABLE 3-3** delineates common exemplars organized by selected Professional Nursing and Health Care Concepts.

Step 7: Write Course Descriptions and Student Learning Outcomes

Chapter 1 described the need to write concise course descriptions to distinguish one course from another. As part of each course syllabus, SLOs need to be developed that align with the course description. The description for the previously mentioned Professional Nursing I (3 credits) course might be as follows:

> This didactic course will introduce the student to nursing concepts needed to develop professional identity and provide safe, patient-centered care. Emphasis will be placed on the role and scope of practice of the professional nurse in

TABLE 3-3 Examples of Professional Nursing and Healthcare Concepts with Common Exemplars in a Prelicensure Nursing Concept-Based Curriculum

Clinical Judgment	Health Care Disparities	Health Care Law
Failure to rescue	Health insurance (United States)	HIPAA
Prioritization	Older adults	ADA
Delegation and supervision	Veterans	Informed Consent
Calling a primary healthcare provider	LGBTQ	Advance Directives
	Language barriers	Nurse Practice Act

ADA = American Disabilities Act; HIPAA = Health Insurance Portability and Accountability Act; LGBTQ = lesbian, gay, bisexual, transgendered, queer.

the healthcare system, therapeutic communication principles, and the nursing process as a tool for developing clinical judgment using best current evidence.

Course SLOs (sometimes called course objectives) outline student expectations by the *end* of the course. Examples for the above Professional Nursing I course might be the following:

1. Describe the primary roles of the professional nurse and members of the nursing team.
2. Explain the purpose of the state Nurse Practice Act and the board of nursing.
3. Utilize basic communication principles as a basis for the nurse-patient relationship and interprofessional collaboration.
4. Differentiate the five steps of the nursing process as a tool for clinical decision making and nursing judgment.

As part of SLO development, it is important to identify how to evaluate student achievement of each course SLO. For example, SLO 2 might be measured by an assignment in which students write a short paper on the purpose of the Nurse Practice Act and the function of the board of nursing. SLO 3 might be measured through a simulated role-play in class with students working in pairs or groups. A grading rubric could be used for both of these assignments. Chapter 4 discusses how to write meaningful SLOs in detail and ways in which they can be evaluated.

Step 8: Determine Where Each Concept Will Be Introduced

The next step is critical so that students have the conceptual building blocks to serve as a solid foundation for understanding and thinking. The faculty work group or full faculty group decides where each concept will be introduced. The introduction is an analysis of the concept, often called a **concept presentation**, described in Step 9. Exemplars should not be taught until the students learn and understand the concept presentation.

Not all concepts should be introduced in the first semester of the nursing program. Gas Exchange (or Oxygenation) is important to learn early in the program because students typically perform respiratory assessments, interpret pulse oximetry readings, and perform skills such as managing oxygen therapy in their first foundational courses. Safety, a Professional Nursing concept, also should be introduced in the first nursing semester because it is the basis for quality care to protect patients and staff members. Conversely, Intracranial Regulation (Health Concept) and Palliative Care (Professional Nursing and Health Care concept) are high-level, complex concepts that should be introduced later in the program.

> **Remember This . . .**
>
> *The introduction is an analysis of the concept, often called a **concept presentation**. Exemplars should not be taught until the students learn and understand the concept presentation.*

Step 9: Develop a Concept Presentation for Each Curriculum Concept

Concepts in each category are presented using a consistent template that illustrates an analysis of the concept. All concepts begin with the definition, but other components of the template vary based on major category. The author has noted some variation in template subheadings throughout the United States and Canada, but generally all templates have the same foundational information. The subheadings for a Health or H/I concept *(italic notations for clarification and explanation purposes only)* typically include the following:

- Definition of concept
- Scope (*continuum, if appropriate* [*see* **FIGURE 3-2** *for an example*]) or categories of concept
- Common risk factors for concept dysfunction or impairment (*can include populations at risk*)
- Physiological (*in some cases, may also include psychosocial*) consequences of concept dysfunction or impairment
- Assessment of concept status (*may include health assessment and diagnostic tests, if applicable*)
- Collaborative interventions to promote the concept or manage concept dysfunction or impairment (*may be divided into primary, secondary, and tertiary prevention*)
- Interrelated concepts (*usually includes 2 to 4 of the most common concepts*)
- Exemplars included in the curriculum

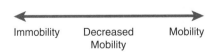

FIGURE 3-2 Example of graphic illustrating the scope of the Health Concept of Mobility

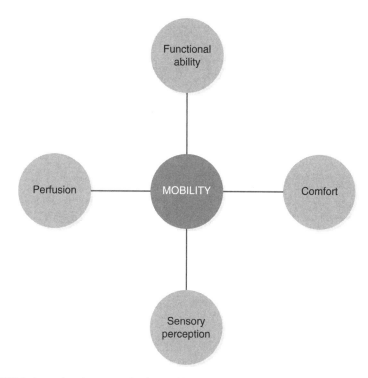

FIGURE 3-3 Interrelated concepts for the Health Concept of Mobility

Interrelated concepts help students make connections between and among concepts. **FIGURE 3-3** illustrates an example of interrelated concepts for the Health concept of Mobility. Appendix B provides an example of how the template is applied for the concept presentation for Mobility.

Health Care Recipient and Professional Nursing and Health Care Concepts are not physiological. Rather they represent attributes, roles, and competencies within the healthcare delivery system. Therefore, the template for these concepts differs from that of the Health Concept template (**BOX 3-5**). Appendix C provides an example of a Professional Nursing Concept presentation for Clinical Judgment.

BOX 3-5 Concept Presentation Template for Professional Nursing and Health Care Concepts/Health Care Recipient Concepts

- Definition of concept
- Categories or scope of concept
- Attributes or theoretic links
- Examples of context in nursing and health care
- Interrelated concepts (*usually includes 2 to 4 of the most common concepts*)
- Exemplars included in the curriculum

Step 10: Determine Where Each Exemplar Will Be Placed in the Curriculum

Once the decisions are made about where to introduce the concept, faculty must determine where to place each exemplar. Ask the following questions to assist in this process:

- Has the concept associated with the exemplar been introduced yet?
- Is the exemplar congruent with the title of the course?
- Is the exemplar congruent with the course focus or description?

To illustrate how to answer these questions, consider the concept of Cognition. Commonly used exemplars for Cognition in a CBC include the following:

- Alzheimer's disease
- Depression
- Seizures
- Traumatic brain injury (TBI)

To address the first question, where could this concept be introduced? Using the plan of study in Box 3-4, Cognition could be introduced in Health Concepts (HCs) I because students need to learn how to assess mental status as part of health assessment. Health assessment is usually taught in the first nursing course if it is not its own stand-alone course. Alzheimer's disease and depression could be placed in HC II because these exemplars are common health problems and are therefore congruent with the course title and focus. Additionally, depression is commonly seen across the lifespan, including as a problem during postpartum. Seizures and TBI are congruent with the title and focus of HC IV. This example illustrates that a concept does not have to appear in every course across the curriculum. There would be no Cognition exemplars in HC III.

After placing all of the exemplars, a final review is helpful to ensure the content for each course can be learned in the credits allocated for the course. Once the course is taught, it will be very important for faculty to assess the need for any changes. Any recommendations for change need to be discussed by the curriculum committee or faculty as a whole, depending on the governance system used by the program or department.

Step 11: Develop Each Course Syllabus and Lesson Plan/Study Guide

At this point in the development of a CBC, faculty members are usually assigned to develop the details of each course, including the course syllabus and lesson plan/study guide. A **lesson plan** provides a guide for faculty as they prepare for class. But, it also can serve as a study guide for students as it delineates learning expectations and assessments. As mentioned in Chapter 1, a lesson plan for a didactic course is a separate document from the official course syllabus and outlines the following:

- Content topics (concept or concept exemplar) with aligned course learning outcomes
- Topical student learning outcomes for each unit, module, or week
- Teaching/learning strategies and activities
- Assignments (preclass, during class, and postclass)
- Assessment of learning methods (formative and summative)

Appendix D is an example of a lesson plan for part of a course in a CBC that introduces a Health concept. Appendix E is an example of a lesson plan for teaching an exemplar. Note that SLOs direct the learning activity and assessment methodology. Chapter 4 discusses how to develop student learning outcomes in detail.

Step 12: Select Appropriate Clinical Experiences and Activities That Are Conceptually Focused

In many programs, clinical experiences are difficult to obtain due to geographic competition for student placement, decrease in acute care beds, and a preference in some areas for BSN students rather than AD nursing students. PN/VN students often spend most of their clinical time in nursing homes, community agencies, ambulatory care, and assisted living facilities where they will likely be employed. RN students also need these community experiences as the number of acute care beds decreases and care moves more into ambulatory care and chronic care settings.

Transitioning to a CBC does not just affect the structure and learning for didactic/theory; it also affects the way laboratory skills, simulation, and outside clinical experiences are planned. The three most important questions for faculty when planning clinical experiences are as follows:

1. Does the clinical experience or simulation allow students the opportunity to meet the course SLOs?
2. Does the clinical agency have enough opportunities for conceptual learning to be successful?
3. Will nurses in the clinical agency support conceptual learning rather than focusing only on skills?

Student experiences in the clinical setting in a CBC are quite different from those in the traditional curriculum. Faculty must plan specific clinical activities that allow students the opportunity to learn conceptually for deep understanding and critical thinking. Chapter 6 describes how to plan, implement, and evaluate conceptual learning in the clinical environment.

▶ Chapter Key Points

- Although the current concept-based curriculum (CBC) model and conceptual learning have been implemented in a number of nursing programs, no two curricula are exactly alike unless a state or province designs a common core curriculum that all of its programs use.
- In nursing education, the most important preplanning considerations for CBC development are similar to Erickson and Lanning's steps, and include the need to 1) obtain faculty buy-in, 2) educate faculty before and throughout the process, and 3) form a curriculum faculty work group.
- A 12-step approach can be utilized for developing the structure of an effective CBC, as delineated in Box 3-3.
- In a CBC, courses are often developed using a lifespan approach rather than dividing the content in several courses based on population.
- The three major Giddens' concept categories are Health Care Recipient Concepts, Health and Illness Concepts, and Professional Nursing and Health Care Concepts.

- Prelicensure nursing programs vary greatly in the number of concepts they choose. There is no evidence that shows how many concepts should be included for a successful and effective CBC.
- Each selected concept requires a definition. Nurse educators can use Giddens' definitions, edit those definitions, or create their own definitions using a variety of resources.
- To select exemplars for Health/Illness or Health concepts, research national, state, and local public health websites for common health problems.
- For Professional Nursing and Health Care Concepts, select exemplars that focus on major issues and concerns in the profession and across the collaborative care team in a variety of healthcare settings.
- To introduce concepts into the curriculum, use concept presentations following consistent concept analysis templates (see Box 3-5 for an example).
- Student experiences in the clinical setting in a CBC are quite different from those in the traditional curriculum. Faculty must plan specific clinical activities that allow students the opportunity to learn conceptually for deep understanding and critical thinking.

▶ Chapter References and Selected Bibliography

*Carrieri-Kohlman, V., Lindsey, A. M., & West, C. M. (2003). *Pathophysiological phenomena in nursing: Human response to illness* (3rd ed.). St. Louis, MO: Elsevier.

Doane, G. H., & Varcoe, C. (2015). *How to nurse: Relational inquiry with individuals and families in changing health and health care contexts.* Philadelphia, PA: Wolters Kluwer Health.

*Erickson, L. (2002). *Concept-based curriculum and instruction.* Thousand Oaks, CA: Corwin Press.

*Erickson, L. (2007). *Concept-based curriculum and instruction in the thinking classroom.* Thousand Oaks, CA: Corwin Press.

Erickson, H. L., & Lanning, L. A. (2014). *Transitioning to concept-based curriculum and instruction.* Thousand Oaks, CA: Corwin Press.

Field, S. C., Aldrich, S. L., Dahlvang, V. K., Fenlason, K. L., Jennissen, S. A., Madigan, K. N., & Thoma, D. M. (2014). Statewide collaborative curriculum project: A shared vision. *Nurse Educator, 53*(12), 699–703.

Giddens, J. F. (2017). *Concepts for nursing practice* (2nd ed.). St. Louis, MO: Elsevier.

Giddens, J. F., Caputi, L., & Rodgers, B. (2015). *Mastering concept-based teaching: A guide for nursing educators.* St. Louis, MO: Elsevier.

Giddens, J. F., Wright, M., & Gray, I. (2012). Selecting concepts for a concept-based curriculum: Application of a benchmark approach. *Journal of Nursing Education, 51*(9), 511–515.

Ignatavicius, D. D., Workman, M. L., & Rebar, C. R. (2018). *Medical-surgical nursing: Concepts for interprofessional collaborative care.* St. Louis, MO: Elsevier.

Keating, S. B. (2015). *Curriculum development and evaluation in nursing.* New York, NY: Springer Publishing.

*Indicates classic reference.

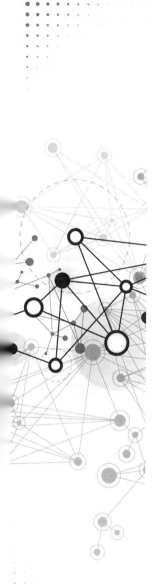

PART II

TEACHING AND LEARNING IN A CONCEPT-BASED NURSING CURRICULUM

CHAPTER 4 Developing Student Learning Outcomes for Conceptual Learning 59

CHAPTER 5 Teaching and Learning in the Concept-Based Classroom 73

CHAPTER 6 Clinical Teaching and Learning in a Concept-Based Nursing Curriculum 95

CHAPTER 7 Teaching in the Concept-Based Online Learning Environment. 125

CHAPTER 8 Using Concept Mapping for Conceptual Learning 147

CHAPTER 9 Using Case Studies effectively in a Concept-Based Curriculum 167

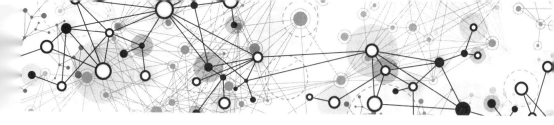

CHAPTER 4

Developing Student Learning Outcomes for Conceptual Learning

Donna Ignatavicius

▶ Introduction to Developing Student Learning Outcomes for Conceptual Learning

As defined in Chapter 1, **student learning outcomes (SLOs)** are the desired expectations regarding knowledge, skills, and attitudes that students are expected to achieve during an educational program. Formerly called "objectives," SLOs organize the curriculum, guide student learning and evaluation, and can be categorized into three levels:

- End-of-program SLOs
- Course SLOs
- Content (unit, modular, or weekly) SLOs

Chapter 1 describes how to develop end-of-program SLOs, also called program learning outcomes (PLOs). This chapter focuses on how to write effective SLOs that measure conceptual learning in a variety of educational environments at the course and modular or weekly level.

▶ Developing Course Student Learning Outcomes

As discussed in Chapter 1, each nursing program must have its own new graduate outcomes written as competency statements while incorporating the program's core organizing concepts or meta-concepts. Each course in the program needs a general description in one or two sentences to briefly provide an overview of the course. Course descriptions should be different for each course in the curriculum. After new graduate outcomes or competencies and course descriptions are written, course learning outcomes, sometimes called course SLOs, need to be developed. The two most important guidelines for writing the course SLOs are that they must be:

- Aligned with the new graduate competencies (also called end-of-program SLOs)
- Consistent with the course description

For example, if writing course SLOs for a Health Concepts I course in a prelicensure nursing program, the nurse educator would first review the organizing themes or meta-concepts for the curriculum (e.g., safety, patient-centered care, evidence-based practice [EBP]). Then review the relevant end-of-program SLOs for new graduates, such as:

- Provide safe, evidence-based nursing care for patients and families in a variety of health inpatient and community care settings.
- Collaborate with the interprofessional healthcare team using informatics and technology to facilitate communication and improve care.
- Participate in quality improvement initiatives to promote optimal clinical outcomes for diverse patients and families.

Remember This . . .

The two most important guidelines for writing the course SLOs are that they must be:

- *Aligned with the new graduate competencies (also called end-of-program SLOs)*
- *Consistent with the course description*

This hypothetical course could have three learning components: a didactic portion, a laboratory skill portion, and a clinical experience portion that could be partly simulation. The course would likely occur early in the nursing curriculum and have a course description similar to this one:

> Built on the Introduction to Health Promotion course, this course focuses on safe, evidence-based nursing care of children, adolescents, and adults experiencing common chronic health problems. Students will have the opportunity to apply professional nursing skills and health concepts in collaboration with the interprofessional health care team in acute and community-based clinical agencies.

Examples of course SLOs for this course that are aligned with the end-of-program graduate competencies and consistent with the course description might include:

- Utilize clinical judgment supported by best current evidence to provide whole-person collaborative care for patients across the lifespan experiencing common chronic diseases.
- Demonstrate professional nursing behaviors within legal and ethical standards of care.
- Formulate clinical questions that need to be addressed to improve safety and quality care for the clinical unit or agency.

All SLOs and other competency statements outline student expectations regarding how they learn concepts and use nursing judgment based on deep conceptual understanding at each level. They reflect student learning in the cognitive, psychomotor, and affective domains.

▶ Developing Conceptual Content Student Learning Outcomes by Learning Domain

After course SLOs are written, conceptual content SLOs are developed and course topics are selected. Content SLOs outline the nurse educator's expectations of the students. They are also essential to help direct or guide the:

- Method of, or setting for, instruction or delivery to meet the SLO
- Learning activities to meet the SLO
- Evaluation method to measure achievement of the SLO

This section describes instruction methods and learning activities for content SLOs in each learning domain; evaluation methods are discussed later in this chapter.

Although SLOs for each domain are presented in the following section, keep in mind that they are often interrelated. For example, learning in the psychomotor domain in nursing requires learning in the cognitive domain. Caring for patients requires a combination of all three domains for whole person collaborative care.

Cognitive Domain

From his classic research, Bloom (1956) developed a **taxonomy**, or classification system, to describe the levels of cognition (thinking) that occur in the **cognitive domain**. This taxonomy is hierarchical, meaning that learning in this domain occurs in ascending order of complexity of thinking. Anderson et al. (2001) revised the

TABLE 4-1 Examples of Verbs for Each Level of the Revised Bloom's (Anderson and Krathwohl's) Cognitive Taxonomy

Cognitive Level (from Lowest to Highest Level)	Examples of SLO Verbs
Remembering	Recall, Define, Label, Select, State, List, Recognize, Identify
Understanding	Explain, Illustrate, Distinguish, Summarize, Translate, Classify
Applying	Apply, Compute, Demonstrate, Interpret, Solve, Construct
Analyzing	Analyze, Compare, Contrast, Differentiate, Categorize, Classify, Prioritize
Evaluating	Evaluate, Critique, Appraise, Justify, Assess, Conclude
Creating	Create, Design, Develop, Formulate, Devise, Plan, Generate

original Bloom's taxonomy as outlined in Table 2-1 in Chapter 2. These researchers changed the noun terminology of Bloom's taxonomy to verbs that more specifically identify the cognitive processing that occurs in one's brain; they also inverted the two highest levels by placing creating (synthesis) at a higher thinking level than evaluating.

Nurse educators need to develop cognitive SLOs when conceptual learning is expected in the classroom or online. Start each SLO with a verb that is consistent with its cognitive level. **TABLE 4-1** lists examples of verbs that are appropriate for each of the six taxonomic levels.

After the appropriate cognitive level is determined and the verb selected, clearly state the expectation of the student. For example, when a concept such as Nutrition is introduced as discussed in Chapter 3, the prelicensure student is expected to define the concept and identify risk factors for decreased or inadequate Nutrition. To articulate these expectations, consider these cognitive SLOs:

■ Define the concept of Nutrition.
■ Describe the scope of the concept of Nutrition.
■ Identify common risk factors for impaired or inadequate Nutrition.

These SLOs are at the lowest cognitive taxonomic level of Remembering. At this level, the student can memorize the information and no thinking is required. Therefore, the following guide applies:

■ Method of, or setting for, instruction or delivery to meet the SLO: Classroom or online
■ Learning activities to meet the SLO: Reading, discussion, pair activity to illustrate the scope of Nutrition, gaming (such as *Jeopardy*)

Knowledge is needed as the foundation for thinking. Anderson et al. (2001) delineated four types of knowledge needed for any discipline or profession:

- Factual Knowledge: Facts and terminology (e.g., medical terminology for nursing)
- Conceptual Knowledge: Classifications, principles, and models (e.g., nursing process, health concepts, professional nursing concepts, health care delivery models)
- Procedural Knowledge: How to perform skills, procedures, or techniques (e.g., sterile procedures, physical assessment)
- Metacognitive Knowledge: Awareness of one's problem-solving skills and self (e.g., reflective processing, analytical abilities)

The Remembering level SLOs listed for introducing Nutrition as a concept could be categorized as Factual and Conceptual Knowledge.

As the student progresses in the nursing program, the expectations regarding the concept of Nutrition increase. For example, in a later course, the student learns about Obesity as an exemplar of the concept of Nutrition. In this course, students are expected to apply the foundational knowledge of Nutrition to learn about Obesity. Consider these SLOs that relate to Obesity:

- Apply knowledge of Nutrition and pathophysiology to determine common assessment findings for the patient with Obesity.
- Prioritize safe, evidence-based collaborative care to promote Nutrition in the patient who is diagnosed with Obesity.
- Apply knowledge of Nutrition and pathophysiology to reduce potentially life-threatening complications of Obesity that have an impact on the interrelated concepts of Mobility, Gas Exchange, and Perfusion.
- Plan health teaching for the patient and family to manage transitions in care to promote Nutrition, Mobility, Gas Exchange, and Perfusion.

These SLOs require students to recall basic knowledge of Nutrition and the pathophysiology of Obesity to meet the expectations for conceptual learning and "thinking like a nurse." All of these SLOs are at the Applying level or higher, which requires clinical reasoning to promote deep learning. Therefore, this guide applies:

- Method of, or setting for, instruction or delivery to meet the SLO: Classroom or online
- Learning activities to meet the SLO: Case study, concept mapping, practice test items

These SLOs require the students to recall facts and principles (e.g., definitions, principles of health teaching, and prioritization) and apply them in complex activities to meet the expectations for deep conceptual learning.

Psychomotor Domain

Learning in the **psychomotor domain** involves the development of skills, including competencies associated with informatics and technology. Although several taxonomies for skill performance can be found in the literature, the classic psychomotor levels published by Dave (1970) are the most commonly used and best fit with nursing skills. The levels of Dave's psychomotor taxonomy are delineated and described in **TABLE 4-2**.

Prelicensure students begin by functioning at the lowest levels of Imitation and Manipulation when learning how to perform a skill in the laboratory setting. In this

TABLE 4-2 Levels of Dave's Psychomotor Taxonomy

Psychomotor Level (from Lowest to Highest Level)	Description of Level
Imitation	Ability to observe a skill demonstration and then attempt to perform the skills.
Manipulation	Ability to perform a skill following instructions rather than after observing a demonstration.
Precision	Ability to perform a skill independently with accuracy and exactness without instructions.
Articulation	Ability to modify a skill to fit a new or unexpected situation; can combine several skills in sequence with consistency and proficiency.
Naturalization	Ability to complete one or more skills with ease by making skill performance automatic with limited physical and mental exertion.

setting, peers and mannequins are used for practicing the skill. Examples of SLOs written at these lower levels include:

- Locate all major peripheral pulses.
- Take an accurate apical pulse.
- Document the apical pulse rate in the appropriate EMR.

All of these skills require psychomotor performance, and require conceptual and procedural knowledge as described in the last section. The concept related to these skills is Perfusion. This guideline applies when developing these psychomotor SLOs:

- Method of, or setting for, instruction or delivery to meet the SLO: Skills laboratory, simulation, or community clinical setting
- Learning activities to meet the SLO: Reading about how to perform the skills, watching a video on skill performance, or practicing the skills in the laboratory

Higher-level cognitive SLOs related to skill performance also may be appropriate. For example, consider this SLO: *Interpret assessment findings related to locating and documenting the strength of peripheral pulses.* Palpating pulses and interpreting the findings are two different levels of expectation. Interpretation requires thinking and represents the Applying level of the Cognitive taxonomy. Unlicensed assistive personnel may obtain a pulse reading, but it is the professional nurse who interprets the findings.

When possible, it is important that students recognize the importance of connecting each skill with a concept. For example, when learning about Nutrition, an important intervention is often providing supplemental or complete enteral nutrition. Students learn the skills associated with this concept. For example, an appropriate psychomotor SLO might be: *Perform enteral nutrition via a feeding tube (nasogastric and G-tube) to promote patient Nutrition.* This SLO helps the student recognize the relationship of the skill to the concept.

In the clinical setting after perhaps weeks or months of skill practice and application, the student is expected to function at least at the level of Precision, or independence. When given different patient assignments, the student may move to Articulation because there are new situations for each patient that may require skill procedure modification. Naturalization occurs after a student graduates and gains confidence as a practicing nurse (Billings & Halstead, 2016).

> ## Remember This . . .
>
> *In the clinical setting after perhaps weeks or months of skill practice and application, the student is expected to function at least at the level of Precision, or independence.*

Affective Domain

Perhaps the most challenging and often ignored learning domain in which to teach and facilitate learning is the affective domain. The **affective domain** involves developing attitudes, values, and beliefs. In nursing, those values are ideally consistent with standards of professional nursing and health care (Oermann & Gaberson, 2017). Based on the classic work of Krathwohl, Bloom, and Masia (1964), the lowest level of the affective taxonomy (Receiving) is synonymous with awareness of one's attitudes, values, and beliefs. As the learner matures in affective learning, professional nursing values are internalized and the student becomes socialized into the profession. **TABLE 4-3** lists the classic levels of affective learning and their description.

Professional Nursing, Health Care, and Health Care Recipient concepts are the most essential foci for affective learning. Professional Nursing concepts include, but are not limited to:

- Professionalism
- Leadership
- Ethics

TABLE 4-3 Levels of Affective Learning Domain

Affective Level (from Lowest to Highest)	Description of Level
Receiving	Ability to be aware of own values, attitudes, and beliefs.
Responding	Ability to react to a situation reflecting own choice.
Valuing	Ability to accept a value and commitment to use that value.
Conceptualizing and Organizing	Ability to develop a value system.
Characterizing	Ability to internalize the value system.

Affective learning domain SLOs that address these concepts might be:

- Formulate own philosophy of Professionalism and professional behaviors (Conceptualizing and Organizing level).
- Differentiate three styles of Leadership in nursing practice (Valuing level).
- Discuss the major principles of Ethics and ethical behavior (Responding level).

Examples of Health Care concepts include Health Policy and Health Care Law. Affective learning domain SLOs that address these concepts might be:

- Select a Health Care Policy that has an impact on nursing practice (Receiving level).
- Read your state's (or province's) Nurse Practice Act to determine the RN scope of practice (Responding level).

A major Health Care Recipient concept is Culture. Examples of affective learning domain SLOs that relate to this concept include:

- Develop a culturally sensitive plan of care for the transgender client (Conceptualizing and Organizing level).
- Discuss the impact of Culture on the care of pregnant Amish women (Responding level).

For affective domain SLOs, these guidelines could apply:

- Method of, or setting for, instruction or delivery to meet the SLO: Clinical conference, seminar, classroom
- Learning activities to meet the SLO: Online discussion forum, concept map, journaling

As in the case of other learning domains, knowledge is also needed to meet affective domain

Factual, Conceptual, and Meta-Cognitive Knowledge are required to meet the two previously listed SLOs that relate to the concept of Culture. The student has to know what transgenderism is and understand the related issue of health care disparity and inequity (Factual Knowledge). The student also has to understand the definition and attributes of Culture (Conceptual Knowledge) and his or her own analytical and reflective abilities (Meta-Cognitive Knowledge).

▶ Measuring Achievement of Course SLOs

Chapter 3 introduced the need for measuring achievement of course SLOs. When developing SLOs at any level, be sure to plan how they will be measured at the specified level. Some of the possible course SLOs for the Health Concepts I course described earlier in this chapter were:

1. Utilize clinical judgment supported by best current evidence to provide whole person collaborative care for patients across the lifespan experiencing common chronic diseases.
2. Demonstrate professional nursing behaviors within legal and ethical standards of care.
3. Formulate clinical questions that need to be addressed to improve safety and quality care for the clinical unit or agency.

The nurse educator plans how each of these course SLOs will be measured at the end of the course because they are not expected to be achieved by students until the course is completed. Several methods are commonly used in prelicensure nursing education to measure achievement of course SLOs, including comprehensive final examinations and commercial standardized tests. For the course SLOs listed earlier, the SLOs in 1 and 2 could be measured by testing.

The most commonly used standardized tests are:

- HESI® (Available through Elsevier)
- Kaplan (Available through Kaplan)
- ATI™ (Available through Assessment Technologies Institute)

Standardized tests are used by most programs for both course assessment and as a method to predict NCLEX® success. However, these tests are not conceptually based. Most companies can provide a report that links concepts with student scores, but the content of the tests at this time is not based on concepts. As discussed in Chapter 10, the NCLEX-RN® and NCLEX-PN® are based on nursing concepts rather than medical diagnosis. As a result of the concept-based curriculum movement for nursing curricula, nursing faculty are being more selective in the use of standardized testing.

The National League for Nursing (NLN) and nursing accrediting/regulatory bodies do not support the use of standardized testing for "high stakes" purposes. For example, in some programs, students who do not meet a certain score on a standardized test cannot progress in the program, even if they pass the course associated with the test. In other programs, students may not graduate or receive a grade for their last course unless they meet a national benchmark score on a standardized test. In both cases, this high stakes approach is not an appropriate use of commercial testing. Research indicates that these tests may not be predictive of NCLEX® pass rates (Sosa & Sethares, 2015). The appropriate use of standardized testing is discussed in Chapter 12.

Remember This . . .

The National League for Nursing and nursing accrediting/regulatory bodies do not support the use of standardized testing for high stakes purposes.

For SLO 3 in the previous list, an examination is not the best method for measuring student achievement. Instead the student may be asked to submit meaningful and appropriate clinical questions using the PICOT format to the nurse educator as an assignment.

▶ Measuring Achievement of Conceptual Content Student Learning Outcomes by Learning Domain

This section provides examples of how to evaluate student achievement of content SLOs by learning domain. A more detailed discussion of evaluating conceptual learning in the classroom and clinical setting may be found in Chapters 10 and 11.

Cognitive Domain

Measuring achievement of cognitive SLOs varies depending on the level of expectation. For example, expectations at lower cognitive levels (Remembering and Understanding) can be easily assessed by quizzes or games such as *Jeopardy*. For higher-level SLOs that require application of knowledge and thinking, more complex evaluative methods are appropriate, such as examinations, graded case studies, scholarly papers, posters, and projects. Examinations are more objective and thus easier to grade (see Chapter 10). However, case studies and scholarly papers can better measure achievement of analyzing, evaluating, and creating SLOs. Scholarly papers are particularly challenging for RN-to-BSN students. Tyndall and Scott (2017) reported a successful framework for their RN-to-BSN students to help them value writing and teach them how to write a scholarly paper.

Projects and papers can be especially useful to help students meet higher-level cognitive SLOs. For example, consider this SLO: *Develop a quality improvement plan to optimize patient outcomes on an assigned unit or agency.* Student achievement of this SLO cannot be measured by an examination. Rather, students would complete a project in which they would first examine nursing practices to select an area that needs improvement. Then they would develop an evidence-based plan for improvement for the selected area to optimize patient outcomes. Examples of quality improvement (QI) projects might be pressure injury prevention, fall reduction, deep vein thrombosis reduction, catheter-associated urinary tract infection (CAUTI) prevention, or C-section complication reduction. The project could be presented as a paper or poster (**FIGURE 4-1**). A grading rubric would be needed to score the project.

Novotny, Stapleton, and Hardy (2016) reported a strategy to enhance and measure critical thinking in graduate nursing students using online asynchronous discussions. The authors found that the students were better able to critically think about concepts being discussed as measured by critical thinking scores before and after the learning strategy. Students stated they learned how to think at a deeper level by analyzing and bringing relevance into their thinking process. Analyzing is a high cognitive level needed for deep conceptual learning and thinking.

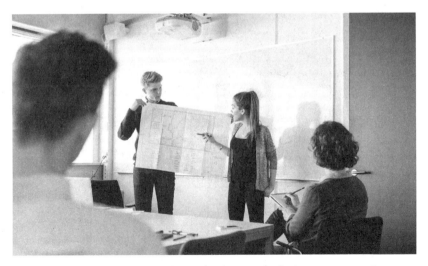

FIGURE 4-1 Students presenting a poster to the class on a quality improvement project
© Kentaroo Tryman/Maskot/Getty

Pierce (2016) reported the use of e-posters in meeting cognitive SLOs for an online graduate nursing research course. The primary concepts taught in the course were EBP and research methods and analysis. The cognitive SLOs that were measured included:

- Appraise data collection and analyses methods.
- Critique published research studies.

Selected research posters were collected from a variety of sources to post online for the students. Some of the posters had an accompanying short presentation by the researcher, but most did not. Using a structured discussion board thread, students applied their knowledge of EBP and research methods and analysis to meet the SLOs. The students not only met the SLOs but found the information provided by the posters helped them improve practice in their own clinical settings.

Psychomotor Domain

Nursing psychomotor skills are most often evaluated by the nurse educator during return demonstrations. A checklist of predetermined criteria sequencing the steps of the skills or procedure is used for grading student performance. A concern for this type of evaluation is that the evaluators using the same criteria may not interpret student performance the same way, thus reducing interrater reliability. To avoid this potential problem, be sure to pilot the evaluation checklist with multiple faculty to achieve at least an 90% agreement on assessment of student performance.

Many programs use a "skills checkoff" as a high stakes assessment, meaning that if a student does not meet the predetermined criteria after two or three attempts, he or she fails the course in which the skill is evaluated. High stakes testing is not recommended by the NLN and nursing accrediting bodies.

Better methods for assessing psychomotor SLOs have been developed and are being used in some nursing programs at both the prelicensure and graduate levels. One of these methods is the use of digital standardized patients. At this time, the most commonly used vendor for this purpose is Shadow Health®. This company is the first to develop and validate clinical reasoning within a virtual patient simulation (www .shadowhealth.com). A number of avatar patients represent diverse opportunities for students to learn assessment skills. A Student Performance Index scores the student's clinical reasoning skills in six areas:

- Subjective data
- Objective data
- Therapeutic communication
- Documentation
- Information process
- Self-reflection

Nurse educators can use this product as an assignment for formative evaluation or as a culminating method for summative evaluation or both. Additionally, other content areas such as Pharmacology knowledge and application also can be evaluated.

Another effective evaluative method for assessing skill competence is the Objective Structured Clinical Examination (or Evaluation). Used in other health professional education programs, nursing programs have begun to incorporate OSCEs as part of their evaluative methods to assess student learning, especially in graduate clinical education for advanced practice RNs.

Brighton, Mackay, Brown, Jans, and Antoniou (2017) reported the results of a qualitative study on the first implementation of a medication administration OSCE in an Australian undergraduate nursing program. The grading criteria and evaluation framework were based on an evidence-based tool found in the literature. Two stages of the study were developed. Stage 1 found three emerging themes prior to OSCE implementation: student anxiety, student preparedness, and the effectiveness of this style of assessment. Most students were prepared for the OSCE, but almost all had high anxiety prior to the assessment. Only a small part of the sample rated effectiveness of the assessment prior to its implementation. Stage 2 after the OSCE yielded another three key themes: feelings toward the OSCE, assessor interaction, and the OSCE environment. Most students found the OSCE useful and liked the interaction of their assessors (evaluators). However, some evaluators were not as helpful and kind as others. The students thought the environment for the OSCE in the simulation laboratory was realistic and, in general, valued the experience.

Affective Domain

Simulation also can be used to assess affective learning. Cantey, Randolph, Molloy, Carter, and Cary (2017) reported the development of simulations to enhance cultural awareness and understanding of social determinants of health. Although this activity was designed primarily for conceptual learning about Culture and Health Care Disparities, student development of simulation scenarios in groups to meet the expected affective SLOs also could be used for formative evaluation. The authors reported that the five scenarios created by the students met these objectives:

- Students learned about health and health care disparities and the community resources they could offer their patients.
- Students' cultural awareness was improved, and they had opportunities to practice communication skills.
- Students learned about various roles of nurses and gained experience working as a team to develop their scenarios.

Another way to evaluate student achievement of affective SLOs is journaling. Using this method, students are evaluated individually rather than in groups. Journaling can be done as part of a theory/didactic course or more commonly as part of the clinical practicum. Consider this affective SLO: *Demonstrate respect for cultural differences when caring for adult patients.* This SLO about the concept of Culture cannot be measured by a test or quiz. Journaling would be better options for evaluation. For a journal entry, students might be asked to share at least two examples of how they demonstrated respect for their patient's cultural preferences and values during care. They would need to support why they felt their actions demonstrated respect, using the literature if possible.

Reflective papers are also effective methods for measuring achievement of affective learning. For example, the author of this text had students write a short reflective paper about caring for older adults in a senior living facility. The paper was intended to meet SLOs related to understanding the nature of older adulthood and appreciate their life experiences. Three parts of the reflection were part of the paper:

- Feelings and perceptions about older adults prior to going to the clinical site.
- Summary of experience with older adults in the senior living facility.
- Feelings and perceptions about older adults after going to the clinical site.

A number of students admitted in their papers that they were guilty of ageism and thought that older adults were naturally confused, incontinent, and needed physical care. They were surprised at the wellness of the older population and their active lives. Many older adults in the facility continued to work part-time, volunteer, return to college, and/or drive a vehicle. In addition, the students were amazed at the wisdom and life experiences of their clients. Many students admitted they thoroughly enjoyed the experience and hoped to have more opportunities to work with this population.

▶ Chapter Key Points

- All SLOs and other competency statements outline the expectations of the students regarding how they learn concepts and use nursing judgement based on deep conceptual understanding at each level.
- Course content SLOs are also essential to help direct or guide the method of, or setting for, instruction or delivery to meet the SLO, learning activities to meet the SLO, and evaluation method to measure achievement of the SLO.
- Nurse educators need to develop cognitive SLOs when conceptual learning is expected in the classroom or online (cognitive domain) (see Table 4-1).
- Learning in the psychomotor domain involves the development of skills, including competencies associated with informatics and technology (see Table 4-2).
- The affective domain involves developing attitudes, values, and beliefs. In nursing, those values are ideally consistent with standards of professional nursing (see Table 4-3).
- Several methods are commonly used in prelicensure nursing education to measure achievement of course SLOs, including comprehensive final examinations and commercial standardized tests.
- Standardized tests are used by most programs for both course assessment and as a method to predict NCLEX® success. However, these tests are not conceptually based.
- Online discussion boards and e-posters are effective ways to evaluate student learning in graduate nursing programs.
- Better methods for assessing psychomotor SLOs have been developed and are being used in some nursing programs at both the prelicensure and graduate levels. One of these methods is the use of digital standardized patients.
- Nursing programs have begun to incorporate Objective Structured Clinical Examinations (OSCEs) as part of their evaluative methods to assess student learning, especially in graduate clinical education for advanced practice RNs.
- Examples of effective ways to evaluate student achievement of affective SLOs are simulation, journaling, and reflective papers.

▶ Chapter References and Selected Bibliography

*Anderson, L. W., Krathwohl, D. R., Arasian, P. W., Cruikshank, K. A., Mayer, P. E., et al. (Ed.). (2001). *A taxonomy for learning, teaching and assessing: A revision of Bloom's taxonomy of educational objectives.* San Francisco, CA: Jossey-Bass.

Billings, D. M., & Halstead, J. A. (2016). *Teaching in nursing: A guide for faculty* (5th ed.). St. Louis, MO: Elsevier.

*Bloom, B. S. (1956). *Taxonomy of educational objectives. Book 1: Cognitive domain.* New York, NY: Longmans.

Brighton, R., Mackay, M., Brown, R. A., Jans, C., & Antoniou, C. (2017). Introduction of undergraduate nursing students to an objective structured clinical examination. *Journal of Nursing Education, 56*(4), 231–234.

Cantey, D. S., Randolph, S. D., Molloy, M. A., Carter, B., & Cary, M. P. (2017). Student-developed simulations: Enhancing cultural awareness and understanding social determinants of health. *Journal of Nursing Education, 56*(4), 243–246.

*Dave, R. H. (1970). Psychomotor levels. In R. J. Armstrong (Ed.), *Developing and writing behavioral objectives.* Tucson, AZ: Educational Innovators.

Keating, S. B. (2015). *Curriculum development and evaluation in nursing.* New York, NY: Springer Publishing.

Krathwohl, D., Bloom, B., & Masia, B. (1964). *Taxonomy of educational objectives. Handbook II: Affective domain.* New York, NY: Longman.

McDonald, M. (2014). *The nurse educator's guide to assessing learning outcomes* (3rd ed.). Brooklyn, NY: JBL Learning.

Novotny, N. L., Stapleton, S. J., & Hardy, E. C. (2016). Enhancing critical thinking in graduate online asynchronous discussions. *Journal of Nursing Education, 55*(9), 514–520.

Oermann, M. H., & Gaberson, K. B. (2017). *Evaluation and testing in nursing education* (5th ed.). New York, NY: Springer Publishing.

Pierce, L. L. (2016). The e-poster conference: An online nursing research course learning activity. *Journal of Nursing Education, 55*(9), 533–535.

Sosa, M.-E., & Sethares, K. A. (2015). An integrative review of the use and outcomes of HESI testing in baccalaureate nursing programs. *Nursing Education Perspectives, 36*(4), 237–243.

Todd, M., Hawkins, K., Hercinger, M., Matz, J., & Tracy, M. (2014). Creighton Competency Evaluation Instrument. Creighton University School of Nursing. Retrieved from www.creighton.edu/nursing/simulation/.

Tyndall, D. E., & Scott, E. S. (2017). Writing development in associate degree in nursing-to-baccalaureate degree in nursing students: Moving out of the comfort zone. *Journal of Nursing Education, 56*(3), 182–185.

---

*Indicates classic reference.

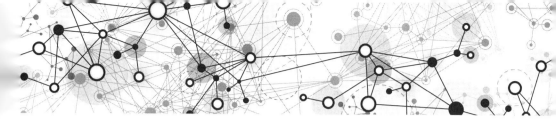

CHAPTER 5

Teaching and Learning in the Concept-Based Classroom

Donna Ignatavicius

CHAPTER LEARNING OUTCOMES

After studying this chapter, the reader will be better able to:

1. Identify four student variables that affect learning.
2. Differentiate four common student learning preferences based on the VARK classification.
3. Describe the importance of active collaborative learning to promote an effective concept-based flipped or scrambled classroom.
4. Explain how to use selected teaching/learning strategies and activities appropriate for the concept-based classroom.

▶ Introduction to Teaching and Learning in the Concept-Based Classroom

As described earlier in this book, a **concept-based curriculum (CBC)** is a structure or model in which selected content is organized around identified program concepts (Giddens, Caputi, & Rodgers, 2015). *A typical pitfall for nursing programs that develop a CBC is the lack of planning for how to deliver or operationalize the curriculum in a variety of learning environments.* Learning how to teach conceptually is an essential skill for a successful CBC.

As discussed in Chapter 2, the effective nurse educator facilitates student learning (learner-centered) rather than focusing on teaching (teacher-centered). Using a learner-centered approach is essential to ensure a meaningful CBC. In the CBC learning environment, learner-centeredness means that students engage in active conceptual learning and thinking rather than being exposed to lengthy lectures in which instructors often "spoon feed" excessive amounts of content. Identifying concepts and key exemplars in a CBC helps eliminate the "nice-to-know" and "nuts-to-know" content.

Changing the traditional classroom and teaching strategies is often a challenge for nurse educators due to lack of time, lack of self-confidence, and/or organizational/program culture (Herrman, 2016). Yet, in their program philosophy, faculty often describe adult learners as being independent, discovering new knowledge, and connecting new knowledge to previous knowledge and experience. These characteristics are very compatible with conceptual learning.

Some students may be challenged in a conceptual learning classroom because they are used to attending lectures to memorize content in prenursing liberal arts and science courses. For example, anatomy and physiology content is typically memorized, and tests measure the ability of the student to regurgitate knowledge. Students who can memorize the information often do well in this type of course. However, in nursing courses, students are challenged to think, make connections, and use clinical judgment. This shift in expectations often results in student complaints and poor student performance.

Nurse educators need to help students learn how to make the transition from memorizing to thinking. Public information about the nursing program needs to include the expectations of students in a CBC and the faculty's philosophy of adult learning. Students need to be held accountable for their own learning and actively participate in the learning process to develop critical thinking and clinical judgment skills.

This chapter discusses how to promote student learning and thinking in a nursing CBC classroom. Examples of specific learning activities and strategies are described and applied to concepts and exemplars. The success of a CBC depends on your ability to help students gain meaningful learning and understanding as they develop patterns of knowing and thinking.

▶ Characteristics of Today's Learners

To facilitate meaningful deep learning, educators need to know who their learners are and what student variables could have an impact on that learning. Consider these four student variables to assess:

- Learning preferences
- Thinking styles
- Developmental stages
- Demographic characteristics

Remember This . . .

To facilitate meaningful deep learning, educators need to know who their learners are and what student variables could have an impact on that learning.

Learning Preferences

Although most adults can learn using a variety of methods, each student has a preferred learning style that best meets his or her needs. A number of learning styles are cited in the literature; however, many educators are familiar with and use the VARK classification of learners (www.vark-learn.com):

V = Visual learners

A = Aural learners

R = Read/write learners

K = Kinesthetic learners

Most nursing students tend to be visual and kinesthetic, but learning preferences can vary among cohorts.

In some nursing programs, new students complete a learning preference tool (such as the VARK Inventory) to determine how they best learn. This assessment helps them select appropriate study methods geared to their preferred learning style. For example, if the student is a *visual* learner, graphic organizers such as concept maps, Venn diagrams, and flow charts are helpful (discussed later in this chapter). If the student is an *aural (auditory)* learner, he or she might want to record classroom discussion (with permission of the instructor) for listening later or request that voice-over lectures be provided on the school's learning management system (LMS). The student who is a *read/write learner* may make copious notations in the reading material, create flash cards, or outline the reading. The *kinesthetic* learner prefers to be active and hands-on. This student prefers practicing psychomotor skills and clinical care experiences as the best way to learn. This is sometimes referred to as "learning by doing."

If your program does not formally assess student learning preferences, begin your course by asking the group to identify what learning styles they prefer. Once you have conducted this assessment, you can better select the teaching/learning methods that are the best fit for the class. **TABLE 5-1** lists examples of teaching/learning activities that are appropriate for each VARK preference.

Thinking Styles

For many years, brain dominance was considered a determinant of how learners think. *Right-brain dominant* learners were described as creative, flexible, and holistic. *Left-brain dominant* learners were classified as analytical problem-solvers. However, more recent research in educational psychology identified three common thinking styles that are not solely based on brain dominance. Interestingly, these styles correlate to the three branches of the U.S. government (Cano-Garcia & Hughes, 2010):

- Legislative
- Executive
- Judicial

Legislative thinkers desire to choose their own learning activities and prefer assignments that allow them to be flexible and creative, similar to right-brain dominant learners. *Judicial* thinkers like to evaluate situations and rules and solve problems that require analyzing multiple concepts, similar to left-brain dominant learners. *Executive* thinkers enjoy carrying out actions and implementing plans either self-created or developed by others.

TABLE 5-1 Appropriate Teaching/Learning Activities Based on VARK Classifications	
Learning Style Preference	**Examples of Appropriate Learning Activity**
V = Visual learners	Video clips Graphic images Graphic organizers, such as Venn diagrams and concept maps
A = Aural (Auditory) learners	Class lecture Online voice-over lecture Storytelling Pair/Group discussions Collaborative testing Sound clips
R = Read/Write learners	Note-taking guides Concept maps Venn diagrams
K = Kinesthetic learners	Concept maps Gaming Venn diagrams Social media

Determining the thinking styles of your students can be very useful when planning teaching/learning strategies. For example, if the class tends to have more *judicial* thinkers, case studies and debates would be most appropriate. If the class tends to have more *legislative* thinkers, graphic organizers such as concept maps would be helpful in the learning process.

Developmental Stage

Nursing students also vary by developmental stage. Students in some prelicensure nursing programs (such as those typically in large public universities) are admitted directly from high school to higher education to obtain their nursing degree. Other programs, especially those in community colleges, private colleges and universities, and career schools, have a mix of students who may range in age from 20 to over 50 years of age and represent several developmental groups. These groups include:

- Baby Boomers
- Generation Xers
- Millennials

Baby Boomers (born 1946 to 1964) represent the smallest group in prelicensure nursing programs, but many are enrolled in graduate nursing programs. In the United States, they are the largest group of consumers of services and products. Because Baby Boomers were born prior to the computer age and Internet, they may or may not embrace learning using technology. Online learning and assignments may be frustrating for them, especially if the technology tools do not properly function. Baby Boomers want to be respected for their life experience and education and build on that foundation. They do not want to waste time with meaningless activities and assignments they perceive do not help them learn.

Generation (Gen) Xers (born 1965 to 1980) were introduced to computers during their adolescence and easily embrace technology to help them learn. They usually respond well to creative and innovative learning activities because they want learning to be enjoyable (Herrman, 2016). Unlike their Baby Boomer parents, Gen Xers tend to work toward achieving a work-life balance.

The *Millennials* are in their 20s and early 30s and are sometimes referred to as "Generation Why" or Gen-Y. These learners usually embrace group work and technology of all types and tend to use a variety of study methods to help them learn quickly (Herrman, 2016). However, as children of Baby Boomers who worked to give them a better life than they had, Millennials may feel entitled to pass or be successful without necessarily putting in the required effort. This characteristic often conflicts with the work ethic value of their parents.

The nurse educator needs to identify which developmental stages are represented in his or her class to help plan the most effective student learning activities. If students vary in their developmental stages, plan a variety of activities that collectively appeal to all subgroups. Examples of these learning strategies and activities are discussed later in this chapter.

Demographic Characteristics

Other student demographic characteristics that may influence how nurse educators plan their classroom conceptual teaching/learning include:

- Gender
- Educational background
- Primary language
- Life experience

A number of articles and books have been published over the years about *gender* differences in brain development. One of the most important differences occurs in the hippocampus of the brain, which is the center of emotions, learning, and memory. Girls develop their hippocampus earlier than boys. This physiological difference may mean that girls are stronger in vocabulary, reading, and writing compared to boys. However, recent research shows that the *adult* male and female brain become more similar and learning differences are minimal (Voyer & Voyer, 2014).

Nursing cohorts are very diverse in their *educational background, primary language,* and *life experience.* Some students attend college shortly after high school graduation, whereas others have a time lapse of many years before college entry. Students also differ in where and how they received their K to 12 education. For example, many minority students in the United States attend schools in very poorly funded educational systems and are consequently at high risk for college attrition. Generation X and Millennial students from any school district or region may have inadequate basic reading, writing, and math skills. The author has found that many students from a variety of educational systems have inadequate vocabulary skills and do not recognize common lay terms that might be used in conversation or on a test. Examples of these words are concurrently, consequent, subsequent, and contraindication. If these terms are important for students to know, the students need to be assisted in learning them.

Some students were educated in countries other than the United States or Canada where learning and evaluation methods are different. For instance, many international students are unfamiliar with multiple-choice testing because their tests were primarily essay questions in which they had to analyze and synthesize multiple concepts to demonstrate critical thinking skills.

International students also learn English as a second (or third or fourth) language and are often referred to as ESL students or **English language learners (ELL)**. These students typically struggle with lay and healthcare terminology because many English words have multiple meanings. For instance, an international nursing student missed a test question regarding appropriate foods for a particular patient because she did not select the correct answer of "tossed salad"—she did not understand why a salad would be thrown out!

Regional differences among students whose primary language is English also may affect understanding of certain words. For example, "pop" is a carbonated beverage in the Midwest. That same beverage may be called a "soda" or "soft drink" in other parts of the United States or Canada. Other regional foods include grits (southeastern United States), Frito pies (southwestern United States), and scrapple (mid-Atlantic states).

Assess the student demographics in your class to help plan appropriate and effective teaching/learning strategies. Incorporate these differences to ensure inclusivity. Be aware that students can learn from each other as they work in pairs or groups in the flipped or scrambled classroom described in the next section.

▶ The Role of Collaborative Learning

Another difference among students is that some prefer learning individually and others prefer learning in groups. Collaborative learning (sometimes referred to as cooperative learning) has been touted as being the best approach for students in the classroom and other educational environments (Sandahl, 2009). Collaborative learning is a critical component of a CBC classroom and occurs best in groups of 2 to 4 students. Students who dislike group activities are usually able to learn from a pair activity. Characteristics of collaborative learning are outlined in **BOX 5-1**.
Forming groups can be conducted in one of several ways:

- Have students select who they want to work with.
- Assign students randomly to groups (A random assignment chart, deck of cards, counting off, or other method can be used.)

BOX 5-1 Characteristics (and Benefits) of Collaborative Adult Learning

- Positive interdependence
- Face-to-face interaction
- Individual accountability
- Sense of common learning goal
- Group processing
- Creation of new knowledge

- Purposefully place students in groups such that they are mixed by performance (e.g., test grades) and English language ability (ELL students who work with native English speakers often benefit because they learn the idiosyncrasies of the English language.)

Another consideration about forming groups is to determine if the groups stay the same for a prolonged period or if group composition changes for each class session or online module. The author has found that changing group membership has advantages over maintaining the same groups because it allows students to network, learn to work with a variety of people, and ensure that no one group has an advantage over another.

▶ The Flipped Versus Scrambled Classroom

For many years, lecture has been the mainstay of traditional classroom teaching. **Lecture** has been considered a one-way experience in which the instructor talks and the students are expected to listen and learn. Homework *after* lecture is designed to help clarify concepts and reinforce learning. This direct instruction strategy supports passive student learning rather than active engagement and in recent years has been regarded as an inadequate way to learn. Nurse educators often use PowerPoint slides to accompany their lecture.

Many prelicensure nursing students request lecture PowerPoint slides to use as study guides. However, faculty tend to use publisher-provided slides that for clinical courses tend to focus less on nursing concepts and more on review of anatomy and physiology, pathophysiology, and medical diagnosis and treatment. Audiovisual and other learning aids in any nursing learning environment should emphasize nursing concepts and related patient, family, and/or population-based care.

Barnett (2014) noted that not all lecturers use the same teaching technique. The best lecturers incorporate relevant concrete examples that clarify and elaborate on course content. Oermann and Gaberson (2017) defend lecture as a viable teaching strategy for large classes (**FIGURE 5-1**). Lecture is often preferred by many aural (auditory) learners. PowerPoint slides also appeal to visual learners.

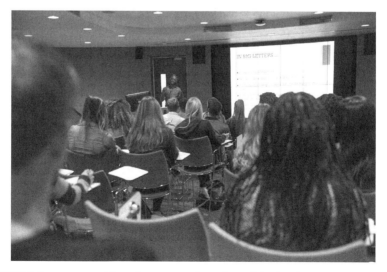

FIGURE 5-1 Instructor providing a lecture using PowerPoint slides for a large class
© Monkey Business Images/Shutterstock

Instead of relying solely on lecture, educators in a variety of fields have called for implementing the flipped classroom. A **flipped classroom** is a model in which lecture and homework are reversed; that is, the lecture occurs *before* class and homework that engages students in active learning is done in the classroom. This approach incorporates peer-to-peer interaction and collaboration as students apply, analyze, and synthesize concepts using a variety of learning activities. The success of a flipped classroom depends on students, who must be accountable for preparing prior to each class.

Holman and Hanson (2016) compared the traditional lecture model with the flipped model using two large groups of students in the last semester of an AD in nursing program. Consistent with previous research, the authors found that the flipped model improved student-instructor interaction, student-centered instruction, and student preparation and learning. Students thought they could apply new concepts immediately through active learning activities. However, more students than not stated that they preferred the traditional lecture model.

The flipped classroom also has been used in graduate nursing education. Critz and Knight (2013) found that NP students liked the online lectures before class to help prepare them for learning activities that were active and engaging. They also thought the flipped model was more student-centered than the traditional lecture model and helped them become more self-directed.

The author has noted that students in prelicensure nursing programs are often resistant to a purely flipped classroom approach, particularly as beginning learners. Students expect the expert nurse educator to provide information that helps them understand class content and highlight the most important concepts. As an alternative, the author and others advocate a scrambled classroom. A **scrambled classroom** is a model in which learning is facilitated by mixing engaging collaborative student activities with multiple short periods (5 to 10 minutes each) in which the instructor clarifies, updates, and prioritizes class content (Barnett, 2014). As nurses, educators often provide timely and relevant examples or stories that enhance understanding and thinking. These periods may be referred to as "lecturettes."

Regardless of how classroom learning occurs or in what model, the nurse educator needs to include time for debriefing. Debriefing is a term that has been largely associated with clinical simulation in the laboratory setting. However, **debriefing** is an important part of learning during which the educator clarifies, highlights, summarizes, and updates class content at various points during class and other learning environments.

▶ Fostering Clinical Imagination

In 2010, a large national nursing education study published by Dr. Patricia Benner and her colleagues found that students did not realize the relationship between theory/didactic content in the classroom and clinical experiences in which they cared for patients. As a result of this lack of connection for students, the research team recommended that classroom time represent a time for clinical imagination in which clinical situations and issues are discussed and clinical concepts are applied (Benner, Stephen, Leonard, & Day, 2010). Classroom teaching/learning activities need to be designed to focus on nursing and health care of patients in a variety of clinical settings.

▶ Relationship of Student Learning Outcomes to Conceptual Learning

As discussed in Chapter 4, the nurse educator develops student learning outcomes (SLO) as part of the lesson plan or student study guide to help determine the learning environments or modalities, learning activities, and evaluation methods. For example, consider the following SLO for a class on the concept of Clotting: *Identify health promotion strategies for the nurse to prevent increased Clotting*. As shown in Table 4-1, the verb "Identify" is at a Remembering level on the revised Bloom's cognitive taxonomy. Therefore, the best learning environment in which students can achieve this SLO is either the classroom or online. Examples of activities that would help students learn the health promotion strategies might include:

- Having students look up the health promotion strategies on their mobile devices
- Games, such as Student Feud or Jeopardy (described later in this chapter)

Ways to formatively evaluate whether students have met the SLO in the classroom or online might include practice NCLEX®-style questions or a case study. The following NCLEX®-style item can provide either formative or summative evaluation about the students' achievement of the sample SLO. The * indicates the correct answers.

The nurse is teaching a woman about how to prevent developing a clot. Which health teaching will the nurse include? **Select all that apply.**

    a.   *"Avoid prolonged sitting or standing if possible."**

    b.   *"Perform ankle pumps every hour while sitting."**

    c.   *"Restrict fluid intake if sitting for a long time."*

    d.   *"Wear supportive stockings when standing for a long time."**

    e.   *"Seek a smoking cessation program if you smoke."**

▶ Selected Strategies and Activities to Promote Active Conceptual Learning

Many teaching/learning strategies and activities, sometimes referred to as **pedagogies**, that have been used in a traditional classroom can be adapted for the CBC classroom. However, the focus or purpose of those activities may be different to ensure conceptual learning and thinking. Some of these activities also may be used in online or clinical environments, especially in clinical postconferences. Be sure not to overuse any one activity or strategy in one class session or use too many different activities in one class session. Otherwise, there will no time for debriefing.

One of the concerns of many nurse educators is the time needed to use pair and group learning activities. However, these activities should *replace* usual lecture time, not supplement it. Nursing students need multiple opportunities to learn how to apply course content such that they can develop critical thinking and clinical reasoning skills for nursing judgment and decision making. The following selected learning strategies and activities are appropriate for achieving this desired outcome.

> **Remember This . . .**
>
> *One of the concerns of many nurse educators is the time needed to use pair and group learning activities. However, these activities should replace usual lecture time, not supplement it.*

Pair Discussions

Hermann (2016) describes the **Let's Discuss** learning strategy in her book on creative learning activities. In her description, she states that the instructor (learning facilitator) initiates discussion of a topic or statement with the entire class. However, this same activity can be used with student pairs to discuss the topic; for example, "Let's discuss the physiological consequences of decreased Mobility on normal body system functions. Talk with the person next to you for 3 minutes and list at least 5 ways that decreased mobility can cause body system complications." This "two heads are better than one" approach promotes conceptual learning about Mobility with peers. At the end of 3 minutes, the instructor asks the entire class to share their answers and may write the responses on a white board, being sure to clarify or correct any misperceptions. Then the instructor might ask the class to determine which nursing interventions help prevent these potential complications. This entire exercise could be used to help initially introduce a concept as shown in Appendix B. It also may serve as a review of previous content prior to new learning about a concept exemplar such as Fracture.

Another variation of this strategy is the more structured Think-Pair-Share activity. For **Think-Pair-Share**, the instructor presents a topic or statement to the class but each student first writes his or her own response on paper or a mobile device within a 2- to 3-minute timeframe. After this time elapses, students in each pair share and compare their answers for another 2 to 3 minutes. Finally, the instructor summarizes the students' responses and may record them on a white board to ensure that any misperceptions are clarified or corrected. Students are often surprised that they have the same responses, but note differences that can enhance or improve their thinking.

During a discussion about patient care, a good question to ask is "What if . . .?" The **What If . . .?** approach provides an opportunity for students to critically think and then discuss the action they would take. This question could be asked for the entire class to consider or used as a pair discussion either in the classroom or online. For example, consider this scenario:

> *A young woman was in a vehicular crash that severely damaged her lower right leg. She has multiple tibia and fibula fractures and severe soft tissue damage. On admission, her neurovascular assessment showed adequate perfusion to her right foot after placement of an external fixator. The primary healthcare provider requested hourly monitoring of her circulation.* **What If** *her lower leg becomes very swollen?*

A follow-up question might be "What Would You Do?" or "What Would You Do First?" Some students may respond that they would notify the primary healthcare provider, rapid response team, or charge nurse. Instead, encourage them to consider what other action they would take as nurses to help the patient waiting for help. Help them clarify how the nurse might prioritize the necessary follow-up assessments and interventions.

A variation of this strategy is to use the "What Would You Do?" question for ethical or controversial issues or situations to help them learn the concept of Ethics. For example:

> *When entering the medication room in the nursing home unit where you work, you observe a nurse taking an opioid drug intended for a patient on your unit.* **What would you do?**

Students could discuss their answers first in a pair or small group and then share with the entire class. Herrman (2016) labels this strategy as "What's the Right Thing to Do?" Any of these questions could be followed with another question: "Why?" "Why?" explains the rationale that is important for concept understanding and thinking.

Structured controversy is also an excellent thinking activity when exploring controversial issues or ethical dilemmas. It can be set up as a group debate or as a pair activity (the author's preference). Students form pairs before the activity begins. The issue or dilemma is presented by the instructor for student deliberation; for example, "All terminal patients should have the right to make decisions about assisted suicide." The following sequence is used for pair discussion of this dilemma related to the concept of Ethics:

- First minute = Student 1 spends 1 full minute arguing the "pro" stance for the statement. Student 2 must actively listen and be quiet during this time.
- Second minute = Student 2 spends 1 full minute arguing the "con" viewpoint while Student 1 listens attentively and is quiet.
- Third minute = Student 1 spends 1 full minute arguing the "con" stance but may not use anything that Student 2 discussed. Student 2 listens attentively and is quiet.
- Fourth and final minute = Student 2 spends 1 full minute arguing the "pro" viewpoint but may not use anything that Student 1 discussed. Student 1 listens attentively and is quiet.

At the end of the 4 minutes, the instructor summarizes the students' responses and may record them on a white board. Students' personal beliefs are usually not obvious during the discussion.

The benefits of a structured controversy activity are its ability for students to:

- Recognize one's own biases, preferences, and values
- Be aware and appreciate others' biases, preferences, and values
- Critically think about both sides of a situation
- Create one's own knowledge
- Refine listening skills

Case Studies

One of the most useful teaching/learning activities is case studies—either as single or unfolding cases. **Case studies** are written simulated learning experiences in which a clinical or healthcare situation is followed by questions for students to answer. *A single case study* presents a clinical or healthcare situation at one point in time. An *unfolding case study* presents a situation that occurs over time in varying stages—hours, weeks, or months.

A single case study, sometimes referred to as the case scenario or quickie case study (Herrman, 2016), presents only a one- or two-paragraph situation. *Avoid the*

BOX 5-2 Example of a Single Case Scenario with Inappropriate Questions

A 61-year-old man was diagnosed with chronic obstructive pulmonary disease (COPD) as a result of a 120 pack-year smoking history last year. He reports that for the last 3 weeks he has had increasing shortness of breath when he works each day as a carpenter. He states that he developed a frequent "wet" cough earlier this week and feels very tired all the time. Today he is visiting his nurse practitioner for an evaluation.

1. What is COPD?
2. What are the most common risk factors for COPD?
3. What acute medical diagnosis does this patient likely have?
4. What medications will the nurse practitioner likely prescribe?

---

pitfall of providing too much information so that students can determine what else they need to address the case. Follow the case information with critical thinking and clinical reasoning questions rather than pose questions in which the answer is embedded in the case. For example, consider the case in **BOX 5-2** for prelicensure nursing students. In this case, questions 1 and 2 can be answered without using a case study. Therefore, these are not appropriate questions and do not require thinking. Questions 3 and 4 are not nursing-focused questions. Instead they ask the student to make a medical diagnosis and determine which medications might be prescribed for the patient. These questions are beyond the scope of practice for a generalist nurse and are therefore not appropriate.

Remember This . . .

Avoid the pitfall of providing too much information so that students can determine what else they need to address the case. Follow the case information with critical thinking and clinical reasoning questions rather than pose questions in which the answer is embedded in the case.

Better questions that require critical thinking and application of knowledge for conceptual learning might include:

- What is the priority concept in this case? What are the interrelated concepts?
- Based on these health concepts, what nursing history questions would you, as his office nurse, ask?
- What focused physical assessment will you perform?
- What adventitious breath sounds might you expect when auscultating the patient's lungs and why?
- What health teaching might this patient need and why?

None of the answers to these questions are provided in the case situation as presented, and all are within the scope of the nurse generalist.

Case studies may be used as a preassignment for class, done in class (or online), or used as a follow-up to class as homework. Students may complete them as individuals, in pairs, or in larger groups. Remember that collaborative learning is often more effective than individual learning. Chapter 9 discusses the use of case studies in detail.

Graphic Organizers

The term **graphic organizers** refers to a group of learning tools in which concepts are presented visually to show relationships, and are particularly helpful for visual learners. Concepts may be shown by the nurse educator to students in a graphic organizer, or students may create them in pairs or larger groups. Student development of these tools can be very useful for those who prefer read/write or kinesthetic learning. If students or the educator verbally explain the content of the graphic organizer, students who prefer aural learning also can benefit. Common examples of these learning tools include, but are not limited, to:

- Decision-making trees/flow charts
- Venn diagrams
- Concept maps

Decision-making trees or algorithms allow the user to determine the best decision to make based on answers to a series of questions. Exhibit 10-4 in Chapter 10 is an example of a decision-making tool to determine if a test item is at an applying or higher cognitive level.

Venn diagrams are graphic organizers that use two or more circles to show comparisons between and among concepts. For example, **FIGURE 5-2** demonstrates the similarities and differences between common assessment findings for rheumatoid arthritis (RA) and osteoarthritis (OA). In the overlapping shaded part of the diagram are findings common to both diseases, such as joint pain, stiffness, and muscle weakness. In the left circle are Heberden's and Bouchard's nodes, bony nodules of the fingers associated with OA. In the right circle are subcutaneous nodules and finger deformities (such as swan's neck) that are associated with RA. Other content ideas for Venn diagrams might include comparison of:

- Drug classifications
- Drug side or adverse effects

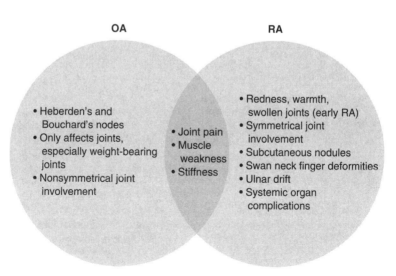

FIGURE 5-2 Venn diagram showing a comparison of typical assessment findings for patients who have osteoarthritis (OA) versus rheumatoid arthritis (RA)

- Disease pathophysiology
- Nursing interventions

Concept mapping is the most complex and often most useful graphic organizer. It can be used in a variety of ways, but is usually used in nursing education for students to present a plan of care for patients in the clinical setting to provide deep learning about selected concepts. Chapter 8 is devoted to discussing how to develop and use concept mapping in nursing education.

Test Item Checks

Students in prelicensure and many graduate programs take a high stakes licensure or certification examination after graduation. Therefore, having students practice taking test items that reflect these examinations is useful in ensuring their success. **Test Item Checks** can be used for learning or formative assessment of learning during face-to-face or online courses. They may be used as an entire class or pair activity, or for individual reflection. Some faculty use smart phone apps or iClickers as an audience response activity for formative evaluation of learning. Consider the following NCLEX®-style test item for the concept of Elimination and its exemplar Crohn's disease:

*The nurse is caring for a client diagnosed with uncontrolled Crohn's disease. Which nursing action is the **priority** for the nurse?*

    A.   Teach the client about foods that should avoided.
    B.   Document the number of stools that the client has each day.
    C.   Assess the client for fluid and electrolyte imbalance.
    D.   Ensure that the client's skin is clean and dry.

*   Note: Answer is C because chronic diarrhea can cause major fluid and electrolyte loss, which could be life-threatening.*

This test item could be introduced at the beginning of class as a springboard for a discussion about the Elimination exemplar. Students could work in pairs to arrive at the correct answer and then provide rationale for their selection. To answer this question, students would need to know from their reading or from a previous Pathophysiology course that patients with Crohn's disease have a chronic inflammatory bowel disease that causes frequent diarrheal stools. They would also have to recall from their basic nursing course that chronic diarrhea can lead to problems with Fluid and Electrolyte Balance. Therefore, the Test Item Check provides the beginning of a discussion about nursing care based on disease pathophysiology. The SLO for this content and Test Item Check might be *Apply the pathophysiology of chronic bowel diseases to prioritize nursing care to ensure patient safety related to Fluid and Electrolyte Balance.*

Test Item Checks are also useful for "soft" concepts such as communication, culture, and caring. For instance, this question assesses learning about communication and an understanding of the care of patients with a cognitive impairment. The major concepts being tested, then, are Communication and Cognition as they apply to the Cognition exemplar of Alzheimer's disease.

*An older client tells the nurse that she is waiting for her mother to come and take her to school. What is the nurse's **best** response?*

    A.   "Your mother is not coming today but might come tomorrow."
    B.   "Tell me about your mother—what does she look like?"

    C.   *"I'll tell the aid to let you know when she gets here."*
    D.   *"I saw her and told her you were waiting to go to school."*

    Note: Answer is B because it is the only statement that reflects validation. The other statements are attempts at reorienting the client, which is not likely given that she has a chronic cognitive impairment.

    Chapter 10 discusses how to write NCLEX®-style test items in detail to promote and evaluate conceptual learning.

Send a Problem

Send a Problem, sometimes called Pass a Problem, is a learning activity in which students individually, in pairs, or in groups of 3 or 4 develop test questions or case studies to share with other students. This strategy is often associated with the problem-based learning model used to educate other healthcare professionals for a number of years. However, it can be used in any curricular model, including the CBC.

    One way to use this activity is at the end of a unit of study and before an examination to review. To begin, place students in planned groups to write two test items or short cases (problems) without keyed answers that focus on one or more selected concepts. Have students place their problems in an envelope and write their names or group number on the outside. Then have them pass their problem to other groups so that each group of students can discuss and collaboratively decide on the answers. After all problems are reviewed and answered, debrief by reviewing the answers with the entire class to ensure accuracy and correct any misperceptions about the concepts being assessed.

Collaborative Testing

Collaborative testing has been used in nursing education for almost 20 years (Lusk & Conklin, 2003), but it is not used as frequently compared to medical education. **Collaborative Testing (CT)** is a strategy in which students work together in pairs or groups to answer test questions. This activity has been reported to enhance learning, promote student success, and increase student retention. CT is an active learning strategy that improves interpersonal skills and enhances clinical reasoning skills based on constructivism learning theory (Duane & Satre, 2014).

    Nursing programs have used CT in several ways. One common method, called *double testing*, allows students to take a test individually and then take the same test as a member of a pair or small group. Most often, if a group achieves an "A" on the group test, each member of the group receives 2 additional points added to their individual test score. If the group achieves a "B," each group member receives 1 additional point added to their individual test score. If the group achieves a "C," no additional points are added. Eastridge (2014) reported an award of 5 points if the group received 100% on the group test.

    Student and faculty responses to CT have been very positive (Parsons & Teel, 2013). **TABLE 5-2** summarizes two recent studies that examined the benefit of CT from different perspectives.

Storytelling

Storytelling can be used effectively by both nurse educators and students. The nurse educator may relate a story that illustrates how one or more concepts are used in

TABLE 5-2 Summary of Two Studies on the Benefits of Collaborative Testing in Nursing Education

Study Citation	Summary of Study Findings
Eastridge, J. A. (2014). Use of collaborative testing to promote nursing student success. *Nurse Educator, 39*(1), 4–5.	■ CT used in AD in nursing program with 90% minority students in New Mexico (primarily from various American Indian pueblos and tribes, Hispanic, Asian, and Arab). ■ Students responses were positive because clinical reasoning was enhanced, group interaction improved, and grades improved. ■ Although CT points allowed one to three students to pass the course, all of those students passed the NCLEX-RN®.
Hanna, K., Roberts, T., & Hurley, S. (2016). Collaborative testing as NCLEX enrichment. *Nurse Educator, 41*(4), 171–174.	■ CT used in a BSN program to determine its benefit to students, impact on comprehensive standardized exit examination scores, and improvement in test scores between individual and group takers. ■ Students responded positively to CT due to development of critical thinking skills and interpersonal skills while interacting as a group member. ■ Fewer students who used CT in the final semester had to retake the final standardized exit examination compared to students who did not use CT over a 3-year period. ■ Students' individual test scores improved when students took the same test as a group.

practice. This story is typically derived from the educator's experience and helps learners gain a deeper understanding of the primary concept and related concepts. For example, the story in **BOX 5-3A** that the author shared with her students relates to the primary concept of Perfusion and the interrelated concept of Clotting. It also demonstrates the role of the licensed practical/vocational nurse in collecting data for a comprehensive assessment by the RN. This potential "failure to rescue" scenario highlights the need for students to focus on the patient experience, as proposed by Benner et al. (2010), and be able to respond appropriately and in a timely manner to changes in a patient's condition (Kavanaugh & Szweda, 2017).

In some cases, the students may be asked to share a story that illustrates critical thinking and nursing judgment related to one or more concepts. For example, in one class, the author was discussing the concept of Sexuality as an interrelated concept to Cognition for the exemplar of Traumatic Brain Injury (TBI). She asked the students to share a story about a patient experience related to Sexuality. This activity is sometimes called *narrative pedagogy*. A student volunteered the story in **BOX 5-3B** to validate the classroom discussion and helped her peers better understand the significance of how TBIs can affect Sexuality. She also explained how she and the staff used critical thinking to help the patient meet her outcome while at the same time ensuring everyone's safety and dignity.

BOX 5-3 Examples of Nurse Educator and Student Stories to Enhance Thinking and Nursing Judgment

A. Nurse Educator Story	B. Nursing Student Story
"When I was Director of Nursing of a continuing care retirement community, I was responsible for both the long-term care (LTC) and independent living residents. One of our LTC residents, Mrs. G., was perceived by my staff as 'demanding.' She frequently reported her unhappiness with the food, dietary staff, and nursing staff. At 89, she was mentally sharp with no signs of cognitive decline.	[Background: As the nurse educator who taught neurological concepts and related nursing care, I focused on major health problems such as spinal cord and traumatic brain injury. I asked the class if they had cared for patients who had neurological damage that affected their Sexuality. I also requested that they explain how that impairment was managed. This is one story that a student shared.]
For 3 to 4 days, Mrs. G. reported sharp pain in her right leg to the charge nurses on each shift, all of whom were RNs. All of them ignored her and no one documented her 'complaint.' On the fourth day, a recently hired 7-to-3 shift LPN (Linda) was giving medications on Mrs. G.'s unit. She examined the resident's leg and reported to me her findings and concern. Linda stated that she had shared her concern with the charge nurse who told her that was 'just the way Mrs. G is.' The LPN stated that the resident's right leg was very pale and cool compared to her left leg. She could not find any pulses in the right leg and was concerned that Mrs. G. might have a problem with her arterial circulation. Upon further comprehensive assessment of Mrs. G.'s leg, I validated Linda's findings and called the physician, who agreed that we should call 911.	"We were in the TBI unit in the rehabilitation center and took care of a prostitute whose pimp beat her with a baseball bat. The patient (I'll call her Lucy) suffered a moderate TBI and was able to ambulate in her wheelchair. Every time she saw a man in the building, whether it was a nursing staff member, visitor, or family member, Lucy would offer to have sex with them. She even solicited one of my peer students! Lucy was always talking about ways to have sex and how much she wanted to have sex. The rehabilitation staff didn't seem to be addressing her issue so we came up with some ideas.
In the emergency department and after several diagnostic tests, Mrs. G. was diagnosed with an acute femoral arterial occlusion. The surgeon stated that if she had waited another day or two that the resident would probably have 'lost her leg.'	Because she was in a private room, we thought it would be a good idea to get her some sex magazines and maybe some sex toys. Then she could pleasure herself and maybe not solicit sex from other people. This would help her physically and protect her dignity at the same time. We shared our plan with the rehabilitation team and they said they would discuss it in their planning meeting the next day. We really don't know if they followed up."
I shared this event with my staff and complimented Linda on her excellent observations and follow-up. I also wrote a letter of commendation for her file. She had been an LPN for only 6 months."	

Each story can be followed up with critical thinking questions. For instance, for the nurse educator story in Box 5-3A, questions for the class might include:

- Why do you think the RN charge nurses ignored Mrs. G.'s report of leg pain?
- Why did Mrs. G. not have palpable pulses?
- What risk factors might Mrs. G. have that contributed to her medical diagnosis?
- What other interrelated concepts do you recognize in this story?
- What would you have done in this same situation as Mrs. G.'s nurse?
- What is the difference in the role of the RN and LPN in this story?

Following class discussion about the story is part of the debriefing needed to develop deep learning and thinking.

Video Clips and Sounds

Numerous video clips, movies, and sounds are available on the Internet from a variety of sources. These tools can help students learn concepts and reinforce previous learning in the cognitive and affective learning domains.

Short video clips can be embedded in the online preclass lecture or Power-Point presentation or viewed during face-to-face class time. They may come from movies, television or Internet shows, or commercials. Before students view the clip, be sure to provide questions or directions that help students frame the purpose of the video. For example, if the purpose of a video is to help students learn about the concept of Safety, video clips available at www.qsen.org are excellent resources. Two examples are *The Lewis Blackman Story* and *The Josie King Story*. *Chasing Zero* is another video that tells the story of how actor Dennis Quaid's infant twins nearly died because of a medication error. These stories illustrate how lack of assessment skills by the entire healthcare team caused multiple errors and unnecessary death of hospitalized patients.

Short video clips also can be very useful to help students gain a deep understanding of "soft" professional nursing and mental health concepts, such as communication, ethics, caring, cultural awareness, and coping. For example, when the author was teaching about Alzheimer's disease as an exemplar for the concept of Cognition, the interrelated concepts of Stress and Coping experienced by family caregivers was discussed. Several YouTube video clips were available so students could hear and see the caregivers' experiences with caring for older parents with Alzheimer's disease. The videos provided a deeper understanding of the strain and grieving associated with patient care at home. Seeing and hearing from the actual caregivers made a bigger impact on the students than any nurse educator explanation of caregiver stress.

During class time, keep video clips at 5 to 10 minutes. *Avoid the pitfall of showing a full-length film during class, especially if it is over an hour*. Longer videos should be assigned as a preclass or postclass activity and are best used with purposeful, guided thinking or reflective questions. For example, the film *The Notebook* is about an older woman who had Alzheimer's disease whose story is told through the lens of her longtime husband. Students might be required to identify which primary concepts are evident in the story and discuss (in class or online) what special nursing care the patient would require if she were hospitalized with a major health problem.

> **Remember This . . .**
>
> *Avoid the pitfall of showing a full-length film during class, especially if it is over an hour. Longer videos should be assigned as a preclass or postclass activity and are best used with purposeful, guided thinking or reflective questions.*

Examples of lung sounds, bowel sounds, and heart sounds are all available on the Internet for preassignment activities or classroom learning. They can be combined with case studies or Test Item Checks. Lung sounds can be used to help students learning the concept of Gas Exchange or Oxygenation. For example, consider this NCLEX®-style practice item. The * indicates the correct answer.

*A client reports feeling out of breath when getting out of bed to go to the bathroom. The nurse hears these breath sounds. (NOTE: Listen to the lung sounds provided.) What is the nurse's **best** action?*

    A.   Document the lung sounds in the electronic health record.
    B.   Notify the primary healthcare provider.
    C.   Start oxygen therapy via nasal cannula.*
    D.   Instruct the client to take frequent rest periods.

Gaming

Gaming is an excellent method for assessing student knowledge (Herrman, 2016). It can be used in a variety of ways, including for review of previously learned concepts or review prior to a test. It is *not* the best learning activity to help students develop critical thinking and deep learning. Gaming can be used in a traditional lecture, flipped model, or scrambled model of teaching/learning. Many games are shown on television, such as *Jeopardy* and *Match Game*, but educators can create their own games if desired. Although the content for a number of courses lends itself to gaming, nurse educators who teach Pharmacology and Pathophysiology, both basic and advanced, commonly use them in their classroom and online. Pharmacology Jeopardy, for example, is appropriate to help students recall drug classifications, side effects, and adverse effects. It also can be used to assess students' knowledge about the nursing implications associated with drug administration. For example, consider these answers and questions:

> *Answer: One of two electrolytes lost when the patient is taking furosemide.*
> Question: What is potassium? (or sodium)
> *Answer: The most important nursing assessment prior to administering amlodipine.*
> Question: What are apical pulse and blood pressure?

Morales (2017) reported the importance of games in her Basic Pharmacology course to help students reinforce knowledge and reduce student anxiety. Games were posted on the LMS for each unit of study in the course. They were also hyperlinked to the drug grid and could be accessed as many times as the student needed using a free software program. Morales recommended that games be used that are familiar to faculty to save time in learning new games or developing their own.

Other familiar games might include the *Match Game, Student Feud* (like *Family Feud*), *Survivor, Who Wants to be a Millionaire?*, and *To Tell the Truth*. Many of these games recently returned to television as new shows with updated approaches. Van Horn, Hyde, Tesh, and Kautz (2014) published an article about using engaging teaching/learning strategies, including gaming, case studies, group projects, and short video clips, to supplement the traditional lecture in advanced Pathophysiology courses in nursing graduate programs. Students found that these activities were student-centered and enhanced their understanding and retention of the course content.

Social Media

Most Millennial and Generation X students use social media for communication with their peers and others. As the nurse educator for students in a Basic Pharmacology course, Morales (2017) reported successful use of social media as a teaching/learning strategy in a Basic Pharmacology course, but stated that it must relate to practice. Facebook served as the social media platform to discuss daily faculty-prepared NCLEX®-style questions and develop test-taking skills. Students also created test items and shared them with their peers. Follow-up discussions and interactions with faculty and peers were viewed very positively by students in the course.

▶ Chapter Key Points

- To facilitate meaningful deep learning, nurse educators need to know who their learners are and what student variables could have an impact on that learning.
- The nurse educator needs to identify which developmental stages and learning preferences are represented in his or her class to help plan the most effective student learning activities.
- Collaborative learning (sometimes referred to as cooperative learning) has been touted as being the best approach for students in the classroom and other educational environments.
- A flipped classroom is a model in which lecture and homework are reversed; that is, the lecture occurs *before* class and homework that engages students in active learning is done in the classroom.
- A scrambled classroom is a model in which learning is facilitated by mixing engaging collaborative student activities with multiple short periods (5 to 10 minutes each) in which the instructor clarifies, updates, and prioritizes class content.
- Many teaching/learning strategies and activities, sometimes called *pedagogies*, that have been used in a traditional classroom can be adapted for the CBC classroom. However, the focus or purpose of those activities may be different to ensure conceptual learning and thinking.
- Debriefing is an important part of learning during which the educator clarifies, highlights, summarizes, and updates class content at various points during class and other learning environments.
- Structured controversy is also an excellent thinking activity when exploring controversial issues or ethical dilemmas.
- One of the most useful teaching/learning activities is case studies—either as single or unfolding cases. Case studies are written simulated learning experiences in which a clinical or healthcare situation is followed by questions for students to answer.

- Graphic organizers refers to a group of learning tools in which concepts are presented visually to show relationships that are particularly helpful for visual learners.

- Venn diagrams are graphic organizers that use two or more circles to show comparisons between or among concepts.

- Test Item Checks can be used for learning or formative assessment of learning during face-to-face or online courses.

- Collaborative testing is a strategy in which students work together in pairs or groups to answer test questions. This activity has been reported to enhance learning, promote student success, and increase student retention.

- Send a Problem, sometimes called Pass a Problem, is a learning activity in which students individually, in pairs, or in groups of 3 or 4 develop test questions or case studies to share with other students.

- Short video clips also can be very useful to help students gain a deep understanding of "soft" professional nursing and mental health concepts, such as communication, ethics, caring, cultural awareness, and coping.

- Gaming is an excellent method for assessing student knowledge; however, it is not the best method for helping students critically think or gain deeper understanding of concepts.

- Social media, such as Facebook, are useful as a teaching/learning strategy for Millennial and Gen X learners.

▶ Chapter References and Selected Bibliography

Barnett, P. E. (2014). *Let's scramble, not flip, the classroom.* Retrieved from www.insidehighered.com/views/2014/02/14/flipping-classroom-isnt-answer-lets-scramble-it-essay.

Benner, P., Stephen, M., Leonard, V., & Day, L. (2010). *Educating nurses: A call for radical transformation.* San Francisco, CA: Jossey-Bass.

Cano-Garcia, F., & Hughes, E. H. (2010). Learning and thinking styles: An analysis of their inter-relationship and influence on academic achievement. *Educational Psychology, 20*(4), 413–430.

Critz, C. M., & Knight, D. (2013). Using the flipped classroom in graduate nursing education. *Nurse Educator, 38*(5), 210–213.

Duane, B. T., & Satre, M. E. (2014). Utilizing constructivism learning theory in collaborative testing as a creative strategy to promote essential nursing skills. *Nursing Education Today, 34*(1), 31–34.

Eastridge, J. A. (2014). Use of collaborative testing to promote student success. *Nurse Educator, 39*(1), 4–5.

Erickson, L. (2007). *Concept-based curriculum and instruction in the thinking classroom.* Thousand Oaks, CA: Corwin Press.

Giddens, J. F., Caputi, L., & Rodgers, B. (2015). *Mastering concept-based teaching: A guide for nursing educators.* St. Louis, MO: Elsevier.

Hanna, K., Roberts, T., & Hurley, S. (2016). Collaborative testing as NCLEX enrichment. *Nurse Educator, 41*(4), 171–174.

Herrman, J. W. (2016). *Creative teaching strategies for the nurse educator* (2nd ed.). Philadelphia, PA: F.A. Davis.

Holman, R., & Hanson, A. D. (2016). Flipped classroom versus traditional lecture: Comparing teaching models in undergraduate nursing courses. *Nursing Education Perspectives, 37*(6), 320–322.

Kavanaugh, J. M., & Szweda, C. (2017). A crisis in competency: The strategic and ethical imperative to assessing new graduate nurses' clinical reasoning. *Nursing Education Perspectives, 38*(2), 57–62.

*Lusk, M., & Conklin, L. (2003). Collaborative testing to promote learning. *Journal of Nursing Education, 42*(3), 121–124.

Morales, K. A. (2017). Active learning strategies to enhance nursing students' knowledge of pharmacology. *Nursing Education Perspectives, 38*(2), 100–102.

Oermann, M. H., & Gaberson, K. B. (2017). *Evaluation and testing in nursing education* (5th ed.). New York, NY: Springer Publishing.

Parsons, S. D., & Teel, V. (2013). Double testing: A student perspective. *Nursing Education Perspectives, 34*(2), 127–128.

Sandahl, S. S. (2009). Collaborative testing as a learning strategy in nursing education: A review of the literature. *Nursing Education Perspectives, 30*(3), 171–175.

Van Horn, E. R., Hyde, Y. M., Tesh, A. S., & Kautz, D. D. (2014). Teaching pathophysiology. *Nurse Educator, 39*(1), 34–37.

Voyer, D., & Voyer, S. D. (2014). Gender differences in scholastic achievement: A meta-analysis. *Psychological Bulletin, 140*(4), 1174–1204.

*Indicates classic reference.

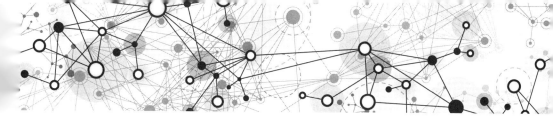

CHAPTER 6

Clinical Teaching and Learning in a Concept-Based Nursing Curriculum

Kristin Oneail and Donna Ignatavicius

CHAPTER LEARNING OUTCOMES

After studying this chapter, the reader will be better able to:

1. Differentiate between learning in the traditional clinical setting and a conceptual clinical experience.
2. Describe the elements of preparing for conceptual learning experiences.
3. Identify the role of a clinical nurse educator (CNE) in a concept-based curriculum (CBC).
4. Explain the benefits of the weekly teaching plan for consistency among clinical sites in a CBC course.
5. Describe examples of appropriate learning activities and assignments in the conceptual clinical experience.

▶ Introduction to Clinical Teaching and Learning in a Concept-Based Curriculum

As discussed throughout this book, nursing education must focus on processes that enable students to develop critical thinking, clinical reasoning, and clinical judgment in preparation for practice in today's collaborative healthcare environment. A concept-based curriculum (CBC) actively engages students in the classroom and/or online to promote deep understanding and meaningful learning. Active engagement is even more important in the clinical setting where students apply concepts from the cognitive, psychomotor, and affective learning domains.

Active engaging learning is necessary to deepen students' theoretical knowledge on a specific concept, enhance their clinical judgment, and improve other essential habits of thought, such as ethical deliberation and reflection (Nielsen, 2009; Tanner, 2010). The clinical experience is the most active component of a nursing curriculum, putting thought to practice while increasing the student's confidence level with each interaction in the clinical learning environment. Clinical practice is important not just for skill development, but also for students to learn about the "norms" of practice and processes in healthcare delivery (Henderson, Cooke, Creedy, & Walker, 2012). This chapter presents strategies and techniques for helping students achieve deep learning and clinical reasoning skills in the clinical environment in a CBC—both in external community healthcare organizations and in internal clinical simulation.

▶ The Traditional Model of Clinical Teaching

Traditional models of clinical teaching that have been used for many years are teacher-centered and are no longer efficient in communicating the complexity of concepts and skill sets required to prepare generalist and advanced practice nurses for contemporary health care (Hardin & Richardson, 2012). Characteristics of a typical *traditional* clinical practicum include:

- Focus on individual student work
- Specific patient assignments (often assigned prior to the scheduled clinical day)
- Random learning based on available patients or clients
- Lengthy preclinical paperwork
- Lengthy postclinical assignments
- Focus on psychomotor skill performance
- No connection between classroom/online learning and clinical learning

---

Remember This . . .

Current traditional models of clinical teaching that have been used for many years are no longer efficient in communicating the complexity of concepts and skill sets required to prepare generalist and advanced practice nurses for contemporary health care (Hardin & Richardson, 2012).

Traditional clinical experiences tend to promote individual student work and are not geared for focused development of collaboration and communication. Student assignments that involve simply going to the agency or unit and doing what the nurse or nurse practitioner does can lead to unpredictable, unfocused, and random clinical learning (Nielson, Noone, Voss, & Mathews, 2013).

▶ Clinical Learning in the Concept-Based Curriculum

In a concept-based clinical experience, the learning outcomes and associated activities are student-centered and focus on:

- The student–clinical nurse educator (CNE) relationship
- The relationship with the unit or agency staff (beginning with shadowing opportunities)
- Peer interactions
- Enhanced interprofessional communication and collaboration
- Professional role integration
- Deep understanding of themes rather than rote memorization (Henderson et al., 2012)

The role of faculty in a CBC clinical environment is to purposefully create opportunities for learning in which students intentionally apply each concept in the context of multiple healthcare settings (Giddens, 2016). To meet this outcome, the concept-based clinical experience shifts from a focus on applying knowledge to an emphasis on promoting clinical reasoning and enhancing clinical judgment through two broad types of activities: direct care activities (DCAs) and focused learning activities (FLAs). Both DCAs and FLAs are connected to concepts being learned in the classroom and/or online. For **direct care activities**, also called direct patient care (DPC), students are assigned to learning activities while providing patient care to achieve one or more competencies related to applying concepts. These competencies are evaluated as either "Met" or "Unmet." DPC may be either total or focused, depending on the learning outcomes for the experience, and may be performed in the simulation or external clinical setting. Focused DPC requires the student to provide partial care to improve meaningful conceptual learning or a skill set. For example, students may perform focused respiratory and cardiovascular assessments on their assigned patients to apply the concepts of gas exchange and perfusion. They then may be asked to interpret the assessment data to identify actual or potential complications for which they can plan and implement care.

Focused learning activities promote learning completed in the laboratory or external clinical setting that support achievement of one or more clinical competencies related to applying concepts for deep understanding. Examples include concept mapping (see Chapter 8), Socratic questioning, data mining, case studies, and interprofessional rounds, discussed later in this chapter. FLAs are completed in small groups and evaluated using grading rubrics. A grading score may be predetermined as acceptable or passing the assignment. Students not meeting the expected score may have the opportunity to improve their work as part of formative evaluation.

Conceptual learning in clinical experiences brings theory to clinical education for deep learning and extends the students' theoretical knowledge to create practical knowledge. Throughout the clinical experience, learners generate pattern recognition and clinical nursing judgment. Practical skills are furthered enhanced through nursing procedures, clinical reasoning, self-reflection, and system thinking. Clinical learning in a CBC also helps students develop an understanding of the culture of health care and nursing, and the effect of this culture on patient care, roles of team members, and

TABLE 6-1 Comparison Between Traditional and Concept-Based Curriculum Clinical Experiences

	Traditional Clinical Experiences	Concept-Based Clinical Experiences
Student assignments	Individualized	Peer and/or group
Focus of clinical assignment	Teacher-centered; skills-centered Total patient care	Student-centered to promote clinical reasoning and judgment Concept focus Clinical unit/agency focus
Shadowing opportunity	Minimal	Nursing/interprofessional
Observational opportunity	Surgery and procedures	Nursing/interprofessional
Community experience	Minimal	Expanded; increased focus on vulnerable populations such as older adults and patients with mental health issues

ways of functioning in nursing and interprofessional teams (Tanner, 2010). Positive learning environments that facilitate students to engage in practice are pivotal if nursing is to shift from traditional "routine" care to practice based on best current evidence.

Clinical learning may be further enhanced when faculty consider placement of courses within the CBC. For example, in a traditional baccalaureate of science in nursing (BSN) program, the community or population-focused course is typically in the last year of the program and often in the last semester. However, placing this course in the beginning of the nursing curriculum can build a foundation for community care and systems thinking. Building on this foundation, students have the opportunity to continue to apply community health concepts. Students then are socialized early to question system factors to enhance patient safety and improve quality of care. **TABLE 6-1** briefly summarizes major differences between clinical experiences in the traditional nursing curriculum and the CBC.

▶ Preparing for Concept-Based Clinical Experiences

In preparation for a change in the focus of the clinical experience, extensive communication and planning with healthcare agencies are essential. A structured partnership between each healthcare agency and the educational institution is needed for a successful curricular shift (Newton, Jolly, Ockerby, & Cross, 2012).

Creating an academic/clinical practice partnership ensures ongoing communication and education before and during the curricular revision. Inclusion of all necessary personnel for the clinical experience change is needed for effective implementation. Collaboration among nursing administrators, clinicians, and nurse educators; support and training for clinicians; peer teaching; and well-planned placement of students in the clinical setting provide the foundational framework for conceptual learning.

Role of the Clinical Coordinator

An important role in the academic institution is the **clinical coordinator** or facilitator, who arranges all clinical experiences and makes rounds in each agency to ensure that students have the opportunity to meet outcomes related to conceptual learning. CNEs for each agency can be either full-time faculty or qualified nurse clinicians who work part-time as adjunct clinical instructors. The clinical coordinator is responsible for frequent interaction and communication with the CNEs during the academic year to obtain ongoing feedback for continuous quality improvement (QI). In some cases, this individual also evaluates the performance of adjunct or part-time clinical faculty.

Role of the Academic-Practice Liaison

To ensure success during the transition to a CBC, a nurse educator (usually a full-time faculty member) serves as a liaison between the nursing program and each healthcare agency. The **academic-practice liaison (APL)** assists in educating leadership and clinical staff in the healthcare agency and advocates for adequate clinical units to meet students' needs each semester or other term. The liaison becomes the coordinator between education and practice, relating to each party the needs and available resources of the other.

The APL also takes on the responsibility of continuing education for staff nurses throughout the clinical experience and answers questions that may arise regarding the curriculum shift. The active role of the liaison with students in the clinical environment includes Socratic questioning as a way to participate in their learning process and assess the learning outcomes of the clinical experience. These interactions build relationships and enhance the level of trust and communication between the academic and clinical practice setting.

Including the staff nurse as integral components of the student-focused clinical learning experience affords the learner a successful and meaningful clinical experience. Staff nurses have an ethical and professional obligation to support students in the clinical setting and provide guidance when necessary (Killam & Heerschap, 2013).

> **Remember This...**
>
> *Staff nurses have an ethical and professional obligation to support students in the clinical setting and provide guidance when necessary (Killam & Heerschap, 2013).*

Assessing characteristics of the clinical practice environment can provide useful insights for further development of learning activities and determine if the clinical site is appropriate for conceptual learning. The APL, with input from leadership and staff nurses, can provide valuable feedback when completing the end-of-term clinical agency evaluation provided by the academic institution. This feedback provides a

BOX 6-1 Role of the Academic-Practice Liaison

- Plan education for clinical agency staff and leadership
- Provide continuing and ongoing education for clinical nursing staff
- Provide clinical support for clinical nurse educators (CNEs)
- Assist with placement of students on clinical units and in community agencies
- Assist with identification of quality improvement issues based on feedback
- Assist with evaluation of clinical units and community agencies and healthcare staff

platform to continually improve the clinical experiences for students, patients, and employees of the practice institution. **BOX 6-1** summarizes the role of the APL.

Role of the Educational Resource Unit

Several new clinical nursing education models have been developed over the past 10 to 15 years, but a limited number of programs have access to these innovations. For example, some nursing programs have partnered with healthcare agencies or clinical units to socialize their students into their culture by developing specialized clinical learning units called educational resource units (ERUs) or dedicated educational units (DEUs). In this partnership, nursing practice informs nursing education, and nursing education influences nursing practice. Instead of the typical 1:8-10 CNE-to-learner ratio, clinical staff nurses serve as mentors for 1 or 2 students for a period of 6 weeks or longer. Some students have the opportunity to stay on the same unit for an entire year to become embedded in the unit culture and have ownership in unit practices and patient care. Staying in one site also helps alleviate the anxiety that is typical each time a student begins a new clinical setting experience.

The ERU experience creates trusting relationships between nursing staff and nursing students, with the CNE maintaining the role as instructor and staff nurses assuming the role of clinical experts. Maintaining the focus on the staff nurse as the clinical expert and the CNE as the learning facilitator not only provides the student with open communication throughout the experience, but allows the staff nurse to be a part of the educational process. The academic-practice partnership, as well as the ERU, begins to develop staff nurses as mentors for the practice environment.

Mentoring the Clinical Nurse Educator

CNEs may be part-time adjunct faculty or full-time faculty. In either case, they have a professional and ethical role in creating an environment conducive for learning that gives the students a platform to clinically reason in the clinical setting (Burrell, 2014). Moving clinical faculty from a content-focused, teacher-centered learning environment to a concept-focused student-centered approach may be the greatest challenge faced by nursing programs (Giddens & Brady, 2007; Hendricks & Wangerin, 2017).

Structured professional development to educate CNEs before and during the transition to conceptual learning in the clinical environment needs to include:

- Components and processes associated with the CBC curricular model
- Comparison between a traditional and CBC clinical experience
- Weekly teaching/learning plans specific for the clinical course

In preparation for a shift to a CBC curriculum, the CNEs must value the benefit of the experience for both the CNE and the student. One of the professional development areas to address is how to create an effective CNE-student interaction time. In a conceptual clinical learning environment, CNEs have time to guide student thinking and facilitate deep learning of key concepts. A concept-based clinical experience enables the CNE to have a stronger presence in the clinical area with a greater impact on student learning and the development of clinical reasoning and judgment.

In addition to professional development sessions, CNE meetings should be scheduled prior to the beginning of the semester (or other term), throughout the semester, and at the end of the semester for debriefing. To ensure communication and collaboration, a course coordinator or lead faculty may be selected to oversee each aspect of the term, including theory, laboratory, and clinical experiences. The coordinator works with all course faculty to ensure their needs are met and that the term is progressing well.

A main focus for the course coordinator is one-on-one communication with the CNE on at least a weekly basis via meetings, phone calls, or email for guidance and support. Communication is also essential when problems or concerns arise in the clinical environment with the student or with the facility. Debriefing meetings usually occur at the end of the term as a faculty group for each clinical course. This method of communication also ensures retention of qualified clinical faculty.

Developing sustainable approaches to enhance the clinical learning environment experience for the student nurses is a primary concern. The best way to achieve a positive learning experience is continuity of CNEs (Newton et al., 2012). In supporting the CNE, as well as the student, weekly teaching/learning plans are provided so all CNEs teaching in the same course help students meet the same learning outcomes and activities. **EXHIBIT 6-1** provides a teaching/learning plan that shows how one program ensured that the same learning experiences were applied to develop clinical conceptual learning in an adult health course in multiple settings. Each week, the same concepts were applied in all learning environments such that there was a strong connection between the didactic and clinical portions of the course.

EXHIBIT 6-1 Example of Weekly Teaching/Learning Plan for NUR 321

Adult Health Weekly Teaching/Learning Plan for Clinical Experience

Theme Six: Protection and Movement
- Concept of Mobility

Theme Three: Homeostasis and Regulation
- Concepts of Fluid and Electrolyte Balance

Students are learning the following exemplars in theory:
- Mobility Exemplars: Osteoarthritis, Hip Fractures/Surgery, Amputations
- Fluid and Electrolyte Balance Exemplars: Acute Kidney Injury, Hyper/Hyponatremia, Hyper/Hypokalemia

(continues)

EXHIBIT 6-1   Example of Weekly Teaching/Learning Plan for NUR 321 (continued)

NOTE: Theory concepts are provided so you can take advantage of any additional learning opportunities that may occur during clinical time to reinforce concepts taught in the classroom.

Clinical Experience Student Learning Outcomes:

1. Students will focus on Quality and Safety Education for Nurses (QSEN) competencies related to Safety, Patient-Centered Care, Informatics, Evidence-Based Practice, Informatics, and Collaboration.
2. Students will develop medication sheets and information related to exemplar diagnoses to assist in evidence-based understanding of patient-centered care for patients affected by mobility and fluid and electrolyte concerns.
3. Students will identify safety concerns specific to the medical-surgical environment in the hospital setting.
4. Students will perform daily care for assigned patients as needed (obtain vital signs [VS], administer bed baths, record intake and output [I&O], and assist in activities of daily living [ADLs]).
5. Students will analyze VS data by identifying abnormal VS parameters and identifying nursing interventions needed.
6. Students will perform focused assessment on areas related to mobility and fluids and electrolytes.
7. Students will review how to collect and document information related to fluids and electrolytes (I&O).
8. Students will assess and manage intravenous (IV) infusion site.
9. Students will perform IV calculations related to infusions or IV medication administration.
10. Students will review patient documentation and identify diagnostic procedures, health history information, and medications that affect the concepts of perfusion and gas exchange in the hospitalized adult patient,
11. Students will identify one patient-specific nursing diagnosis or collaborative problem related to concepts of mobility or fluids and electrolyte balance in the hospitalized adult patient, and develop expected patient outcomes and nursing interventions related to these patient problems.
12. Students will identify and develop a patient teaching plan related to a priority patient teaching need.
13. Students will perform mock/actual medication administration pass with one medication that is administered intravenously.
14. Student will report to nursing staff utilizing the situation, background, assessment recommendation (SBAR) format.

Learning Activities

Make sure you have posted the clinical unit document to the unit nursing station so all staff in the unit are aware of student activities for the day.

This week you can assign the students based on the nursing assignments. Within that nurse's assignment, the students could work either together or separately based upon what you think would be best for those students.

1. Students will obtain VS, collect I&O data, perform assessments, and perform 60-second situational assessments on all assigned patients. Students will document one full assessment on clinical documentation forms for instructor evaluation. Other

EXHIBIT 6-1 Example of Weekly Teaching/Learning Plan for NUR 321 (continued)

assessments may be documented in the electronic health record (EHR). Students will complete a concept map on the patient from the written documentation. Patient education documentation also will be completed on this patient.

Make sure the nursing assistants (NAs) are aware that the students will be obtaining VS on identified patients. Divide them with clear responsibilities. Utilize the clinical documentation form so all communication for NAs is available. Have students enter VS and I&O into the EHR. Students should immediately report abnormal VS. Reinforce with students how/when/etc. I&O is to be collected.

I&Os are totaled related to clinical site polity. The CNE will discuss and review with students the importance of tracking I&O and daily weights and assist students to identify exemplars that are affected by fluid overload and/or dehydration. Also assist students to track I&O and weight trends since admission for an individual patient and discuss relevance of trends.

2. Students will bring evidence of clinical preparation on the exemplar medical conditions, medications, and laboratory studies related to mobility and fluid and electrolyte balance.

You will need to review preclinical paperwork and discuss the conditions and medications the students reviewed, especially discussing patient monitoring related to the medications (i.e., checking blood pressure or heart rate before giving certain medications or ordering certain laboratory work and focusing on explaining/reinforcing the importance of sodium and potassium levels). You could do this prior to having them look for charting/patient information related to these conditions. Ideally, this discussion is early in the clinical day, to tie in concepts as they see them on the clinical unit.

3. Medical administration record (MAR)/chart/laboratory tests reviews: Situation, background, assessment, recommendation (SBAR) and Nursing Diagnoses/Collaborative Problems

Have the students reflect on the patients they assessed and have them review those charts for medications/laboratory data/procedures, etc. related to the concepts of mobility and fluid and electrolytes. Have them reflect on what they would look to be abnormal—what types of medical or personal histories might the patients have that could predispose them to these concerns. Review SBAR related to these patients/concerns.

4. Students will assess and manage IV site, bag, tubing, and calculations of maintenance IV and piggyback IV (IVPB). Students will document IV assessment on at least one patient.
5. Students will practice calculation of maintenance IV solution and IVPB infusions. Students can do IV assessments and change IV tubing for patients on the unit.

Instructor is to assist students with their assessments and management of the IV sites, bags, and tubing. Help students identify nursing inventions that may be needed and to communicate with the patient's nurse any interventions completed.

Instructor to review adult IV maintenance fluid calculations, drug calculations, and IVPB administration calculations with students and do sample calculations. Try to make sure students will be able to calculate at least one of each type during this clinical day. Refer any students who need additional practice to the laboratory via a laboratory referral form.

6. Students will perform mock/actual medication administration: IV medication.

(continues)

EXHIBIT 6-1 Example of Weekly Teaching/Learning Plan for NUR 321 (continued)

Using the MARs the students reviewed, select one medication that they can "pass." You should do this with each student individually. They should perform all steps of medication administration (including patient rights and all significant premedication administration steps). Then have the student verbalize how to complete medication administration (using safety steps, retrieving the information from the EHR). Identify student strengths and any areas for improvement. This would be a good time to fill out a referral if you feel students are not ready to pass medications in real time.

7.   Students will report off to each other and then nursing staff utilizing SBAR format.

In order for students to practice good communication, they should first practice with each other to ease anxiety and "practice" what they want to say. Students should then deliver report on the patients they cared for to nursing staff in this format. Feedback (verbal) from nursing staff should be elicited after clinical (if possible) to provide feedback to students.

Instructor Postconference Discussion and Activities
Review clinical paperwork and give suggestions for documentation (referrals if necessary. Students should be completing well-documented assessments by this time in real time). Discuss concept map, potential primary need, nursing diagnosis/collaborative problems, and teaching needs for the patient they assessed.

Discuss IV calculations related to medication administration. Review any questions/concerns with students.

Debrief on the concepts of the day. Allow the students to reflect on the concepts witnessed in the patient population. Steer the conversation on how these are reflected in the nursing diagnoses and collaborative problems.

Preclinical Paperwork
Review: All forms needed for clinical and bring to clinical: SBAR, 60-second situational assessment, week 3 clinical documentation.
Review: Calculations related to IV medication administration (medication administration IV module)
Review: Assessment points for mobility, IV assessment, integumentary assessment
Review: Standard plans of care for exemplar diagnoses and skills related to identified nursing interventions

All information from exemplars, medication cards, and laboratory information MUST be referenced. You CANNOT "cut and paste" information from text or other sources. You need to read and summarize information into your own words.

Exemplars for MS Week 3: Osteoarthritis, Hip Fracture, Amputation (Below Knee Amputation), Dehydration
■   In a Word (or equivalent) document, complete an "Exemplar Card" for each Exemplar. Information that must be included: Exemplar name, pathophysiology, and risk factors, Diagnostic procedures or surgical interventions related to exemplar, laboratory studies related to exemplar, nursing interventions (evidence based) related to exemplar, and necessary patient education related to exemplar.
■   Print and bring to clinical as preclinical paperwork.

EXHIBIT 6-1 Example of Weekly Teaching/Learning Plan for NUR 321 (continued)

Medication Cards for Adult Health Nursing Week #3
Mobility: Review pain medications.
Fluids and Electrolytes: Potassium chloride, magnesium sulfate; *loop diuretic—* furosemide (Lasix), bumetanide (Bumex); *Potassium sparing—*spironolactone (Aldactone)

Laboratory Cards for Week 3
- In Word (or equivalent document), complete a "lab card" for each laboratory study. Information that must be included: Laboratory test name, specimen or type of test, purpose of test, normal ranges, when the test is used/indicated.
- **Serum:** Sodium, potassium, magnesium, chloride, basic metabolic profile (BMP)
- **Urine:** Complete urine analysis

Clinical Paperwork Due
Preclinical paperwork:
    Exemplars:
    Medications:
    Laboratory tests:
Patient charting on one of the assigned patients:
    Vital signs (VS)
      VS, I&O
    Basic nursing care
      Safety, activity, hygiene/dressing/comfort
      Nutrition and hydration, elimination, skin care
    Significant physical assessment findings
    Specific system assessment
      Musculoskeletal assessment and interventions
      Integument assessment and interventions
      IV assessment
      Morse Fall Scale
      Concept Map
    One nursing diagnosis or collaborative problem with expected outcome and at least five nursing interventions related to outcome
    Patient Education: Teaching plan related to priority teaching need
    If students earn a failing grade on clinical paperwork, this is a reason for the student to have a remediation form completed for failing to fulfill course requirements and must resubmit assignment to your satisfaction.

Courtesy of Kristin Oneail, MS, RN

    The CNE and student have the opportunity to develop a relationship such that the instructor can gain a greater understanding of each student's individual learning needs. CNEs want students to "think on their feet" and make clinical judgments while providing meaningful feedback to each student. The concept-based clinical experience supports the development of clinical judgment and helps students progress along the novice-to-expert continuum.

    The CNE and the student in the clinical settings are equally involved in learning from each other; learning is affected by their culture, values, and background throughout the learning process (D'Souza, Venkatesaperumal, Radhakrishnan, & Balachandran, 2013). The CNE's confidence and competence "can make or break" a clinical experience. He or she needs to be dedicated and approachable, not just by the students but also by anyone employed in the healthcare institution or community agency.

CNEs also must have a sense of belonging at the academic institution. Although their schedules may not always allow for attendance at program or university events, they should be invited so they feel included in the academic milieu. Although many CNEs function as adjunct or part-time faculty in the same practice settings where they work full-time, they are in a different role, which needs to be recognized and respected by the staff nurses. The role of the CNE is one that should be deliberate and intentional with guidance and with a specific focus to the academic institution and the educational skills required for the role (Roberts, Chrisman, & Flowers, 2013).

▶ Connecting Conceptual Clinical Learning with Classroom, Laboratory, and Simulation Learning

Curricular shift to a conceptual focus must occur in all teaching/learning environments to have successful outcomes. Conceptual decisions must be made across the curriculum and with defined plans for all involved. Nurse educators in the didactic, laboratory, and clinical learning environments are all involved in the education and communication process.

Multiple student "check-offs" on every skill is not an appropriate use of time in the laboratory or clinical setting. Instead, faculty need to achieve a consensus on which skills should be included and what can be practiced (not evaluated) or eliminated. Examples of key skills most programs contain for evaluation include IV initiation, urinary catheter insertion, and wound care. All of these skills have a focus on maintaining infection control and sterile technique and reflect the key concept of Immunity and the exemplar of Infection.

Clinical simulation in nursing education has provided a means for students to learn and apply theoretical concepts of nursing care within a safe environment. Focusing the simulation on key components of skills and concepts is the ideal approach for successful learning for the student. Each simulation should be videotaped, to enhance the debriefing process after completion of the experience. Debriefing promotes deep conceptual learning, clinical reasoning, and critical thinking, which are required to ensure appropriate and timely clinical judgments.

Socratic questioning is a technique that nurse educators can use to stimulate thinking and deep conceptual learning in the classroom, laboratory, and simulation (Burrell, 2014). Faculty should pose high-level thinking questions so students are stimulated to reason and not recite facts. These questions probe assumptions and relationships, analyze concepts, and clarify meaning. Examples of Socratic question stems in any learning environment might include:

- What does this mean?
- Why do you think . . .?
- Can you give me an example?
- What do we know about . . .?

- How does that concept relate to . . .?
- Is there be a better way to do that?

Further discussion about using Socratic questioning in the conceptual clinical setting may be found later in this chapter.

Reflection may be utilized as an assignment in the classroom, laboratory, simulation, or the clinical environment to promote self-awareness about the benefit of a learning activity and the impact of the activity on the student to help develop professionalism (Hatlevik, 2012). In the laboratory setting, it affords the student the ability to process when performing a skill or clinical simulation.

Concept mapping is an excellent tool to assist learners in making the connections between concepts and the patient. In the laboratory setting, students may be required to create a map for each procedure to be practiced to include the procedure, rationale for performing the procedure, and expected outcome for each procedure (Burrell, 2014). This assignment assists the student to visualize the logical flow of the procedure and helps emphasize best practices for its performance. Chapter 8 provides detail on the use of concept mapping.

▶ Selecting and Managing a Concept-Based Curriculum Clinical Learning Environment

The purpose of a CBC clinical experience is to ensure that students develop high-level thinking skills and clinical reasoning while performing integrated learning activities within a clinical environment. By gaining a deep understanding of key concepts, students are able to recognize recurring characteristics and apply them to a wide variety of clinical situations and patient/family concerns. Meaningful learning occurs when students make substantive connections between new information and their preexisting knowledge (Getha-Eby, Beery, O'Brien, & Xu, 2015). The CBC clinical experience is student-centered and increases the likelihood of meaningful learning as well as engagement in the clinical experience. The connections that students need to make must be supported by teaching approaches that allow students to construct deep meaning and understanding (Giddens & Brady, 2007).

Remember This . . .

The CBC clinical experience is student-centered and increases the likelihood of meaningful learning as well as engagement in the clinical experience. The connections that students need to make must be supported by teaching approaches that allow students to construct deep meaning and understanding (Giddens & Brady, 2007).

Enhancing clinical learning in a CBC must include multiple diverse internal (simulation) and external experiences. Community sites such as senior centers, schools in underprivileged areas, nursing centers, domestic violence and homeless shelters, and the hospital environment give the student a varied and realistic view regarding the needs of a community or patients. Students' involvement in diversity experiences promote their growth in engagement, motivation, and active complex thinking (D'Souza et al., 2013). The positive outcomes of assimilating students into the community and nursing unit strengthens the skills and thought processes of the student. Effective clinical learning requires integration of nursing students into clinical unit activities, staff nurse's engagement to address individual student learning needs, and innovative clinical teaching approaches.

Nurse educators need to select clinical sites that provide an opportunity for students to meet the course student learning outcomes (SLOs). In some cases, students can use various clinical sites in the same course in which to apply selected concepts. By using a variety of settings, the program is better able to manage increasingly limited external clinical experiences (Higgins & Reid, 2017). For example, if the APL wanted students to apply the concepts of Health Promotion and Immunity in clinical practice, a number of sites could be used, including pediatric immunization clinics, older adult housing centers, and flu clinics. Students would be placed in various settings to apply these same concepts.

Another consideration in conceptual learning is that although patients experiencing the exemplars discussed in class or online may not be available, conceptual learning may be achieved. For example, if the Health concept of Nutrition is being studied in class with the exemplars of Obesity and Protein-Calorie Malnutrition, students could assess patients at risk for these problems and compare and contrast their nutritional status for actual evidence of these health problems or risk for them.

In some courses, depending on the concepts being learned, all students in a course apply concepts in the same type of setting. For example, learning about care of postpartum patients would most likely occur in either a hospital mother-baby unit or in clinical simulation.

Concept-based learning in the clinical environment must integrate theory with practice as conceptual knowledge is translated. Structured clinical time to increase interaction between students and their CNEs in preconference, postconference, and time on the clinical unit optimizes perceived learning (Nielson, 2016). Instructor availability, assistance with problems, and innovations in learning activities contribute to a student-centered clinical learning environment.

Best practices in conceptual clinical education are ones that (D'Souza et al., 2013):

- Encourage student-CNE interactions
- Develop reciprocity and cooperation among students (student-student interactions)
- Encourage active learning
- Provide students with prompt feedback
- Emphasize time on learning activities and assignments
- Communicate high expectations
- Respect diverse abilities of students

Student-student (peer-to-peer) and student-CNE interaction in the clinical learning environment are the two major influences on the effectiveness of clinical learning.

▶ Conceptual Clinical Learning Activities and Assignments

Conceptual clinical learning provides an integrative, interprofessional environment that allows students to engage in planned learning activities that blend knowledge, psychomotor skills, and ethical comportment to focus on Professional Nursing and

Health and Illness concepts. These activities recognize adult learning theory by facilitating student inquiry and allowing for testing of ideas without the responsibility of total patient care for each clinical experience (Nielsen, 2009).

Desired outcomes of the clinical experience using a concept-based approach increases direct contact time for students and CNEs, provides opportunities for faculty to model communication and health assessment skills, and allows students to focus on one main idea at a time without having responsibility for all patient care. CNEs need to learn teaching strategies that address student learning needs and areas for improvement (Suplee, Gardner, & Jerome-D'Emilia, 2014).

Development of theoretical knowledge influences the ability of students to connect theory with practice, especially early in nursing education. Peer-to-peer activities and shadowing experiences promote deeper integration and reorganization of new and existing clinical knowledge, resulting in substantial gains for the student clinical learning and engagement outcomes (D'Souza et al., 2013).

Students need innovative, engaging, and planned clinical experiences to develop understanding of contextual and conceptual factors that influence nursing care to appreciate salience and recognize patterns in findings (Nielson et al., 2013). Planned clinical learning activities move students away for the traditional focus of being task-driven toward a deeper understanding of knowledge application in the clinical environment. The types of learning activities or assignments that need to be created must encourage students to think in a systems or process mode in the practice environment. Selected examples of specific activities are described in the next section of this chapter. Additional ideas are available in many of the references at the end of this chapter and elsewhere in this text.

Remember This . . .

Planned clinical learning activities move students away for the traditional focus of being task-driven toward a deeper understanding of knowledge application in the clinical environment.

Interprofessional Activities and Assignments

Interprofessional education (IPE) is defined as learning that occurs across two or more professions, is interactive, and involves reflection; it requires collaboration among students of these professions (Hudson, Sanders, & Pepper, 2013). IPE assists with developing a collaborative culture in health care to achieve optimal outcomes for patients, families, and populations.

Rounding experiences may occur with primary healthcare providers, rehabilitation therapists, diagnostic testing technicians, dietitians, environment services, social services, and nursing managers. Assign students in 2-hour blocks to round and observe with the healthcare team. Require them to document their observations and complete a reflection about the experience. Postconference discussion promotes an appreciation and respect for team members from multiple health professions or disciplines. Multidisciplinary or interprofessional education also enhances critical thinking, open-mindedness, and flexibility in students that will assist them in their professional careers (Killam & Heerschap, 2013).

Safety-Focused Activities and Assignments

Safety always has been a focus for any nursing curriculum. The development of the QSEN initiative demonstrated the need for utilizing specific safety-focused assignments in the laboratory and clinical experience to solidify the role that individual and systems safety plays in nursing practice. Examples of safety-focused activities include:

- Case studies
- SBAR practice
- 60-second situational assessments

Single- or Unfolding Case Studies that focus on safety are used frequently in the laboratory, simulation, and external clinical site as a focused learning activity (FLA). Chapter 9 describes the use of these learning activities in detail.

In any patient care clinical agency, the SBAR method for communication or other established method is a necessary skill. In many settings, SBAR has been revised to include an introduction component, thus renaming it to ISBAR to remind the staff and students to introduce themselves. In other agencies, an additional R is added for ISBARR to account for the receiver's response to the recommendation. The introduction component helps students increase their confidence level when contacting a physician or other healthcare provider and promotes clinical reasoning. **EXHIBIT 6-2** provides an example of a student script for practicing ISBAR.

The most useful safety-focused assignment in the clinical environment is the *60-second situational safety assessment*. Another term for this type of assessment is a "doorway safety assessment." The situational safety assessment includes components of presence of individuals in the patient's hospital room, the presence of any tubes or lines in the patient, and an environmental survey of the room with a focus on identification of any safety concerns. **EXHIBIT 6-3** provides an example of a situational safety assessment.

EXHIBIT 6-2 Example of ISBAR

Introduction: "Hello, my name is _____, I am an RN from 14 Tower caring for Hilary Jones in Room 16.

Situation: Mrs. Jones has reported pain throughout the night. She was medicated at 4 am with 2 mg of hydromorphone for hip pain 10/10, and 1 hour later her pain was still at 8/10. The current order is hydromorphone 2 mg IV every 6 hours PRN for pain.

Background: Mrs. Jones is a 70-year-old, White female status post-ORIF of the right hip 3 days ago, status post-fall at home. She developed a PE on post-op day 2. She is on a heparin infusion and has NKDA.

Assessment: Her VS are _____ (stable) and wound is _____. Mrs. Jones rates her pain at a 10/10 with a sharp quality. She is refusing to go to physical therapy. Pedal pulses are palpable (students provide VS and wound assessment data—gives students opportunity to critically think about VS and learning to describe a wound— (normal vs. abnormal).

Recommendation: Could the hydromorphone dose and/or timeframes be changed? Every 4 hours?

EXHIBIT 6-3 Example of a 60-Second Situational Safety Assessment

Purpose: This exercise is designed to assist you in the development of *situational awareness*. In the patient care area, situational awareness focuses on the *art of patient observation*. This includes routine use of a general survey (observation) of the patient, family, and environment during every incidental encounter and periodically at planned intervals throughout the day. *Situational awareness* promotes a safer patient care environment and helps the nurse develop care priorities and attention to clinical detail.

Directions: Enter the patient's room and observe the patient, family, and environment for up to 60 seconds while reviewing the following questions in your mind.

- ABC without touching the patient:
  - What data lead you to believe there is a problem with airway-breathing-circulation?
  - Is the problem urgent/nonurgent?
  - What clinical data would indicate that the situation needs immediate action and why?
  - Who needs to be contacted and do you have any suggestions/recommendations?

- Tubes and lines:
  - Does the patient have any tubes or an IV line?
  - Is the IV solution the correct one at the correct rate?
  - Does the patient need these tubes; if so, why?
  - Do you note any complications?
  - What further assessment needs to be done?

- Respiratory equipment:
  - If the patient is utilizing oxygen, what would you need to continue to monitor?
  - How would you know it is functioning properly?

- Patient safety survey:
  - What are your safety concerns with this patient?
  - Do you need to report this problem and to whom?

- Environmental survey:
  - What about the environment could lead to a problem for the patient?
  - How would you manage the problem?

(continues)

EXHIBIT 6-3   Example of a 60-Second Situational Safety Assessment (continued)

- Sensory:
  - What are your senses telling you?
  - Do you hear, smell, see, or feel something that needs to be explored?
  - Does the patient's situation seem "right"?

What additional information would be helpful for further clarification of the situation?
What questions are unanswered and what answers are unquestioned?

Post Conference

After review of each student's patient, which patient would you focus on first? Why?

Reproduced from Struth, D., Grbach, W., Vincent, L., Heil, J., & Simpson, C. (2009, June 25). The 60 Second Situational Assessment. Retrieved November 11, 2011, from www.qsen.org/the-60-second-situational-assessment/

60-Second Assignment

A 60-second assignment may be utilized in the clinical area when there is "down time" for the nursing student. Having a quick clinical reasoning activity provides the student an educational opportunity at all times. Some assignments may last longer than 60 seconds. See **EXHIBIT 6-4** for examples of the 60-second assignment.

Quality Improvement Assignments

Quality improvement (QI) is an essential area of knowledge and understanding that students need to learn to move toward exploring system safety. In this type of assignment, students identify a variety of unit- or agency-specific QI initiatives and link knowledge to practice (Seibert, 2014). The assignment is a group project that highlights teamwork and collaboration, evidence-based literature regarding the QI focus, and patient-centered care initiatives. System and patient safety is the primary emphasis for successful improvement in care. **BOX 6-2** lists examples of QI projects that may be used in the clinical setting.

Concept Mapping

Concept mapping enables the student to make connections in a method that creates knowledge in a way that makes sense to the student. This learning activity promotes critical thinking, creative thinking, and a holistic understanding of patient needs in nursing (Suplee et al., 2014). Utilizing the concept map provides a visual tool to document a student's thought process.

In a conceptual clinical experience, concept maps focus on the connection between the concept and the patients in the unit or agency, not necessarily a specific

EXHIBIT 6-4 Examples of 60-Second Assignments

60-Second Assignment	60-Second Assignment
Find the patient teaching information on this floor regarding _____. (Oxygenation, Safety, Diabetes)	Ask the student to tell you the most important thing he or she will do for the patient and defend this as a priority or tell why it is the most important.

60-Second Assignment	60-Second Assignment
What is your role (student) in a code? Each staff member's and other departments' role in a code?	Safety activity—What would your priority intervention be if you walked into your patient's room and found him or her lying on the floor?

60-Second Assignment	60-Second Assignment
What assessment data are relevant to your patient's cognitive function?	What discharge needs does your patient have and how will you meet those needs?

60-Second Assignment	60-Second Assignment
Identify five health issues in the population you are working with: Look up prevalence rate (on one). Identify how health issues might affect daily life.	Check the internet and find out the rate of (name the disease process) in both various ethnic/racial groups to determine any health disparity.

60-Second Assignment	60-Second Assignment
From the unit report sheet, have one student check all IV solution rates, expiration date for tubing, solutions, and sites for a designated group of patients.	Narrative assessment—Ask the student to write out a head-to-toe assessment on a progress note.

medical focus or diagnosis. The desired outcome is to complete the concept map and conceptual focus prior to the clinical experience and then make changes based on the patient experience. This activity allows the student and the CNE to evaluate the student's understanding of the concept, the exemplar, patient care needs, and interventions for nursing care. Chapter 8 provides more detail regarding concept mapping as a tool for clinical and classroom learning.

BOX 6-2 Examples of Quality Improvement Projects

- Pain reassessment compliance
- Urinary tract infection occurrence
- 2 hour repositioning
- Dressing changes completed on time
- Hand washing from patient room to patient room (include all of interdisciplinary team)
- Isolation carts present for all isolation rooms
- Height/weight present on charts or in computerized charting
- Pressure injury monitoring
- Restraint monitoring
- Fall risk documentation
- Hourly rounding documented
- White board use for communication
- Hand off reporting

Remember This . . .

Concept mapping enables the student to make connections in a method that creates knowledge in a way that makes sense to the student.

Socratic Questioning

Asking questions and having discussions regarding application of concepts to foster the transfer of learning is an expected outcome of every clinical experience. A clinical environment that not only fosters discussions and debates, but also allows the student to make mistakes is an ideal clinical environment. As learners, students are expected to make errors. Confronting those errors with an open discussion framework not only allows for learning to occur, but also helps the CNEs and student evaluate the error and identify changes needed for the future.

Questioning for deep learning involves not just asking for factual recall, but encouraging students to consider the causes of events or situations (Nielson, 2016). An engaged CNE guides the Socratic questioning technique and centers questioning around concepts rather than medical conditions or technical skills. Asking "why?" is a guiding principle in this type of questioning.

High-level questions in a learning environment promote students' thinking at deeper levels. Nursing educators and staff nurses need to ask open-ended higher-level questions to stimulate thinking and help students make connections between their theoretical knowledge and their clinical thinking and clinical reasoning.

Socratic questions can be asked before or after a student shares his or her assessment findings in an effort to redirect the student's interpretation of those assessments if needed. Questioning also enables the student to provide reflection on whether the interventions in the clinical setting were appropriate. Socratic questioning incites the examination of complex issues, assists with characterizing situations, and leads the way for students to describe the meaning of concepts when utilized the clinical setting (Burrell, 2014). Examples of specific questions that relate to patient care experience include:

- Tell about your weekly assigned concept and give an example of a nursing intervention you will perform today focusing on the concept.
- What laboratory or diagnostic data have you utilized to focus on the weekly concept?
- Describe other interventions that might be possible with your patient and why each intervention would be appropriate and evidence-based.
- Describe the concept of _____ and give examples of exemplars for this concept.
- How would the concept of _____ have an impact on the community?

Peer-to-Peer Interaction

Peer collaboration provides opportunities for students to learn teamwork skills needed in their future professional work, builds their confidence level, and decreases their anxiety. Peer learning is associated with increased problem solving, communication, and clinical reasoning skills.

The CBC clinical environment encourages opportunities for both independent and collaborative experiences. Any level of clinical experience can benefit from peer-to-peer learning. Community, mental health, or adult health areas can utilize increasing complexities of peer learning. Examples of peer-to-peer assignments include:

- Communication: interviewing of community individuals
- Community immersion at homeless shelter
- Assessment clinics in community settings
- Medication clinics in community settings
- Patient assignments in acute and long-term care

Reflections

A pivotal goal in the CBC clinical experience is the opportunity for students to reflect on the events that occur in the clinical environment. Reflections written after their clinical experiences are a strategy to help students process and learn from their experiences (Lasater, 2011). Although not a graded assignment, instructor feedback is given to propel students to higher-order thinking within the reflection. Reflection assignments may be required for each clinical learning experience.

Guided reflections are often the best tool to elicit the level of learning students need to develop their thinking. Students vary widely in their ability to be reflective and need guidance to learn what is important to notice to develop their thinking like a nurse. For guided reflections, always provide a focus for student thinking. For instance, one of the QSEN competencies may be a focus for a given week. The CNE may ask students to provide two examples of how they demonstrated the Professional Nursing concept of Patient-Centeredness during their clinical experience.

▶ Organizing Conceptual Clinical Learning Activities and Assignments

As described earlier in this chapter, weekly teaching and learning plans provide structure to promote knowledge application, deeper understanding of concepts and exemplars, and development of clinical reasoning and nursing judgment. Each course in a CBC requires an organized overall plan, sometimes called *scaffolding,* for how each clinical experience will be organized. **EXHIBIT 6-5** provides an example of clinical activities and experiences for a course in a prelicensure BSN program.

EXHIBIT 6-5 Scaffolding Example for Clinical Experiences in NUR 321

Experience Number	Course Week	Concepts	QSEN
1	2/3	Functional ability, pain, Family dynamics, culture, patient education	Patient-Centered Care
2	4/5	Gas exchange, Perfusion	Safety
3	6/7	Mobility, Fluids and electrolytes	Teamwork and Collaboration
4	8/9	Acid/base, Immunity, Inflammation, Infection	Evidence-Based Practice
5	10/11	Glucose regulation, Intracranial regulation	Informatics
6	12/13	Nutrition, Elimination, Tissue integrity	Quality Improvement

Weekly Progression
Vital Signs, Glucose, Intake and Output: Documented by Students

Week	Structure	Clinical Activities
1 Functional ability, pain, family dynamics, culture, patient education	Shadow RN ½ day	Role of Nurse Review patient charting, access patient medical record (all students to access individually patient chart (verify access ability) SBAR 60-second situational assessment Review preclinical paperwork of nonpharmaceutical pain techniques and policy Review assigned medication cards for medications that have an impact on pain: *Nonopioid analgesic*—Acetaminophen; *nonsteroidal antiinflammatory agents*—ibuprofen, naproxen (Naprosyn); *opioid analgesics*—morphine sulfate, fentanyl, hydromorphone (Dilaudid), oxymorphone (Opana); *opioid agonists*—codeine, acetaminophen and hydrocodone (Vicodin), acetaminophen and oxycodone (Percocet), *nonopioid centrally acting analgesic*—tramadol (Ultram) Head-to-toe assessment Functional assessment screen Pain assessment (simulated EHR) Patient education Discharge planning (document either patient education or discharge planning in simulated EHR) **Specifics of documentation to submit for grading Worksheet on roles and responsibilities **Admission chart: Collect data on one patient as if "new admission" and complete patient admission data in simulated EHR, including documentation of head-to-toe assessment

(continues)

EXHIBIT 6-5 Scaffolding Example for Clinical Experiences in NUR 321 (continued)

Week	Structure	Clinical Activities
2 Gas exchange, Perfusion	No nurse-assigned student buddies	VS on all patients SBAR 60-second situational assessment Bed bath: Skin assessment Review preclinical paperwork for diagnoses of chronic obstructive pulmonary disease, heart failure, hypertension, hyperlipidemia, including significant laboratory and diagnostic testing. Review assigned medications that affect gas exchange and perfusion: **Gas exchange:** *Bronchodilators, beta-2-adrenergic agonists*—short acting: albuterol, long acting: salmeterol (Serevent); *anticholinergics*—tiotropium (Spiriva); alpha-1 proteinase inhibitor (Zemaira); dornase alpha (Pulmozyme); *inhaled glucocorticoid*—fluticasone (Flovent) **Perfusion:** *Beta blockers*—carvedilol (Coreg), metoprolol (Lopressor); *angiotensin-enzyme inhibitor*—lisinopril; *angiotensin receptor blocker*—valsartan (Diovan); *cardiac glycoside*—digoxin; *calcium channel blockers*—verapamil (Calan), diltiazem (Cardizem); *potassium channel blockers*—amiodarone, sotalol; *cholesterol-lowering medication*—statins: atorvastatin (Lipitor); ezetimibe (Zetia); *combination drug*—amlodipine and atorvastatin (Caduet); aspirin; ferrous sulfate Review patient documentation in chart: Laboratory results and procedures affected by gas exchange and perfusion Document pulse oximetry and VS in patient chart **Specifics to document for respiratory and cardiovascular (including peripheral vascular) assessment in simulated EHR Mock medication administration for one medicine (listed previously) Diagnostic procedures as able Patient education and discharge planning (simulated EHR)
3 Mobility, Fluids and Electrolytes	Nurse-assigned student buddies	SBAR 60-second situational assessment VS on assigned patients Daily care for assigned patients (bed baths, assist ADLs, etc.) Review preclinical paperwork for diagnoses of osteoarthritis, hip fracture, amputation (BKA), dehydration, including significant laboratory study results and diagnostic testing Review assigned medications cards on medications that affect mobility and fluids and electrolytes

Mobility:

Review pain medications; *fluids and electrolytes*—potassium chloride, magnesium sulfate; *loop diuretics*—furosemide (Lasix), bumetanide (Bumex); *potassium sparing*—spironolactone (Aldactone)

Review patient documentation in chart: Laboratory results and procedures affected by mobility and fluids and electrolytes

I&O: Review how to collect and document in simulated EHR

***Specifics to document for IV site assessment in simulated EHR.

Mock medication administration for one medication (listed previously)

Document physical assessment of IV site assessment, muscle strength, and integument assessment in simulated EHR

Patient education and discharge planning (document one in simulated EHR)

Students practice reporting off to each other on one of assigned patients in presence of the clinical instructor—turn in SBAR form to instructor as clinical paperwork

---

Review of midterm progress

SBAR

60-second situational assessment

Review preclinical paperwork of assigned diagnoses of hypokalemia, hypernatremia, acute renal failure, Crohn's disease, ulcerative colitis, pneumonia

VS on assigned patients, including significant laboratory results, diagnostic testing

Review assigned medication cards on medications that affect acid/base, immunity, inflammation, and infection

Acid/base, immunity, inflammation and infection:

Acid/base balance—sodium bicarbonate; *infection*—fluoroquinolone, levofloxacin (Levaquin), vancomycin; *penicillin derivative*—piperacillin and tazobactam (Zosyn); *third-generation cephalosporin*—cefepime; *beta-lactam antibiotic*—imipenem–cilastatin (Primaxin), rifaximin

Inflammation:

Glucocorticoids—dexamethasone, intravenous immunoglobulin G (IVIG)

4
Acid/base,
Immunity,
Inflammation,
Infection

Nurse-
assigned
student
buddies

(continues)

EXHIBIT 6-5 Scaffolding Example for Clinical Experiences in NUR 321 (continued)

Week	Structure	Clinical Activities
		Immunity: *5-Aminosalicylates*—mesalamine (Asacol), adalimumab (Humira) Documentation Daily care for assigned patients (bed baths, assist ADLs, etc.) Medication administration for one patient (oral medication) Report off to nurse using SBAR format
5 Glucose regulation, Intracranial regulation	Student individually assigned to RN patients	SBAR 60-second situational assessment VS on assigned patients Review preclinical paperwork of assigned diagnoses of diabetes mellitus, Parkinson's disease, multiple sclerosis, and cerebrovascular accident, including laboratory results and diagnostic testing Review assigned medication cards on medications that affect glucose and intracranial regulation **Glucose regulation:** *Insulins*—insulin aspart (NovoLog), insulin glargine (Lantus), insulin detemir (levemir); *second-generation sulfonylurea*—glipizide (Glucotrol); *biguanide*—metformin (Glucophage); *gliptin*—sitagliptin (Januvia) **Intracranial regulation:** *Osmotic diuretic*—mannitol, phenobarbital, lorazepam (Ativan); *antiplatelet*—clopidogrel (Plavix), alteplase (Activase), *Parkinson's disease*—carbidopa-levodopa (Sinemet); *multiple sclerosis*—interferon-beta (Avonex), prednisone, methylprednisolone Daily care for assigned patients (bed baths, assist ADLs, etc.) Glucose monitoring for assigned patients Be prepared to pass all patient medications (time management/organization) and pass medications agreed upon with clinical instructor *** specifics Perform complete patient assessment (document head-to-toe assessment in simulated EHR) Shadow off-unit diagnostic testing if appropriate Discharge planning Patient education Report off to nurse using SBAR format

6 Nutrition, Elimination, Tissue Integrity, Clotting	Students individually assigned to RN patients	SBAR

SBAR
60-second situational assessment
VS on assigned patients
Review preclinical paperwork of assigned diagnoses of urinary tract infection, pyelonephritis, pressure ulcers, deep vein thrombosis, including laboratory results and diagnostic testing
Review assigned medication cards on medications that affect nutrition, elimination, tissue integrity, and clotting

Nutrition:
Multivitamin infusion, ondansetron (Zofran), pantoprazole (Protonix)

Elimination:
Sulfonamide—sulfamethoxazole-trimethoprim (Bactrim); *5-alpha-reductase inhibitor*—finasteride (Proscar); *selective alpha, blocker*—tamsulosin (Flomax)

Tissue integrity:
Review dressing solutions and care: *Clotting*—enoxaparin (Lovenox), heparin, warfarin (Coumadin); *direct thrombin inhibitors*—apixaban (Eliquis); *direct factor Xa inhibitor*—rivaroxaban (Xarelto)
Daily care for assigned patients (bed baths, assist ADLs, etc.)
**Specify documentation to be added to simulated EHR.
Perform focused assessments on all assigned patients: Nutrition, elimination, perfusion, tissue integrity (document one assessment of each in simulated EHR)
Braden Scale assessment: Document one patient in simulated EHR
Be prepared to pass patient medications (time management/organization) and pass medications agreed upon with clinical nurse educator
Report off to nurse using SBAR format
Patient education
Discharge planning
RN work-around assignment (post conference)

Courtesy of Kristin Oneall, MS, RN

As shown in Exhibit 6-5, planned clinical activities and assignments shift the clinical emphasis to concepts of professional nursing and patient care to increase the transfer of knowledge to new situations. Maximizing student engagement is critical to achieving clinical learning outcomes that are central to the clinical curriculum in the CBC.

▶ Chapter Key Points

- The traditional setting has a focus on skills, requires students to perform total patient care, and is teacher centered; the concept-based curriculum setting is student-centered, has a teamwork and collaborative focus, and utilizes interactive teaching/learning strategies.

- For direct care activities, also called direct patient care, students are assigned to learning activities while providing patient care to achieve one or more competencies related to applying concepts. These competencies are evaluated as either "Met" or "Unmet."

- Focused learning activities promote learning completed in the laboratory or external clinical setting that supports achievement of one or more clinical competencies related to applying concepts for deep understanding.

- The elements of preparation for the clinical environment include open communication between the academic institution and clinical sites; education of all healthcare personnel who will have interaction with the student learner, and identification of an appropriate liaison between the academic institution and practice environment.

- The role of the academic-practice liaison includes assisting in educating all healthcare personnel who will be involved in the clinical units or agencies and the students, coordinates between education and practice, provides continuing education opportunities for all nursing staff, questions students in a Socratic method, assesses the effectiveness of the learning experience, and evaluates the educational process.

- The clinical nurse educator communicates consistently with students and staff nurses, provides active teaching strategies for the student, and debriefs each clinical experience to allow the student to learn the most each clinical day.

- The weekly teaching/learning plan provides a detailed explanation of student assignments and expectations to promote continuity and consistency for each clinical site or agency experience.

- Examples of student learning activities utilized in the conceptual clinical experience include safety-focused assignments, reflections, concept maps, interprofessional assignments, 60-second assessments or situations, and quality improvement assignments.

- Peer-to-peer interactions are essential as part of a concept-based curriculum clinical experience to promote the development of teamwork skills, build student confidence, and decrease student anxiety.

- Each clinical course in a concept-based curriculum needs an overall plan to demonstrate scaffolding of clinical experiences as they relate to concepts and exemplars being learned in class or online.

▶ Chapter References and Selected Bibliography

Bartges, M. (2012). Pairing students in clinical assignments to develop collaboration and communication skills. *Nurse Educator, 37*(1), 17–22.

Burrell, L. (2014). Integrating critical thinking strategies into nursing curricula. *Teaching and Learning in Nursing, 9*(2), 53–58.

D'Souza, M. S., Venkatesaperumal, R., Radhakrishnan, J., & Balachandran, S. (2013). Engagement in clinical learning environment among nursing students: Role of nurse educators. *Online Journal of Nursing, 3*, 25–32.

Duncan, K., & Schulz, P. (2015). Impact of change to a concept-based baccalaureate nursing curriculum on student and program outcomes. *Journal of Nursing Education, 54*(3), S16–S20.

Getha-Eby, T., Beery, T., O'Brien, B., & Xu, Y. (2015). Student learning outcomes in response to concept-based teaching. *Journal of Nursing Education, 54*(4), 193–200.

Giddens, J. F. (2016). Underestimated challenges adopting the conceptual approach. *Journal of Nursing Education, 55*(4), 187–188.

Giddens, J. F. (2017). *Concepts for nursing practice* (2nd ed.). St. Louis, MO: Mosby.

*Giddens, J. F., & Brady, D. P. (2007). Rescuing nursing education from content saturation: The case for a concept-based curriculum. *Journal of Nursing Education, 46*(2), 65–69.

Giddens, J. F., Wright, M., & Gray, I. (2012). Selecting concepts for a concept-based curriculum: Application of a benchmark approach. *Journal of Nursing Education, 51*(9), 511–515.

Hardin, P. K., & Richardson, S. J. (2012). Teaching the concept curricula: Theory and method. *Journal of Nursing Education, 51*(3), 155–159.

Hatlevik, I. K. R. (2012). The theory-practice relationship: Reflective skills and theoretical knowledge as key factors in bridging the gap between theory and practice in initial nursing education. *Journal of Advanced Nursing, 68*(4), 868–877.

Haugan, G., Sørensen, A. H., & Hanssen, I. (2012). The importance of dialogue in student nurses' clinical education. *Nurse Education Today, 32*(4), 438–442.

Henderson, A., Cooke, M., Creedy, D. K., & Walker, R. (2012). Nursing students' perceptions of learning in practice environments: A review. *Nurse Education Today, 32*(3), 299–302.

Hendricks, S. M., & Wangerin, V. (2017). Concept-based curriculum: Changing attitudes and overcoming barriers. *Nurse Educator, 42*(3), 138–146.

Higgins, B., & Reid, H. (2017). Enhancing "conceptual teaching/learning" in a concept-based curriculum. *Teaching and Learning in Nursing, 12*(2), 95–102.

Hudson, C. E., Sanders, M. K., & Pepper, C. (2013). Interprofessional education and prelicensure baccalaureate nursing students. *Nurse Educator, 38*(2), 76–80.

Ironside, P. M., & McNelis, A. M. (2010). Clinical education in prelicensure nursing programs: Findings from a national survey. *Nursing Education Perspectives, 31*(4), 264–265.

Khan, B. A., Ali, F., Vazir, N., Barolia, R., & Rehan, S. (2012). Students' perceptions of clinical teaching and learning strategies: A Pakistani perspective. *Nurse Education Today, 32*(1), 85–90.

Killam, L. A., & Heerschap, C. (2013). Challenges to student learning in the clinical setting: A qualitative descriptive study. *Nurse Education Today, 33*, 684–691.

Lasater, K. (2011). Clinical judgment: The last frontier for evaluation. *Nurse Education in Practice, 11*(2), 86–92.

Lasater, K., & Nielsen, A. (2009). The influence of concept-based learning activities on students' clinical judgment development. *Journal of Nursing Education, 48*(8), 441–446.

Marchigiano, G., Eduljee, N., & Harvey, K. (2011). Developing critical thinking skills from clinical assignments: A pilot study on nursing students' self-reported perceptions. *Journal of Nursing Management, 19*(1), 143–152.

Mood, L. C., Neunzert, C., & Tadesse, R. (2014). Centering the concept of transitional care: A teaching-learning innovation. *Journal of Nursing Education, 53*(5), 287–290.

Newton, J. M., Jolly, B. C., Ockerby, C. M., & Cross, W. M. (2012). Student centeredness in clinical learning: The influence of the clinical teacher. *Journal of Advanced Nursing, 68*(10), 2331–2340.

Nielsen, A. (2009). Concept-based learning activities using the clinical judgment model as a foundation for clinical learning. *Journal of Nursing Education, 48*(6), 350–354.

Nielson, A. (2016). Concept-based learning in clinical experiences: Bringing theory to clinical education for deep learning. *Journal of Nursing Education, 55*(7), 365–371.

Nielson, A. E., Noone, J., Voss, H., & Mathews, L. R. (2013). Preparing nursing students for the future: An innovative approach to clinical education. *Nurse Education in Practice, 13*(4), 301–309.

Papathanasiou, I. V., Tsaras, K., & Sarafis, P. (2014). Views and perceptions of nursing students on their clinical learning environment: Teaching and learning. *Nurse Education Today, 34*(1) 57–60.

Roberts, K. K., Chrisman, S. K., & Flowers, C. (2013). The perceived needs of nurse clinicians as they move into an adjunct clinical faculty role. *Journal of Professional Nursing, 29*(5), 295–301.

Seibert, S. A. (2014). Safety consciousness: Assignments that expand focus beyond the bedside. *Nurse Education Today, 34*(2), 233–236.

*Senita, J. (2008). The use of concept maps to evaluate critical thinking in the clinical setting. *Teaching and Learning in Nursing, 3*(1), 6–10.

Suplee, P. D., Gardner, M., & Jerome-D'Emilia, B. (2014). Nursing faculty preparedness for clinical teaching. *Journal of Nursing Education, 53*(3 Suppl.), S38–S41.

Tanner, C. A. (2010). From mother duck to mother lode: Clinical education for deep learning. *Journal of Nursing Education, 49*(1), 3–4.

*Tanner, C. A. (2006). Thinking like a nurse: A research-based model of clinical judgment in nursing. *Journal of Nursing Education, 45*(6), 204–211.

---

*Indicates classic reference.

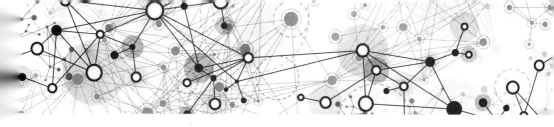

CHAPTER 7

Teaching in the Concept-Based Online Learning Environment

Nicole Heimgartner & Cherie Rebar

▶ Introduction to Online Learning

The American Association of Colleges of Nursing (2014) estimates the number of job openings within the nursing workforce will reach 1.2 million by the year 2020. This projected need, combined with the Institute of Medicine's (IOM's) (2011) call for 80% of nurses to have a BSN degree by 2020, created an explosion in the use of online programs. Additionally, the IOM recognized a need for more nurses to be prepared at the masters and doctoral levels.

Online learning platforms can supplement the face-to-face classroom, exist as a portion of a blended or hybrid class (e.g., 50% face to face, 50% online), or be a stand-alone method of instruction. Numerous nursing education programs at the BSN completion and graduate level are offered fully online. Regardless of the platform, it is important for faculty to gain knowledge to consistently apply evidence-based online learning principles to create effective learning experiences for learners.

An educator's first experience with online learning may occur when he or she is asked to "move" a traditional course that was taught in the face-to-face environment to an online platform. Although it might seem like a natural transition to take a well-developed face-to-face course and simply place it into a learning management system (LMS) online, traditional teaching strategies are not always effective online. The needs of online students require thoughtful and specific online course approaches and development. Both the *quality* of education and the *access* to resources (such as resources available through the Americans with Disabilities Act) provided in any face-to-face environment must be carried over into the online environment. Educators should refer to their institutional policies regarding access and ADA requirements to ensure these processes are followed when designing and delivering online materials.

Online learning by nature is conceptual and rooted in the tenets of constructivism as discussed in Chapter 2. Much of the design emphasis in online learning is to build on what learners already know. In order to build on this foundation, educators must be careful to assess what is known and work with existing understanding to construct more complete knowledge development by effectively planning learning experiences (Boettcher & Conrad, 2016). Once the core concepts are identified within a course, the online structure will help direct the learner toward the core conceptual knowledge. The majority of the online course should push the learner toward application of these concepts. This process leads the learner to deep and meaningful learning as discussed in Chapter 2.

▶ Types of Online Learning

Online learning can be categorized into two primary types: asynchronous and synchronous learning. **Asynchronous online learning** means that learning and/or instruction can occur at any time. Using this approach, students can log in to a course, access the instructional materials, and complete assignments at any time conducive to their schedule. Learning content is divided into "chunks" called *units* or *modules* (which often align with weeks of the class), and assignments have established due dates. However, students may choose to work ahead of these deadlines. When online learning began, asynchronous learning was very popular. However, with the development of advanced technology, including virtual live classrooms and spontaneous collaboration tools, the use of synchronous learning has increased.

Synchronous online learning is learning and/or instruction that occurs at a specific time within the online setting. For example, an educator may schedule set times that class discussions occur and all students are required to log in to the course at that time to participate.

▶ Methods Used in Designing Online Learning

Multiple methods are used to design online learning courses. Traditionally, when at least 80% of a course is delivered online, it is referred to as an **online course**. When 40 to 79% of a course is delivered online, it is referred to as a **blended** or **hybrid** course design. When 15 to 39% of a course is delivered online, it may be considered *lightly* blended or hybrid. Traditional face-to-face courses typically contain less than 14% of the content online (Boettcher & Conrad, 2016).

Most higher educational institutions create their own definitions of what percentages constitute blended versus fully online courses. For example, some colleges and universities state that an online course must be delivered 100% online. In other institutions, a blended course is between 15 and 25% online, with the remainder as face-to-face. Be mindful of an institution's method requirements when determining which course materials will be included within the online environment.

Collaborative learning can be used in any learning environment to promote teamwork and prepare the learner for nursing practice. Online courses are excellent tools to promote interprofessional education (IPE) because students from multiple disciplines can work together within the same course, enriching the opportunities for collaboration. The key to successful collaborative learning is communication, which can bring unique challenges in the online environment.

> **Remember This . . .**
>
> *Be mindful of an institution's method requirements when determining which course materials will be included within the online environment.*

▶ Netiquette and Communication

The term "netiquette," with its core set of associated rules, was originally developed by Virginia Shea and first published in 1994 (Shea, 1994). Although these rules seem dated, they continue to function as a foundation on which to build online behavior expectations. Most online programs have adapted rules of expected online behavior to promote the basic elements of effective online communication. **TABLE 7-1** illustrates how these classic principles apply in today's online learning environment.

TABLE 7-1 Netiquette Principles and Application

Principles	Application Connections in 2016
Remember the human	There is a person on the other side of the screen. It is often difficult to infer tone or meaning, which enhances the importance of effective communication. Although some educators consider the use of emoticons unprofessional, students often use an emoticon to show intention and this can be helpful when providing feedback.
Adhere to the same standards of behavior online that are expected in real life	Ethical behavior is the expectation. Discuss plagiarism. Emphasize the ethical standards and expectations for testing online and use security measures to protect testing integrity when necessary. Many online testing centers are now available to provide proctored testing for online courses.

(continues)

TABLE 7-1 Netiquette Principles and Application (continued)

Principles	Application Connections in 2016
Know where you are in cyberspace	Communication in a discussion forum is different than communication via text messaging with friends. While it seems self-explanatory, this often bears clarification with today's student. C U L8TR may be acceptable to text. It is not acceptable in a course discussion.
Respect other people's time	While the current culture is one of immediacy and email can be sent and received in real time, it is not realistic for students to expect an immediate response to every question. Establishing clear parameters for educator feedback and helping students really understand what to expect will help them respect the educator as well as peers in the collaborative online working environment.
Make yourself look good online	Although students cannot judge by appearance in the online forum, they can judge by writing and presentation. Communication that is unclear or full of misspellings can cause a student to doubt an educator's ability or the competence of a peer. Spell-check within a discussion forum is just as important as it is in written assignments.
Share expert knowledge	Allow opportunities and provide encouragement for students to share their own knowledge. This connects directly to conceptual learning, allowing a natural bridge to be built between new content and acquired skill.
Keep flame wars under control	"Flaming" is a term used to describe communicating an opinion in a manner that is inflammatory. Many times, discussions will center on topics that may be controversial. Opinions can and should enter into the discussion. However, an opinion must always be supported by research and voiced in a manner that is respectful.
Do not abuse your power	While the educator may be very comfortable in the online classroom, the student may not be. Establishing online expectations is important, as are having strategies for easing anxiety in the online learning environment (see section "Delineating the Role of Nurse Educators in Online Course Development").
Be forgiving	This principle seems to apply throughout the test of time.

Data from Shea, V. (1994). *Netiquette*. Albion Books: San Francisco, CA.

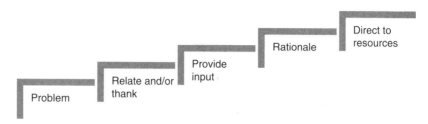

FIGURE 7-1 The feedback pathway

One of the biggest issues that new online educators experience is an inundation of email from students. This behavior often stems from lack of guidance in the classroom as well as ineffective communication within the online environment. Be sure to create a safe place (forum) within the course for students to post questions. This step allows all students to benefit from the answers to the questions, encourages students to help each other, and decreases the number of individual responses needed. This process is also an excellent way to establish boundaries. Assure students that the forum will be checked daily, Monday through Friday, so they understand when their questions will be answered. Then, be sure the forum is assessed daily because follow-through is a critical element in establishing teaching presence online.

When responding to a student individually, it is important to respond completely. Although it takes a bit longer initially, a complete response will allay anxiety and prevent further individual emails. The goal is to redirect the learner back into the online environment for problem solving and direction. This process is learning-centered because it presents communication in a manner that allows the student to learn through doing.

The feedback path outlined in **FIGURE 7-1** can be very helpful for new nurse educators during online communication with students. When a student contacts the educator, first address the problem. Emailing an instructor, especially one that a student has never seen or met, can be very intimidating. Therefore, relate to the student and thank the student for "reaching out." Provide input with a rationale, and conclude with directing the learner to resources to assist him or her within the course.

One helpful technique is to develop a list of email response stems that can be tailored for each student. This plan prevents writing the same responses for multiple students. Many times, student questions are very similar. Be sure, that when using a stem, to apply personalized response information to the student. Remember to always use the student's name in the communication to increase personalization. *Timely student feedback is essential!* **TABLE 7-2** provides an example of the feedback pathway process applied when communicating with a student online.

▶ Online Presence

Establishing nurse educator presence in the online learning environment is an essential component to teaching success. In a traditional classroom, educator presence is established when an instructor walks into the room. Students assess the educator in terms of professionalism, organization and presentation, and competence, based on what they see. In the online environment, students assess educators through their comments, the structure of the course, the verbiage in the syllabus, the quality and timeliness of their feedback, and overall online presence (**FIGURE 7-2**). **Online presence**

TABLE 7-2 Application of the Feedback Pathway Process in a Communication Example

Problem (Student)	Feedback Path	Example (Educator)
"When is the discussion post due in this course?"	Address problem	"I received your email."
	Relate or thank	"Thank you for your question."
	Provide input	"The initial post to the discussion forum is due on Wednesday by midnight."
	Rationale	"Every discussion will be set up in the same way, and posting due on Wednesday allows plenty of time for group discussion."
	Direct to resources	"Discussion forum guidelines are located in Module One to provide details of the assignment."

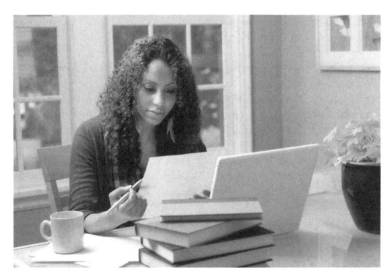

FIGURE 7-2 Student looking at the home page of a course in a learning management system
© YinYang/E+/Getty

begins when the nurse educator establishes the first contact with students. During this contact, the students assess the organization, competence, professionalism, and presentation of the educator. This initial contact often sets the tone for how students perceive that the course will be conducted throughout the term.

In preparation for establishing online presence, the educator must be aware that four generations of learners will be present in the online environment: Baby Boomer, Generation X, Millennial, and Generation Z students. Each generation is unique; however, establishing connections and creating an engaging learning community is a need for all generations. It is also important for the educator to recognize and appreciate the knowledge and experiences that each student brings to the learning environment. When educators use constructivist theory to establish online presence, they are taking the first steps in fostering a healthy learning community that produces student engagement, the overall goal of online learning. Engagement fosters critical thinking and judgment, which in turn increases the application of knowledge in nursing practice (Hampton & Pearce, 2016).

> **Remember This . . .**
>
> *Online presence begins when the nurse educator establishes the first contact with students. During this contact, the students assess the organization, competence, professionalism, and presentation of the educator. This initial contact often sets the tone for how students perceive that the course will be conducted throughout the term.*

Three types of educator presence have been discussed in the literature: social presence, cognitive presence, and teaching presence. These types are briefly described in the following section as they apply to online learning today.

Social Presence

Social Presence Theory, as classically designed by Short, Williams, and Christie (1976), can help with understanding how learners interact. **Social presence** asserts that a consequent relationship is yielded by the degree of connectivity between people (Gunawardena, 1995, in Rebar, 2010). The ability to feel connected can influence how educators interact with students (and vice versa) and how students engage with material and each other during the learning process, particularly when they cannot physically see the other learners (Gunawardena & Zittle, 1997, in Rebar, 2010). Consequently, in an online environment, the intention, body language, and inflection of both students and educators cannot always be accurately interpreted (Rebar, 2010). Tu and McIsaac (2002) validated that demonstrating social presence increases interlearner and learner-facilitator (educator) interactions, which in turn enriches the educational process (in Rebar, 2010).

Examples of ways to demonstrate social presence in the online environment include the following:

■   Effective use of ice-breaker forums, in which the facilitator creates a discussion forum at the onset of the online course where students and faculty post informal information to get to know each other. For example, the facilitator may ask the students to post where they are from and one unique characteristic about themselves. The faculty member also would post where he or she is from and a unique self-characteristic.

■   Designation of virtual office hours, in which the facilitator uses the LMS to host office hours in which the students may virtually "drop by" to interact with the faculty member. This involves the use of a webcam for both parties, as well as auditory software.

Cognitive Presence

Cognitive presence was originally defined as "the extent to which learners are able to construct and confirm meaning through sustained reflection and discourse" (Garrison, Anderson, & Archer, 2001). Since its inception, this definition has been expanded to include the process of building knowledge throughout an online course. In order to understand cognitive presence, nurse educators must consider the impact of reflection and communication. An open awareness to the potential impact of an online response is critical. Student responses should be questioned to promote growth and discussion, yet balanced with positive feedback to promote positive discourse. As educators begin to assess the students' depth of knowledge and interact through discussion, they begin to shape their cognitive presence within the course.

Teaching Presence

Teaching presence is defined by the elements of instruction that make up the course. Although they are separate from the nurse educator, the manner in which they are discussed or presented affects teaching presence. A classic example of teaching presence is the course syllabus, which should set the expectations for each course. A syllabus for an online course should *not* be exactly the same as the syllabus for a face-to-face course. The course outcomes may be the same, but the expectations may be different based on the course environment. A syllabus that is poorly organized or that presents dated information can affect the educator's ability to establish teaching presence in the online classroom. Additionally, a syllabus that does not present the importance of a collaborative learning community in the online environment will make achievement of that sense of community very difficult.

The culture of immediacy is embedded in today's student. When educators are not clear regarding expectations, students can make assumptions based on their perceptions. For example, clarifying that faculty will be involved in every discussion but may not respond to every online post gives the student a clear idea of what to expect. This communication prevents the student from drawing inference from a response or a lack of response. Remember that in a traditional face-to-face classroom, students know that they come into class, take a seat, and are directed by the educator. In the online environment, the student does not know what defines being "in class," so the educator needs to help the student understand the flow of education within the online setting. Teaching presence is also established though email communication to help provide individualized instruction and response, as previously discussed.

▶ Learning Management Systems

A **learning management system (LMS)** is a type of software or application that is used to structure an online or hybrid course. It can also be used to host a MOOC—a Massive Open Online Course—which gives limitless numbers of people the ability to take an online course (usually without charge) (Educause, 2016). Most nurse educators use an LMS for their own institution's nursing courses; however, expert nurse educators may host MOOCs to provide ongoing education to other nurse educators.

Within the LMS, the nurse educator stores and presents learning materials in an organized location, provides feedback on online assignments, and manages the grade book. The LMS can be used to support face-to-face traditional courses, as well as to deliver hybrid or fully online courses (Schnetter et al., 2014). The LMS may be used by the educator to store the course syllabus, post interesting information such as articles or web links, or test or quiz students. Robust LMSs have built-in test analysis software so that nurse educators can review statistical data and make any desired modifications directly in the online test to update student grades.

Many LMS options are available (such as Blackboard, CANVAS, Moodle); some are free (called "open access"), whereas others require institutions to pay subscription or user fees. The free versions of LMS can be upgraded if an institution wishes to pay for additional features that can be unlocked.

Using Learning Management System Tools for Classroom Preparation

Depending on the specific type of LMS that an institution utilizes, the educator has access to a variety of functions that help organize classroom preparation. These functions may be sorted by "tabs" on the left side of the screen or may be organized from top to bottom. Whether teaching in a face-to-face, blended, or online course, LMS can be useful for course organization. Examples of these functions may include any mix of the items listed in **BOX 7-1**.

BOX 7-1 Examples of Learning Management System Functions

- Assignments*
- Attendance roster
- Blogs
- Calendar*
- Certificates of completion or attendance
- Chat rooms
- Discussion forums*
- Files*
- Folders*
- Grade book*
- Group rooms*
- Interactive lessons
- Interactive platforming (e.g., Hot Potatoes)
- Journals
- Pages
- Photo (or clipart) repositories
- Quizzing and testing*
- Surveys/Questionnaires
- Syllabus repository*
- Website (external) access*
- Wikis*

*Those functions listed with an asterisk are common to most learning management systems.

Before using any of the LMS functions, think about methods of maintaining this type of information in a face-to-face environment. Then, think about how that could be modified for the online environment. For example, are assignments photocopied and passed out during class? Or perhaps are Word documents emailed to students or uploaded into a current LMS? How is work collected? Do students print their submissions and hand them in, or do they email documents that must be downloaded, graded, and then uploaded again? In an *Assignment* function of an LMS, educators experience a much more robust way of creating an assignment, one in which directions can be given, completed assignments can be obtained, feedback can be provided online, and grades can be recorded. Students may be given the option (as individuals or as groups) to directly type an answer to the assignment or to upload a file that they have created offline. The educator can record marked-up feedback that the student can view, and translate that feedback into customized grading based on a created rubric. Many LMSs have incorporated visual and auditory capability, which allows the educator to verbally record feedback in addition to written feedback on submitted work.

LMSs with **Attendance** functions give the nurse educator the ability to record each student's attendance behavior. The instructor may choose to set up this function to allow tracking whether students are present, tardy, absent (excused), absent (unexcused), or have another status. This data can be easily trended for reporting purposes or for counseling students who may be struggling yet have not consistently been present for class, laboratory, and/or clinical experiences. *Certificates* may be generated to demonstrate attendance or completion of an assignment, survey, or other course-related task.

Blogs, chat rooms, group rooms, and Wikis are collaborative functions within an LMS that work much like they work on the Internet. **Blogs** are websites or web pages created by learners or groups in which student comments and opinions are posted in a conversational style. The **chat room** function can be personalized so that teams, groups, or students and educators can interact synchronously via text. This feature can be beneficial when using collaborative learning strategies or when a written exchange needs to be formally maintained for the duration of the course or thereafter. **Group rooms** give groups places to store files that are exclusive to their work but not necessary for the rest of the class to access. **Wikis**, a collaborative effort created by different members of the course, give students opportunities to collectively share notes or study tips or creatively present work.

The **Calendar** feature of an LMS is usually attached to other functions of the course. When creating Assignments, the Calendar feature automatically populates to show when the Assignment is due. The educator can enter other important dates into the Calendar that are not course-specific, such as institutional registration or drop dates, or reminders to be preparing for a test or quiz. Complementing the Calendar feature, a To Do List allows students to create their own list of tasks they need to accomplish as they participate in the course. For example, students may wish to put a reminder to check out the online library while researching information for a written paper. This reminder would show up only for the student requesting it, because it is a personalized function within the LMS.

Discussion boards, a hallmark of online education, provides "threaded" forums in which students and the educator can engage asynchronously. The educator typically poses a "discussion question," for which students must individually synthesize material (from theory bursts, viewing material, class notes, assigned reading, etc.) and create a response that addresses the question. It is common practice to require students to make one initial posting (their own answer) by a certain day of the week, and then to require them to engage with other students and/or the nurse educator at least several times during the rest of the week or module. These conversations, in a blended or online course, often take the place of a traditional face-to-face classroom lecture experience. The discussion forum is a valuable tool in the development of conceptual learning. Faculty can help students build upon previous learning and refine understanding and transferability of concepts as newer material is introduced.

> **Remember This . . .**
>
> *The discussion forum is a valuable tool in the development of conceptual learning. Faculty can help students build upon previous learning and refine understanding and transferability of concepts as newer material is introduced.*

Learning materials are organized within the LMS into Folders, which may reflect different modules, Files (such as Word, Excel, PowerPoint, or PDF documents) that pertain to content and concepts, and Pages, which are web pages that allow the educator to create text and picture communication to the class. Pages are often used within Folders to introduce the week's or module's learning material and activities, assignments, and due dates. Within Folders, the educator also can upload website (external) links, photos (which may be stored in an LMS Photo repository), and the course Syllabus (which may be linked to the Syllabus Repository). Interactive lessons created within the LMS or on platforms such as Hot Potatoes™ can be included within Folders. Hot Potatoes™ is an interactive educational technology used to create quizzes, short-answer or crossword tasks, scrambled word exercises, and matching or ordering activities (www.hotpot.uvic.ca).

Journals allow the student a place to record reflective thinking. Depending on the LMS, journals may be set to be viewable only by the student or by the student and educator. This feature is an exceptional place for the student to reflect on exemplars that have been presented, while allowing the educator to get a first-hand glimpse into the learner's conceptual understanding.

Quizzing and testing functions allow the nurse educator to create assessments directly within the LMS for formative or summative evaluation. Just like a test given via paper and pen, online quizzes or tests can be constructed to include multiple-choice, matching, or short-answer questions. Some institutions utilize a third-party online proctoring service such as Examity® to minimize breaches in academic integrity during the quizzing or testing process. Another feature that minimizes cheating allows the educator to randomize the order of questions and/or answers. The educator can preset the quiz or test to be taken only once or multiple times and can predetermine a time limit. Some LMSs allow the faculty to review how long the student participated in an activity such as quizzing or testing. If academic integrity compromise is suspected, the educator can immediately see if the student spent time on the activity or clicked answers within seconds.

Grading of multiple-choice or matching questions in online quizzes or tests can be done manually by the nurse educator or by the LMS. If desired, the educator can allow students to view their results immediately (or later) with the correct answers, and grades can immediately be translated into the Grade Book. These automated functions increase the ease of testing and the opportunity to give immediate feedback about grades. However, this feature should never replace meaningful discussion about student test performance, whether face-to-face, via email, in a chat room, or by telephone. Students often have questions for instructors about specific quiz or test questions or about their approach to test-taking.

Ensuring Course Consistency Within the LMS

Having consistent terminology and reference points for online learning language is important for course development within the LMS. Asynchronous or synchronous learning can be used in any course design. The type of learning, as well as the method of online learning, determine the strategies for successful online course design. A standard course template to use within the LMS is suggested to ensure course consistency. A standardized format does not mean that every course is the same or that every course has to contain the same type of activities. Rather, the format presents the syllabus, course resources, and overall course structure consistently, so that each time students open a new course, they will be able to find learning materials in the same place from course to course. This process is critical because students have a finite learning time. It is more important that they spend their time engaged in learning rather than looking for the resources that they need within a course. A standardized course format like the one in **FIGURE 7-3** can alleviate student anxiety and create ease of use for the nurse educator and student alike.

It also can be extremely helpful if the institution or nursing program has a checklist to use when setting up a course, whether the course will be used to supplement the face-to-face learning environment or to deliver a blended or fully online course. This guide helps ensure consistency and quality in setting up a course within an LMS. Another important way to ensure quality of an online course is to consider membership in Quality Matters (QM), a nonprofit organization that is "continuous, centered, collegial, and collaborative" (Quality Matters, 2016, para. 1) to ensure of online quality. QM offers exclusive evidence-based rubrics and standards that are the "benchmarks for evaluating the design of online and blended courses" (Quality Matters, para. 3). Training can take place so that institutions have their own QM reviewers. QM also offers expert external peer reviewers that can help institutions gain QM Certification for courses, demonstrating to learners, parents, faculty, staff,

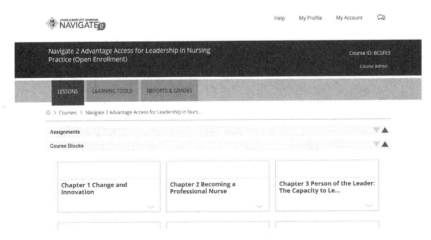

FIGURE 7-3 An example of a standardized nursing course format

and providers of accreditation that national and internationally recognized standards have been achieved.

Designing and Structuring the Course

The design of an online course should begin with program student learning outcomes (SLOs) (also known as program learning outcomes or new graduate competencies) followed by course learning outcomes. Ideally, an online course should have four to seven course learning outcomes (depending on the credits of the course) that connect directly to selected program SLOs. Every assignment and element within the course should align with the course outcomes. Further, objectives can be established in a weekly unit or module. A modular approach is very popular and may span 1 week or several weeks, depending on learning outcomes, assignments, and content. Each module should have three to five learning objectives that connect to specific course learning outcomes. More learning outcomes do not equate to more learning. Modules should center on a given concept and lead the learner to application of the concept. This learning is often accomplished by the use or one or more exemplars. When concepts versus content are used, content saturation is less likely to occur, as described earlier in this text.

Keeping students engaged within current discussions is essential rather than having them focused on what is coming next in the course. If multiple discussions are open at one time, the depth or level of discussion can be hindered. Creating a clutter-free learning environment is essential in online education. The Internet has an endless supply of information that can be linked to an online course. However, just because something relates to a particular concept does not mean that it belongs within the course. One of the most important roles of online nurse educators is to find engaging learning resources that help students connect and apply materials that fit into the context of the overall course. It is common practice to evaluate a course based on the amount of content the course contains. However, it is more important to look at the overall picture of the course and help students gain a salient understanding and meaningful conceptual learning and thinking. See **TABLE 7-3** for checklists to keep in mind when creating an online course.

▶ Fostering Conceptual Thinking in Interactive Discussion Forums

Educator feedback plays an integral role in moving learners forward in conceptual thinking, particularly within discussion forums that take the place of the traditional face-to-face classroom environment. When constructing discussion topics, begin with the end in mind. Start with the concept and develop the query with the vision of where the discussion should go. **TABLE 7-4** gives examples of types of questions that can be used in different types of online discussions. The key element when designing a discussion is to consider the purpose it will serve in meeting the course outcomes and the modular learning objectives.

In a concept-based curriculum, the nurse educator presents information conceptually and serves as a facilitator to help students connect numerous concepts as learning progresses. As in the face-to-face environment, helping students tie information together is often best accomplished by a facilitated discussion between the educator and students. In a blended or online environment, the discussion may take place asynchronously instead of synchronously.

TABLE 7-3 Section 1: Course Information			
This section refers to the online course syllabus and course information, including objectives, student learning outcomes, course requirements, and academic integrity.	✓	**N/A**	**COMMENTS**
Syllabus is easily located.			
Syllabus is available in a printer-friendly format.			
Course catalog information is provided: Description, units, prerequisites.			
Instructor contact information is available.			
Instructor office hours are available (online/on-campus).			
Required and supplemental textbooks, readings lists, and course materials are listed.			
Learning objectives are clearly stated.			
Course student learning outcomes are stated.			
Course communication instructions and guidelines are stated (i.e., Instructor email guidelines).			
Grading policy is clearly stated.			
Directions are *clear* and easy to understand for tasks and assignments.			
Academic integrity policy is clearly presented.			
Specific technology requirements are stated (if needed).			
Late and makeup work policy is clearly stated.			
Student support: Course contains extensive information about being an online learner and links to campus resources.			
An orientation for the course is offered, online or on campus.			

Reproduced from Palomar College. (2012). Online course best practices checklist (validation of preparedness to teach online). Retrieved March 2017 from www2.palomar.edu/poet/BestPracticesChecklistSP12.pdf

TABLE 7-4 Types of Discussion Forums with Examples		
Discussion Type	**Overview**	**Example**
Factual	Definitive answers. Difficult to generate lengthy discussion. Ideal for basic concepts or introduction.	What are the current guidelines for the treatment of hypertension?
Problem-solving	Encourages relevancy and application to concepts. Encourages critical thinking.	As a nurse manager, how will labor laws affect your daily decisions or staffing plans?
Socratic	Challenges students to clarify what they know in conjunction with data and potential assumptions. Forces students to challenge previously held assumptions. Many Socratic discussions start with a factual element and progress to a Socratic exploration. These discussions lend themselves to controversial topics and can produce healthy interaction and discussion.	If you were a nurse manager, how would you feel about unions? Why? Have you ever felt powerless in the workplace?
Supportive	Frequently set up for students to engage informally with each other or with the educator.	What expectations do you have within this course?
Icebreakers	Initial course discussions in which students introduce themselves and begin to connect with each other and with the course.	Introduce yourself to the class and share your most recent experience with hospital administration.

Giving students feedback in any environment is multifaceted. Doing so in the online environment is no different. The nurse educator needs to be mindful of all students who are engaging in discussion forums, not just the ones who post the most responses or with the most frequency. When class sizes are small (fewer than 15 students), learner participation is easier to monitor and facilitate (Parks-Stamm, Zafonte, & Palenque, 2016). The educator can draw from each student's post and synthesize it to formulate further questions or summarize the information to facilitate conceptual thinking. As the class size increases, participation in online discussion forums increases, research shows that it becomes easier for students to "hide" by posting infrequently or contributing little meaningful information (Kim, 2012). Educators may skim over multiple posts, missing opportunities to help some students synthesize learning. When this oversight happens, the need for deliberate instructor feedback directed at conceptual learning increases. The educator must encourage students to take ownership for the learning while carefully and methodically giving them reasons to want to engage in the learning.

▶ Delineating the Role of Nurse Educators in Online Course Development

Boettcher and Conrad (2016) divide an online course into four phases, with specific foci during each phase. The *first* phase, or course beginning, should focus on establishing presence within the online environment. The course beginning should focus on clear expectations, including the concepts of netiquette.

The *second* phase of the online course is the "early middle" and is characterized by solid teaching presence and learners finding their place within the course discussions (Boettcher & Conrad, 2016). The *third* phase, referred to as the "late middle" should be filled with coaching, assessment, and empowering the student. The *final* phase is the closing weeks of the course. The phase should be characterized by pruning and refining students' thought processes, with planned elements of reflection and evaluation.

Using these stages of online course development, nurse educators can identify their respective role within the online environment (**TABLE 7-5**). In the beginning

TABLE 7-5 Role of the Nurse Educator During Each Phase of Online Course Development

Phase of Online Course Development	Role of the Nurse Educator
First phase (course beginning)	■ Begin to establish online presence. ■ Outline clear course expectations.
Second phase (early middle)	■ Establish solid online teaching presence. ■ Use various LMS elements, such as PowerPoint presentations and collaborative learning tools. ■ Provide feedback to students.
Third phase (late middle)	■ Shift emphasis from presence to coaching. ■ Promote discussion and application of new concepts. ■ Continue to provide feedback and encourage conceptual thinking.
Fourth phase (closing)	■ Provide summary and conclusion. ■ Encourage students to showcase their growth and leadership through collaborative projects.

phase of an online course, establishing presence is essential. As discussed earlier in this chapter, establishing connections and an element of trust from the *very beginning* of the course can have a dramatic impact on the progression of learning and interaction throughout the course. When students are confused or feel isolated in the beginning stages of the course, it can be difficult to build or restore a community learning environment. Thus, the first week of a course is the most critical.

Research has shown several effective strategies to reduce anxiety associated with online learning. Incorporating some of these ideas in the first week of the course can be very beneficial to the student. According to St. Clair (2015), there is a widely held belief that if students are seeking an online program, they must be technologically savvy. This assumption is a major misconception because the technological experience and knowledge of online learners varies widely. Even if a student is technologically savvy, the LMS is often a new experience that takes time and understanding as students learn to effectively navigate it.

St. Clair (2015) suggests developing an online check-in quiz that is not course related and nonthreatening. This assessment gives students an opportunity to try submitting and discussing information without fear of doing something incorrect. Although the quiz takes time at the beginning of the course, it is an important foundation to allow true conceptual learning to develop as the course progresses. Discussion forums should be maintained throughout the course, inviting questions and comments as described earlier in this chapter. This tool helps the student ask questions and allows others to learn from the question as well as from peer and educator's responses. Remember to maintain and readily respond to the questions posted.

In the *early middle* phase of the course, learners are starting to feel more comfortable and there is an established rhythm in the course. Teaching presence is developing during this phase, and often new elements of the LMS are being employed (such as PowerPoint presentations, Google documents, and collaborative learning assignments). In the *late middle* phase of the course (as defined by Boettcher & Conrad, 2016), the educator begins to shift from teaching presence to a coaching and empowering presence. Desirable difficulty in this stage is important to promote discussion and application of new concepts. At this point within the course, the educator helps students transition toward synthesis of content-driven materials introduced earlier. This new understanding then can be transferred by the learning into different situations. While the educator's role begins to shift, the importance of feedback does not. Strong feedback is needed throughout the course, particularly to empower students to think conceptually. Guiding the learner toward the answers to thinking questions is preferred rather than providing all of the answers. Consider the development of each student and how the course is progressing, and then tailor feedback based on this information.

For example, at this stage within the course, hypothesize that the nurse educator is planning to create a Module to teach about ethics in nursing. The educator who is a *novice* in teaching hybrid or online courses may choose to include a variety of materials that he or she thinks is necessary to adequately cover this topic. These materials may include, but not be limited to, the following:

- A pretest to assess students' knowledge about the topic
- A web link or LMS page that explains ethical definitions
- A reading assignment from a textbook
- Links to supplementary websites that explore ethical dilemmas in health care
- A quiz about ethical terminology
- A discussion board to interact about ethical issues

- A paper about an ethical issue in nursing
- A posttest to assess learner understanding of the material

Easily, this grouping of material could provide learners with the "content" needed to gain a beginning understanding of ethics in nursing. However, does it foster salience of conceptual understanding, or does it simply lead to content saturation?

By contrast, the *experienced* nurse educator recognizes that quantity of resources and assignments does not necessarily yield quality conceptual understanding. Learning materials within a Module should follow a predictable standard format, just as the overall LMS presentation should adhere to a consistent format. First, key learning materials and reading assignments would be presented. Then, any additional or recommended materials can be included. Within these elements, exemplars may be identified so learners gain the essence of the key learning needed for this Module. Finally, a method of assessment would be included. It is helpful to group each of these elements (required learning materials, optional materials, learning activity, and assessment methods) into three separate Folders within the Module.

For this particular topic, the experienced nurse educator may prepare the learning materials with a link to the American Nurses Association (ANA) Code of Ethics for Nurses (2015) and give directions about the areas on which the learner is to focus. This assignment may include reading the entire (easy-to-read) 64-page document. The educator may then determine that for students who wish to have additional interpretive support may benefit from the three ANA Course Slides Set that accompanies the Code of Ethics. These slide sets could then be placed within the Folder for optional materials, with a Page that emphasizes to the learners that viewing of these slide sets is optional. Instead, this resource simply clarifies content in case students think they need more assistance in the learning process. Finally, the educator could seek or develop an exemplar-based learning activity with an appropriate rubric assessment method to help the learners conceptualize the material and demonstrate learning. When teaching conceptually, *quantity* of materials does not translate to *quality*. Carefully select and plan exemplar activities to underscore conceptual learning.

The nurse educator also might choose a prewritten case within the ANA Faculty Pak (2016) on ethics, or write their own (**BOX 7-2**). A sample case is included within the Folder for the learning activity with the corresponding assessment method.

The educator explains the learning activity on a Page. It also may be helpful to students to provide a brief comparison and contrast between ethical and moral dilemmas on this Page.

BOX 7-2 Ethics Case Exemplar

An RN has been assigned to care for a patient who is a ward of the state that lives in a local prison. This patient was recently convicted of rape and felony assault. His medical history includes pancreatic cancer. When asked about his end-of-life wishes, the patient expresses that he does not wish to undergo extensive lifesaving measures, but wants to be kept comfortable at all costs. He says to the nurse, "I have a right to remain free of pain." As the evening progresses, the patient expresses that he is experiencing pain at a level of "8" on a "1-10" scale. The nurse is torn. On the one hand, the nurse recognizes the Patient Bill of Rights and knows that he is to act as an advocate for the patient; however, he also has strong feelings about the patient's status as a convicted felon because his sister is a rape survivor.

BOX 7-3 Ethics Case Exemplar Questions

- Is this an ethical dilemma or a moral dilemma? Provide rationale.
- Apply the concepts of justice and beneficence to this case.
- How does the nurse reconcile his own acknowledged bias with his accountability in the role of the nurse?
- When, if ever, does the nurse have a right to refuse provision of care?
- With whom should the nurse consult?

The Assignment could then follow, with instructions for the learners to answer the questions (**BOX 7-3**) in a discussion post and to respond to a minimum of two peers and/or educators, after reading the case. The educator provides a due date and time for each learner's individual post to be made. Finally, the educator would post a grading rubric that correlates with the learning objectives for this assignment. It is important to remember that each assignment within a course needs to have a clear, definitive rubric so learners will know exactly how they are being evaluated.

Remember This . . .

When teaching conceptually, quantity of materials and activities does not translate to quality. Carefully select and plan exemplar activities to underscore major conceptual learning.

This type of exercise facilitates learning of content, yet gives the learners an opportunity to tie materials together conceptually in the Assignment for purposes of assessment. The nurse educator can use this opportunity within the discussion post to facilitate and direct (or redirect) the learning, as needed, based upon learner initial posts and responses. Following is an example of how a novice educator may respond in a discussion thread related to ethics and a better example of how an experienced online educator facilitates conceptual learning about ethics:

> **Instructions:** In the threaded discussion below, provide your initial response to these questions by 11:59 PM EST on Wednesday, April 9. Respond to at least two peers and/or instructor by 11:59 PM EST on Sunday, April 13. Please see the rubric for discussions located in the Rubrics Folder for grading criteria.
> - Is this an ethical dilemma or a moral dilemma? Provide rationale.
> - Apply the concepts of justice and beneficence to this case.
> - How does the nurse reconcile his own acknowledged bias with his accountability in the role of the nurse?
> - When, if ever, does the nurse have a right to refuse provision of care?
> - With whom should the nurse consult?
>
> **Nursing student John's initial response:** "This is both an ethical and moral dilemma. The nurse has an ethical and legal obligation to care for the patient, but also has a moral obligation to stand up for what is right. Rape and assault are not right. Justice means being fair and showing respect for all people, and beneficence is done for the benefit of others. The nurse is supposed to treat all patients the same, so it doesn't matter if the nurse has a bias. He has to put that

aside and still take care of the patient. The nurse can never refuse to care for someone because that is not right. The nurse could talk with other nurses who have taken care of this patient when he was admitted before, and ask what they did in the same circumstance."

Novice online educator response: "Good answer, John. You are correct by saying this is an ethical and moral dilemma. I agree that rape and assault are not right. This has to be a difficult situation for the nurse to find himself in, since his sister was a rape survivor. Just remember that all nurses have bias and have to work through that when they care for different patients. The nurse may be able to request a reassignment. Also, remember that the nurse shouldn't violate the patient's privacy by talking to other nurses."

Experienced online educator response: "Thank you for your initial post, John. You have identified beginning points to consider in this ethical and moral dilemma that the nurse faces. Consider including a reference for the definitions of justice and beneficence, and exploring how these definitions are reflected (or not reflected) in the case. When caring for patients, it is inevitable that the nurse will at some point experience bias. In some cases, the nurse can reconcile their bias and still be able to provide safe, competent, patient-centered care. When the nurse feels he or she is unable to reconcile that bias, it is important that they seek out their nurse manager to discuss the possibility of reassignment so that the patient can be assured of objective care. This is very important, as the nurse-patient relationship could certainly be compromised based on the nurse's actions or inactions. Can you think of ways in which the nurse could communicate with the nurse manager about his feelings, under these circumstances? Is it appropriate for the nurse to discuss his or her own feelings about this dilemma with other nurses who are not immediately involved in the patient's care? Think about HIPAA law when considering your answer to this question. To assist you in future discussions, be sure to include appropriate scholarly references to substantiate your points."

Notice that the *novice* online educator commends the student's work and provides concise, unilateral feedback that does little to acknowledge the student's misconceptions. Instead of fostering conceptual thinking, the novice online educator has simply provided a limited amount of isolated, content-directed understanding while overlooking important opportunities to guide the student's conceptual understanding.

The *experienced* online educator still acknowledges John's input and provides direction about using references to substantiate points. He or she then uses the following sentences as an opportunity to redirect the student's thinking by correcting misunderstandings, and fostering deeper levels of concept integration. The educator has effectively pointed out the content-driven thinking that is inaccurate and encourages the student to think conceptually about how the nurse's subsequent actions will be affected based on that information. This gives the student an opportunity to synthesize individual pieces of information—the essence of conceptual thinking.

The *closing* weeks of the course are a time to provide a summary and conclusion. Part of providing a conclusion is allowing learners to assess what they have learned and how they can use this information to move forward. Often, in an online course, the closing weeks will feature students' collaborative projects, allowing learners to showcase their own leadership and growth. As with any course, evaluation is an integral part of future course revision and design.

▶ Chapter Key Points

- Online learning by nature is conceptual and rooted in the tenets of constructivism.
- Online learning can be categorized into two primary types: asynchronous learning and synchronous learning.
- Online learning can be delivered fully online or as part of a blended or hybrid course design.
- When communicating in the online environment, use the feedback path; timely student feedback is essential.
- Discussion boards, a hallmark of online education, provides "threaded" forums in which students and the educator can engage asynchronously.
- Online presence begins when the nurse educator establishes the first contact with students.
- Online educator presence includes social, cognitive, and teaching presence.
- Learning management systems (LMSs) contain multiple features that support online, blended, or hybrid learning.
- A standard course template to use within the LMS is suggested to ensure course consistency.
- Conceptual presentation of materials in modular components reduces content saturation.
- When constructing discussion topics, start with the concept and develop the query with the vision of where the discussion should go.
- Educators modify their respective role within the online environment dependent upon course phase.
- Experienced educators tailor resources and assignments to yield quality conceptual understanding versus quantity of work.

▶ Chapter References and Selected Bibliography

American Association of Colleges of Nursing. (2014). *Nursing shortage.* Retrieved from www.aacn.nche.edu/media-relations/fact-sheets/nursing-shortage

American Nurses Association. (2015). Code of ethics for nurses with interpretive statements. Retrieved from www.nursingworld.org/DocumentVault/Ethics-1/Code-of-Ethics-for-Nurses.html

American Nurses Association. (2016). Faculty pak. Retrieved from www.1440n.com/ANA/15-335/3/

Boettcher, J., & Conrad, R. (2016). *The online teaching survival guide: Simple and practical pedagogical tips* (2nd ed.). Jossey-Bass: San Francisco, CA.

Educause. (2016). What is a MOOC? Massive Open Online Course. Retrieved from https://library.educause.edu/topics/teaching-and-learning/massive-open-online-course-mooc

Garrison, D., Anderson, T., & Archer, W. (2001). CoI Model. Retrieved from https://coi.athabascau.ca/coi-model/

*Gunawardena, C. N. (1995). Social presence theory and implications for interaction and collaborative learning in computer conferences. *International Journal of Educational Telecommunications, 1*(2/3), 147–166.

*Gunawardena, C. N., & Zittle, F. J. (1997). Social presence as a predictor of satisfaction within a computer-mediated conferencing environment. *American Journal of Distance Education, 11*(3), 8–26.

Hampton, D., & Pearce, P. (2016). Student engagement in online nursing courses. *Nurse Educator, 41*(6), 294–298.

Institute of Medicine (IOM). (2011). *The future of nursing: Leading change, advancing health.* Washington, D.C.: National Academies Press.

Kim, J. (2012). Influence of group size on participation in students' participation in online discussion forums. *Computers & Education, 62*(3), 123–129.

Odell, J., Abhyankar, R., Malcom, A., & Rua, A. (2014). Conscientious objection in the healing professions: A reader's guide to the ethical and social issues. Retrieved from https://scholarworks .iupui.edu/bitstream/handle/1805/3929/conscientiousobjectionethicalanalyses.pdf?sequence=1

Quality Matters. (2016). Why QM? Retrieved from www.qualitymatters.org/why-quality-matters

Palomar College. (2012). Online course best practices checklist (validation of preparedness to teach online). Retrieved from http://www2.palomar.edu/poet/BestPracticesChecklistSP12.pdf

Parks-Stamm, E., Zafonte, M., & Palenque, S. (2016). The effects of instructor participation and class size on student participation in an online class discussion forum. *British Journal of Educational Technology.* doi: 10.1111.bjet.12512

Rebar, C. (2010). *Perceptions of community of associate degree nurse learners in an RN-to-BSN online program* (Doctoral dissertation). Retrieved from www.proquest.com/en-US/products /dissertations/individuals.shtml

Schnetter, V., Lacy, D., Jones, M., Bakrim, K., Allen, P., & O'Neal, P. (2014). Course development for web-based nursing education programs. *Nursing Education in Practice, 14*(6), 635–640.

*Shea, V. (1994). *Netiquette.* Albion Books: San Francisco, CA.

St. Clair, D. (2015). A simple suggestion for reducing first time online student anxiety. *MERLOT Journal of Online Teaching, 11*(1). Retrieved from www.jolt.merlot.org/vol11no1/StClair_0315.pdf

*Short, J. A., Williams, E., & Christie, B. (1976). *The social psychology of telecommunications.* New York: John Wiley & Sons.

*Tu, C., & McIsaac, M. (2002). The relationship of social presence and interaction in online classes. *American Journal of Distance Education, 16*(3), 131–150.

*Indicates classic reference.

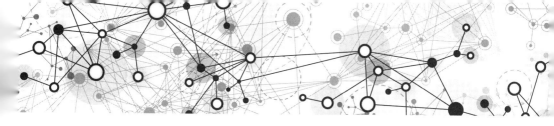

CHAPTER 8

Using Concept Mapping for Conceptual Learning

Deanne Blach

▶ Introduction to Concept Mapping

Concept mapping is an instructional strategy that can be used for many different types of learners, including those who learn by visual, auditory, read/write, and kinesthetic styles. A **concept map (CM)** is a hierarchical graphic organizing tool that does the following:

- Engages the student in the learning process
- Allows opportunities for collaborative learning
- Increases critical thinking and scientific reasoning

Concept mapping is an innovative approach in healthcare education that creates meaningful learning because students are better able to organize knowledge, create connections, and develop clinical judgment skills that ultimately improve patient safety and quality care (Erickson, 2008; Schuster, 2016). Concept mapping emerged in nursing education in the early 1990s as a student-centered active learning strategy, linking classroom knowledge to clinical practice with an increase in learner engagement (Daley, 1996). This strategy also has been used in nursing clinical practice settings to improve critical thinking and clinical reasoning, especially among new nursing graduates (Schuster, 2016).

In the early 2000s, concept maps (CMs) in nursing education were introduced as a replacement for the traditional nursing care plan in the clinical setting and are sometimes referred to as *care maps* (Daley, Morgan, & Black, 2016; Schuster, 2016). The expansion of concept mapping in nursing education continues through the work of the National League for Nursing, using high-fidelity simulation and CMs to cultivate self-confidence in nursing students (Kinchin, 2015).

Most of the published studies on CMs are not recent, but are cited frequently as classic research. Classic nursing education studies suggest that CMs improve critical thinking and clinical reasoning by helping students make connections between newly learned information and preexisting knowledge (Daley, 1996; King & Shell, 2002). Thus, this learning activity is grounded in constructivist theory, as described earlier in this text. Daley, Shaw, Balistreiri, Glasenapp, & Piacentine (1999) evaluated CMs progressively for students during a single clinical rotation by using the scoring system developed by the founders of concept mapping—Joseph Novak and Bob Gowin. These nursing researchers found significant differences in the students' first and last CM scores and recommended this educational tool to improve critical thinking when providing patient care. The researchers' students also suggested that concept mapping be incorporated into the nursing curriculum as a tool to help them develop their thinking.

Other health professions' educational programs also utilize CMs in their curriculum. A systematic review of 35 studies by Daley and Torre (2010) showed that concept mapping served the following four functions:

- Promoting meaningful learning and thinking (often in collaborative with other students)
- Providing additional resources for student learning
- Enabling instructors to provide student feedback
- Assessing student learning and performance

This study also found that CMs were excellent tools for developing critical thinking and clinical reasoning.

Assimilation Theory as a Basis for Concept Mapping

Concept mapping was developed in 1984 by Novak and Gowin based on educational psychologist David Ausubel's classic assimilation theory of meaningful learning. According to Ausubel's educational theory (1963), meaningful learning integrates new information into a preexisting foundation of relevant knowledge. This information is rearranged and reordered to develop new meaning and a better understanding of the concepts. Understanding requires concept connections and synthesis into a learner's existing network of knowledge rather than rote memorization. A CM, then, is a visual roadmap of ideas that represents a set of concepts that are embedded into a network of knowledge to develop meaningful relationships.

Terminology Associated with Developing Concept Maps

Novak and Gowin (1984) defined a *concept* as "a regularity in events or objects designated by a label" (p. 15). It can range from being limited to complex. The updated definition for this text is somewhat different in that concepts are classifications or categories of information or knowledge that can be ideas or mental images. They are not objects or things and can be flexible and dynamic.

Novak and Gowin (1984) proposed a CM hierarchical structure with the main concept as the most general concept and other concepts that are more specific. In nursing education, the main concept can be the "focus question" or central focus; basic need that identifies the concept being explored; a patient problem, situation, or issue; or a short patient scenario. The main concept is followed by other concepts representing the components of the nursing process or clinical judgment. The concepts are tied together with **linking words** that are often verbs essential to demonstrate their connections. These linking words provide the meaning of the *relationships* between two or more concepts. *Lines with arrows* show direction and must include linking words that describe the relationships among the concepts.

As shown in **FIGURE 8-1**, the central focus of this basic CM is Measuring Vital Signs in an Adult. The individual vital signs (Core Body Temperature, Pulse, Respiratory Rate, and Blood Pressure) are connected to the main focus with lines with arrows that contain linking words to show relationships. For example, characteristics of vital signs include the rate, rhythm, and quality of the pulse. These linking words are written on the line between Measuring Vital Signs in an Adult (main focus) and Pulse (sub-concept). Students often have the most difficult time in concept mapping with linking the words to depict a specific meaningful relationship.

Propositions, the building blocks of knowledge, are formed when two or more concepts are connected with linking words and lines to establish meaning. Propositions become the fundamental units in the learner's cognitive structure. The richness of the meaning increases exponentially with the number of valid propositions as the concepts relate to other concepts (Novak, 2010). The propositions can either be valid (the grass is green) or not (the ocean is purple). This relationship leads to a discussion about whether a proposition is valid or invalid, providing an opportunity to exchange views and recognize missing linkages between concepts. Cognitive meanings cannot be transferred from learner to learner, but each learner puts the information together in his or her unique way. Learning new information requires conversation, an exchange of dialog, a sharing of information, and sometimes compromise (Novak & Gowin, 1984).

Remember This . . .

Cognitive meanings cannot be transferred from learner to learner, but each learner puts the information together in his or her unique way. Learning new information requires conversation, an exchange of dialog, a sharing of information, and sometimes compromise (Novak & Gowin, 1984).

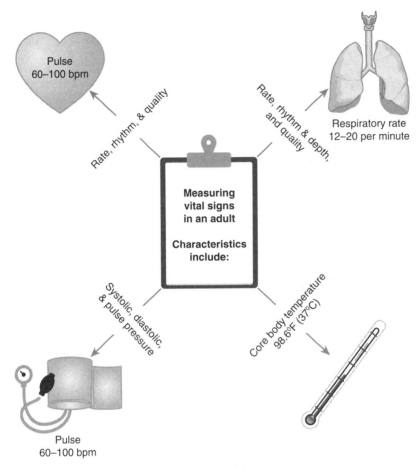

Pulse
60–100 bpm

Rate, rhythm, & quality

Rate, rhythm & depth, and quality

Respiratory rate
12–20 per minute

Measuring
vital signs
in an adult

Characteristics
include:

Systolic, diastolic,
& pulse pressure

Core body temperature
98.6°F (37°C)

Pulse
60–100 bpm

FIGURE 8-1 Basic concept map for vital signs in an adult

The CM is an effective tool to provide the nurse educator an opportunity to correct misconceptions either as a missing link or an error in a connection. The misconception (the expressed meaning) of the learner is not necessarily wrong or unacceptable, but holds a functional meaning to the learner. It is not uncommon for misconceptions to persist for years. When the nurse educator can assist the student in integrating one or more missing concepts, the misconception can be corrected and clarified. The student's prior knowledge influences the new learning; both the educator and learner are able to negotiate new meaning (Novak & Gowin, 1984).

▶ Use of Concept Mapping in the Concept-Based Nursing Curriculum

Concept mapping promotes conceptual learning by helping the learner see the big picture and events that contribute to the main concept or focus problem. A CM helps the learner break down the big picture into smaller parts, defining the relationships among nursing concepts and promoting conceptual understanding (Novak, 2010). This process makes it an appropriate tool within a concept-based curriculum in any type of nursing education program.

As an active learning strategy, concept mapping can be used in the classroom or online for introducing a concept or exploring concept exemplars. CM work fosters the development of group and collaborative learning. In a classic study, Boxel, Linden, Roelofs, and Erken (2002) found significant learning gains when concept mapping was used for a group project. Each learner's work is unique, though, and is based on his or her own understanding of the content. As learners work together on a concept mapping project, they are engaged and benefit from each other's perspective. Students become full partners in the learning process and take responsibility for their own learning experience.

Using Concept Maps in a Prelicensure Nursing Program

When beginning to assist students in learning CM development, make the assignment simple. Future assignments can build upon previous work. The nurse educator's role is to be an encourager and facilitator in CM construction. Recognize that some students will take longer than others to understand CM development. For instance, creative and visual learners may more easily adapt to CMs than more linear, concrete, and auditory learners. Concept mapping in a concept-based curriculum can be used for many purposes, including the following:

- Substitutes for traditional written assignments
- Visual representations of basic pathophysiology and pharmacology concepts
- Replacements for traditional nursing care plans
- Tools for patient education and health teaching

For example, convert traditional written assignments into concept mapping projects to ease learners into the conceptual learning and thinking process. Basic concepts in the first nursing course might include mobility, tissue integrity, gas exchange, perfusion, and ethics. **FIGURE 8-2** illustrates a CM on risk factors for inadequate perfusion and health teaching to prevent inadequate perfusion. The nursing process is another early concept learners can explore. Concept mapping can clarify the components of the nursing process and the relationships of the parts to the whole.

Remember This . . .

When beginning to assist students in learning concept map (CM) development, make the assignment simple. The second assignment can build upon previous work. The nurse educator's role is to be an encourager and facilitator in CM construction.

Another use for CMs is in a basic pathophysiology or pharmacology course. For example, students may develop CMs using an exemplar or drug classification as the central theme or focus to link nursing implications for medication administration. The concreteness of these topics lends them to CM development early in the curriculum.

CMs often replace traditional care plans in the clinical setting because they create meaningful learning for learners as they organize their thoughts in a different way to promote deep learning. Students can plan care for their assigned patients and show

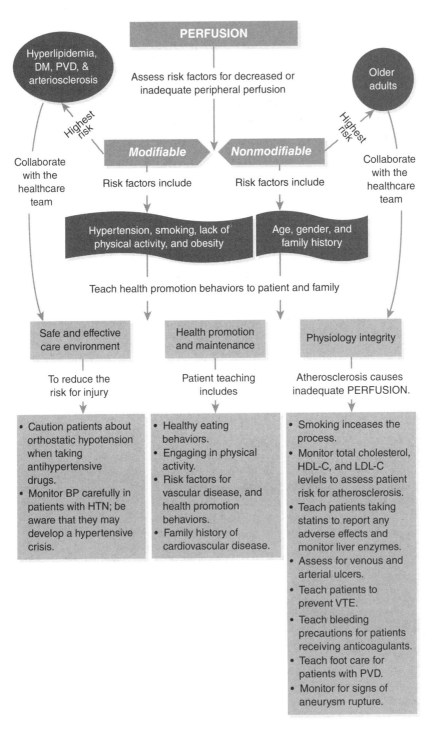

FIGURE 8-2 Concept map for risk factors for inadequate perfusion

© Deanne Blach. Used with permission.

how their plans can meet patient outcomes. Or, in the postclinical conference setting, students can work collaboratively to develop a CM about an interesting clinical patient as a case study review, ideally related to concepts recently explored in the classroom. As new ideas are brainstormed, new connections can be made.

Clinical educators often prefer clinical CMs because they are easier and quicker to evaluate than the traditional care plans and allow them to see the misperceptions about specific nursing care more quickly. Although Pam Schuster's work did not include connecting the concepts with lines and words for linkages, Schuster (2000) noted that nursing students were better able to document care in a CM, better able to organize care, and thought that CMs were less cumbersome than traditional care plans. Students usually respond very positively to CMs. In an evaluation of using concept mapping as a tool to replace care plans in the clinical setting, students reported that they recognized new relationships with drugs, why they were taken, what the adverse effects were, and how they affected laboratory values (Caputi & Blach, 2008). These connections were not recognized within the traditional care plan format.

As a paired assignment in the clinical setting, learners can share the care of a complex patient. For this collaborative assignment, one student provides direct patient care and the second student develops a CM as a focused learning activity (see Chapter 6) to document the patient's assessment and relevant nursing care. During the second clinical day, the students might switch roles. Collaboration throughout the clinical experience provides an opportunity to discuss patient assessment findings, such as laboratory values related to the clinical condition, fluid volume status, and cardiac function. Nursing interventions and how medications affect a patient's condition also can be compared between students (Caputi & Blach, 2008). The clinical educator is able to determine if important concepts or interventions have been missed.

CMs are also effective teaching tools for patient education. For example, students can develop a CM for a patient with a low reading level and incorporate images as a visual representation of the content. The teaching plan can then be presented to the class or incorporated into a simulation activity (Samawi, Miller, & Haras, 2014). Examples of topics for patient education include drug therapy, self-management, and transition management. Learners can work in pairs or small groups to develop these maps. If the entire clinical group develops a CM using the same concepts, each CM will be different and reflect each student's interpretation of content linkages. This activity helps students realize there is more than one right way to do the project as long as the concepts are present and the linkages are valid.

Using Concept Maps in a Graduate Nursing Program

CMs can be used in graduate nursing programs in a number of ways, including the following:

- Substitutes for traditional written assignments
- Visual representations of advanced pathophysiology and pharmacology concepts
- Tools for learning complex concepts

For example, the central focus or core concept for a graduate program CM is Health Policy and Advocacy (Master's Essential VI) (American Association of Colleges of Nursing, 2011). The educator may present a map to help students learn the main concept and sub-concepts or require students to create a CM that shows the concept relationships as an assignment.

> **Remember This . . .**
>
> Concept maps can be used in graduate nursing programs in a number of ways, including the following:
>
> - Substitutes for traditional written assignments
> - Visual representations of advanced pathophysiology and pharmacology concepts
> - Tools for learning complex concepts

▶ How to Develop a Meaningful Concept Map

The educator could begin with a simple first assignment. For example, in a beginning prelicensure course, the CM might be related to vital signs. Beyond the normal parameters in adults, as shown in Figure 8-1, a more in-depth analysis of vital signs in a CM could incorporate factors that affect the vital sign values. These factors might include perfusion issues, safety issues, assessment of circulation or neurovascular checks, different routes and sites for measurement, factors that affect regulation, and differences in ages, equipment, and methods (**FIGURE 8-3**). A CM also could be developed for other concepts and their specific exemplars, such as Fluid and Electrolyte Balance (hypovolemic shock), Perfusion (chronic heart failure), Gas Exchange (chronic obstructive pulmonary disease), and Intracranial Regulation (traumatic brain injury).

Concept mapping can be very useful to help students understand Professional Nursing and Health Care concepts. Examples include role of the nurse, interprofessional collaboration, healthcare organizations, and healthcare disparities. Each of these concepts could be the central focus of a CM.

Setting up a successful learning environment is important for learner success when developing CMs. Nursing faculty should know what concept mapping is, how to facilitate learning, and how to be consistent with each other when reviewing the CMs with students (establishing interrater reliability). Most CMs are evaluated as either a pass or fail grade. If a more detailed grading system is required, a rubric should be developed so that all educators are measuring the same elements. A care plan rubric can be modified to include the linkages and clarity required for a CM.

As with any learning activity, there is more than one way to introduce the learner to concept mapping. In the classroom, the nurse educator can create a CM on a whiteboard or electronically display the work on a screen for the class to view. Concept mapping also can be introduced online or in clinical postconference. Regardless of how concept mapping is introduced, provide learners with a hands-on learning experience. Acting as a role model, the nurse educator may choose to create a CM and share copies with all students as the content is presented. The learning environment can be set up to provide tools for student success in understanding the development of a CM by providing classroom tools (colored paper, markers, scissors, sticky notes, and pictures) or instructions or guidance for computer software, if used.

Computer-assisted concept mapping (CACM), available from many sources, uses computer software to develop an individualized CM for a variety of electronic devices, including the iPad. The advantages of using CACM are numerous and include an increased flexibility and fewer limitations when adding content, changing

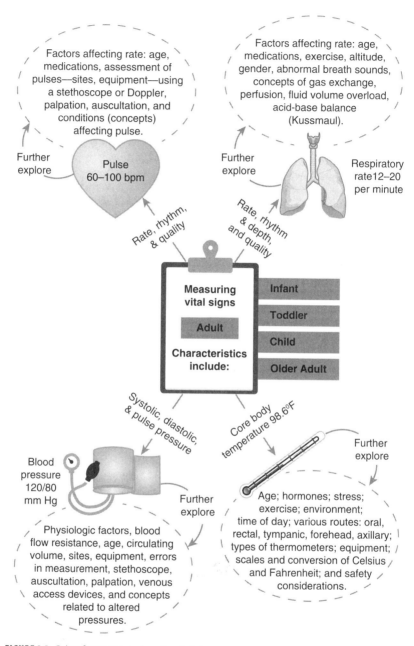

FIGURE 8-3 Other factors to explore for vital signs concept map

colors, or rearranging content when compared to the traditional paper method of concept mapping. Students can appreciate the ease of creation and the unlimited digital abilities of space, revision, collaboration, and sharing with CACM (Mammen, 2016). Visually organizing and reorganizing the information leads to retention and clarification of the content.

Many of the CACM software programs are *free*, including the following:

- Virtual Understanding Environment (VUE) Version 3.2.1
- XMind Version 3.4.1
- MindMaple Version 3.4.1 (smartphone and iPad features)

Cmap Version 6.01.01, designed by Novak's Institute for Human and Machine Cognition, is also free but requires registration. It, too, has iPad features that make mobility convenient. Prezi, most often used for presentations, is set up like a CM, allowing for integration of pictures, video links, and documents. Images "fly in," areas of focus are emphasized, and relationships can be labeled. The free version of Prezi requires the final document to be posted online for sharing (Mammen, 2016). Simple to use, Inspiration® has concept mapping software for purchase that will create the shapes, colors, lines, and spacing on the line to add the linking words. This software is also useful for developing other types of graphic organizers, outlines, and graphs.

▶ The Step-by-Step Approach to Concept Map Development

The process of developing a CM can be broken down into a series of steps (**BOX 8-1**). It is important that both educators and students are provided clear instruction and facilitated practice time for CM development. This process ensures consistency in the teaching/learning approach and values the CM as a tool to process connections that foster deep learning. Educator-designed CMs provide an example for students as a basis for their own CMs. The nurse educator uses the CM to explain the details of the concept and as a guide for making connections in the classroom or online learning environment. Students can then expand on the concept by developing a patient-specific CM using the presented concept with a short case scenario provided by the educator. Be sure to provide clear expectations of what students must include on the CM.

The main concept or focus question is based on the content provided in the didactic portion of the course, a patient scenario, or actual assigned patient in simulation or external clinical environment. Regardless of its focus or central theme/concept,

---

BOX 8-1 Ten-Step Approach for Developing a Concept Map

Step 1: Determine the main concept or focus question.

Step 2: Clarify/define concepts and sub-concepts.

Step 3: Create a parking lot for sub-concepts.

Step 4: Organize and prioritize the information.

Step 5: Arrange the sub-concepts around the central focus or concept.

Step 6: Draw lines using arrows to connect sub-concepts.

Step 7: Label the lines with linking words that show concept relationships.

Step 8: Add pictures and color for visual appeal and clarity.

Step 9: Make a key and include references.

Step 10: Revise the CM as needed.

a stepwise approach to CM development can help ensure consistency and assist with grading if the educator desires. In this section, the 10-step approach for developing a CM as a group learning activity in prelicensure programs is applied to the exemplar of Chronic Heart Failure for the concept of Perfusion. As defined in Chapter 2, exemplars are specific content topics that relate to and represent identified concepts.

Step 1: Determine the Main Concept or Focus Question

In this first step, using Tanner's Model of Clinical Judgment (described earlier in this book), the nurse educator guides the learners (often in groups) in deeper understanding of the concept of Perfusion. After students are first introduced to this concept, the nurse educator may create a short scenario to help students start making connections to determine who may be at risk for inadequate perfusion (the Noticing phase in Tanner's Model of Clinical Judgment). Providing a scenario allows students to design the CM to focus on the whole person in the patient situation. The group can print their scenario in the center or top of a large poster-size paper or electronic CM as either a face-to-face or online activity. An example scenario might read as follows:

> 66-year-old Marty Engels has a history of chronic heart failure (CHF); is admitted today to the emergency department for a weight gain of 5 pounds in 3 days, shortness of breath, and change in LOC (restlessness).

Step 2: Clarify or Define Concepts and Sub-Concepts

Learners need to be clear on the definitions of the concept(s) and exemplar. The main concept of Perfusion is defined as "the flow of blood through the arteries and capillaries delivering nutrients and oxygen to cells" (Giddens, 2017, p. 167). The exemplar for Perfusion, Chronic Heart Failure, is defined as a common chronic health problem with episodes of acute failure causing hospitalization (Ignatavicius & Workman, 2016). Learners may determine other priority concepts related to perfusion (interrelated concepts), such as Gas Exchange and Fluid and Electrolyte Balance. These interrelated concepts are part of the CM sub-concepts.

As part of the learning, students need to review closely related terms such as ischemia, hypoxia, anoxia, and hypoxemia. The scenario provides just enough information for learners to recognize problems as they occur (the Interpreting phase of Tanner's Model of Clinical Judgment) and be able to add additional elements to the scenario to make it more interesting and complex. The bulleted parking lot list can be written on a sheet of paper or entered into an electronic document, as described in the next step.

Step 3: Create a Parking Lot for Sub-Concepts

Placed in small groups, learners are guided into brainstorming as they consider what would be relevant to the patient in the scenario and the identified sub-concepts. One person is the record keeper and lists the ideas that are derived from brainstorming. An example of ideas generated by the chronic heart failure could include the following:

- Signs and symptoms of right-sided heart failure
- Signs and symptoms of left-sided heart failure

- Systolic and diastolic heart failure
- Considerations for older adults
- Priority patient problems
- Common drug therapy
- Nursing interventions
- Diet and lifestyle
- Patient education
- Diagnostic studies
- Decreased cardiac output
- Inadequate perfusion
- Staging of heart failure
- Common causes
- Assessment and history
- Acute exacerbation
- Interprofessional collaboration
- Patient outcomes
- Pulmonary edema
- Home care management
- Positioning
- Fluid volume overload

This process of brainstorming all potential information related to patient care is part of Tanner's (2006) phase of Noticing, which triggers additional data collection.

Step 4: Organize and Prioritize the Information

Often the learner lists very specific thoughts in the parking lot, such as daily weight, breath sounds, digoxin, furosemide, pulse rate, edema, tachycardia, and B-type natriuretic peptide (BNP). These ideas can be grouped under broader categories such as medications, assessment data, and laboratory work. With the educator's guidance, not all elements in the parking lot will be placed on the CM.

The nurse educator may request elements of the nursing process or phases of clinical judgment. This process of "pruning" the parking lot allows the group to determine priorities. In this process, the learner can recognize problems when they occur (Interpreting), according to Tanner's Model of Clinical Judgment. The educator needs to be available to discuss this process with each group and lend clarity about what information to keep or leave behind.

The small group's next step is to organize the parking lot information in some sort of order to categorize and prioritize the information. The learners can take the list from the parking lot and transfer the main categories onto colored sticky paper. These sticky notes can be placed anywhere on a large poster-size paper and moved around until the organization makes sense to the group. Digital content using computer CM software can be easily moved or rearranged.

Step 5: Arrange the Sub-Concepts Around the Central Focus or Concept

The next step is to arrange the sub-concepts determined as most important from the parking lot for the CM around the central focus (in this case, the patient scenario).

The learner takes previous knowledge and arranges and rearranges it in a way that is logical and makes sense. This creates a more integrated cognitive knowledge structure (Abel & Freeze, 2006). Once learners rearrange the sub-concepts, they are demonstrating they know what to do (the Responding phase of Tanner's Model of Clinical Reasoning). Priorities of care should be evident at this point in the process of designing the CM.

Step 6: Draw Lines Using Arrows to Connect Sub-Concepts

The concepts and sub-concepts are then connected by lines using arrows to determine the direction of the relationship and describe the relationship. When the learner shows connections between the concepts with lines and arrows, it helps clarify the concepts. These solid lines can be one-directional or bi-directional, indicating the flow of relationships. A potential relationship could be demonstrated by a dotted line.

To reduce clutter on the CM, Novak and Gowin (1984) suggest arrows are not needed if the CM has a hierarchy to it or if there is one major concept with all other sub-concepts subsumed underneath. Nursing care and interprofessional collaboration, however, cannot usually be mapped in a hierarchical structure.

Sometimes the learner is unclear where to put the information or how to connect it to other sub-concepts. One solution is to put this information on the edge of the CM and seek assistance in incorporating that information. The lines are essential to show the connections among concepts. The lines help the learner understand the impact on other variables (the Reflecting phase of Tanners' Model of Clinical Judgment).

Step 7: Label the Lines with Linking Words That Show Concept Relationships

Labeling the lines with linking words is a critical step that demonstrates what the relationship is between and among concepts. As mentioned earlier in this chapter, this step tends to be the most difficult for students. If there are too many words on the line, it may indicate the information should be its own concept.

Step 8: Add Pictures and Color for Visual Appeal and Clarity

Pictures and other visual images can enhance the look of the CM and clarify its content. If using paper material and markers, clip art can be printed to use, as well as color advertisements from newspapers. Old nursing magazines have advertisement photos and other nursing and medical pictures that can be incorporated. Learners can be very creative and have fun adding the visual piece. Art is also available within computer CM software programs. Many times, the main concept can be depicted as a picture rather than as words. For example, for chronic heart failure, a sick heart caricature can be used. Although not in full color for this book, the CM shown in **FIGURE 8-4** includes pictures to help students understand the pathophysiology of CHF.

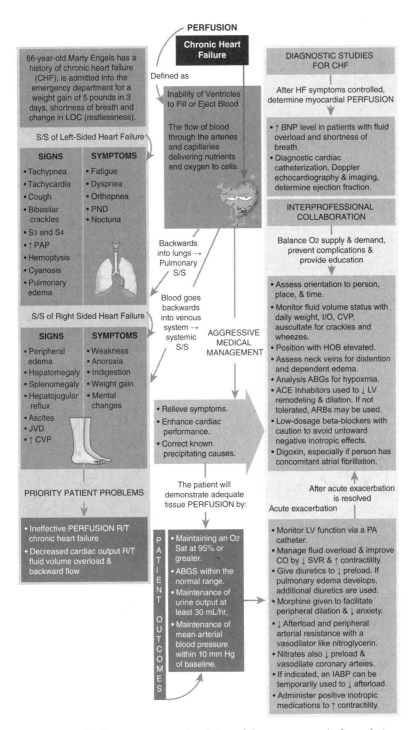

FIGURE 8-4 Example of concept map on chronic heart failure as an exemplar for perfusion

Step 9: Make a Key and Include References

While not always needed, a CM key may provide understanding for the educator reviewing the CM of the learner's intention for using specific colors and shapes. This information can be placed on the edge or bottom of a CM. References can be included on the back of hard-copy CMs or as a separate electronic document. Providing evidence for safe, quality nursing practice is essential for the student to include.

Step 10: Revise the Concept Map as Needed

Revision improves clarity, allows the learner to "clean up" the CM, and reduces cluttering and overcrowding. Learners who complete a CM and review it again later often find different connections and are able to rearrange the content for added or improved understanding. The first CM is certain to have flaws, but a second map usually shows key relationships more clearly. As an option, a draft CM may be turned in for review by the nurse educator. If the CM is weak, the learner may need to resubmit a revision. Providing another opportunity for clarity can be very helpful to the learner to make connections that were missed during the first draft. The revision process further enhances understanding and meaningful learning.

Remember This . . .

Revision improves clarity, allows the learner to clean up the concept map, and reduces cluttering and overcrowding.

▶ Faculty and Student Development

Lack of knowledge is often the main reason why there may be resistance to concept mapping as a strategy to engage students and improve critical thinking abilities. Providing a faculty workshop for all educators to have the same instruction provides a consistent approach for student success and faculty buy-in. Students can attend the workshop, so everyone receives the same set of instructions and guidance. Designing a CM in a collaborative work group can further clarify CM development and organization because each team member considers the ideas of group members.

Students can be introduced to CMs by using a nonnursing topic for their first assignment. Examples could include putting together the steps of a vacation, changing of a tire, or the etiquette of eating. This exercise allows them to later use the skill set to work on a more complex nursing topic. For example, pathophysiology content lends itself to concept mapping. The students can select a concept and exemplar to diagram on a CM. This assignment assists students in learning the typical assessment findings associated with selected diseases and health conditions. **FIGURE 8-5** shows a CM on Hypovolemia, which is an exemplar for Perfusion.

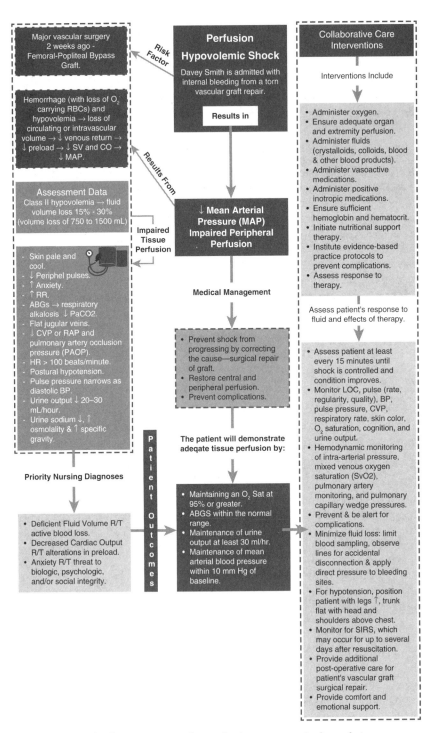

FIGURE 8-5 Example of concept map on hypovolemia as an exemplar for perfusion

© Deanne Blach. Used with permission.

Learning Tool or Graded Assignment: Evaluating a Concept Map

To determine the type of evaluation of a CM, the educator must decide on the purpose of the CM. Is it a learning tool or a graded assignment? Students typically take a graded assignment more seriously. According to Oermann (2017), CMs are best used for *formative* evaluation, but can be evaluated and graded as a *summative* tool based on predetermined criteria. Some of the same criteria can be used for a care plan as a CM, for example, if the correct assessment data are provided, if the information is linked with the correct diagnoses and problems, whether the interventions and treatments are specific and relevant, and if relationships among the concepts are accurate (Oermann, 2017).

One major advantage of CMs is the reduced time required to review them compared to traditional care plans. An important element to accurately understand what the connections are is to have students discuss their thought process in making connections as they move their hands around the map. When reviewing a CM as a clinical care map, the educator evaluates the following:

- Weekly progression (Students' maps get more complex as they practice and revise.)
- Creativity (Given a few points, the core content must be on the CM.)
- Relationships between ideas (These ideas must have a line with linking words.)
- Links in the nursing process or clinical judgment (These phases must be present and correct.)
- Presence of errors or misperceptions (These corrections can be made immediately.)

The other part of CM evaluation is to elicit the students' perceptions of the learning experience. The author's last-semester nursing students completed an evaluation for using concept mapping in the clinical setting for the first time. When these students were asked "How did the CM clarify patient information?" the students' responses included the following:

- "It put pieces of a puzzle together."
- "I considered aspects of the nursing process and patient care that get overlooked on a busy day."
- "I saw new connections."
- "I saw relationships with drugs, why they are taken, their adverse effects, and how they affect lab values." (Caputi & Blach, 2008)

Nursing education research validates that students value concept mapping as a learning and critical thinking tool. Students surveyed in a study by Harrison and Gibbons (2013) found that concept mapping helped them connect theory (knowledge) to practice, which facilitated clinical judgment when providing patient care.

Adding Concept Maps to a Portfolio

CMs help confirm clinical competencies and demonstrate new connections. They can be added to a portfolio as documentation of how well the student achieved mastery of the concepts. The progression in complexity can be seen as students are able to build upon previous experience. Portfolios can be used for students' self-assessment of their progress in developing CMs to meet their goals. The nurse educator should be able to determine whether the student met the outcomes of the course by assessment of the portfolio (Oermann, 2017). Usually there is a major difference between early course CMs and CMs produced in the last semester or quarter of their program.

▶ Chapter Key Points

- Concept mapping is an innovative, student-centered learning approach that fosters meaningful learning by organizing content in a way that makes sense, creates connections, and develops critical thinking skills.
- Concept mapping is an active collaborative learning strategy in which brainstorming is beneficial.
- Novak and Gowin's work with concept mapping is based on David Ausubel's assimilation theory of meaningful learning.
- Novak's theory proposes a hierarchical structure with the main concept as the most general concept and other concepts that are more detailed and specific. The concepts are tied together with linking words that clarify the meaning of the relationships between two concepts.
- Propositions, the building blocks of knowledge, are formed when two or more concepts are connected with linking words to establish meaning.
- Concept maps (CMs) are effective tools to determine if the student has misperceptions that can be clarified immediately.
- The lines that are drawn with an arrow indicating direction must include a few descriptive words that detail the relationships between the concepts.
- Concept mapping can be used in a classroom, online, or in clinical or simulation learning environment in which concepts can be identified, explained, and connected.
- Start simple, providing a basic CM as a guide for the students.
- Learners can use paper, markers, and pictures or use a computer-assisted concept mapping (CACM) software to design CMs.
- CM development can be learned by using a 10-step approach.
- Revision of a CM provides clarity in making connections that were missed in the first draft.
- The grading of a CM is usually formative; if CMs are graded, evaluation criteria must be developed to delineate student expectations and ensure educator consistency in grading.

▶ Chapter References and Selected Bibliography

*Abel, W., & Freeze, M. (2006). Evaluation of concept mapping in an associate degree nursing programme. *Journal of Nursing Education, 45*(9), 356–364.

American Association of Colleges of Nursing (AACN). (2011). *The essentials of master's education in nursing.* Washington, D.C.: AACN.

*Ausubel, D. P. (1963). *The psychology of meaningful verbal learning: An introduction to school learning.* New York, NY: Grune & Stratton.

*Boxel, C. V., Linden, J. N., Roelofs, E., & Erken, G. (2002). Collaborative concept mapping: Provoking and supporting meaningful discourse. *Theory Practice, 41*(1), 40–46.

Burrell, L. A. (2014). Integrating critical thinking strategies into nursing curricula. *Teaching and Learning in Nursing, 9*(2), 53–58.

Caputi, L., & Blach, D. (2008). *Teaching nursing using concept mapping.* Glen Ellyn, IL: College of DuPage Press.

*Daley, B. J. (1996). Concept maps: Linking nursing theory to clinical nursing practice. *Journal of Continuing Education in Nursing, 27*(1), 17–27.

Daley, B. J., Morgan, S., & Black, S. B. (2016). Concept maps in nursing education: A historical literature review and research directions. *Journal of Nursing Education, 55*(11), 631–639.

*Daley, B. J., Shaw, C. R., Balistreiri, T., Glasenapp K., & Piacentine, L. (1999). Concept maps: A strategy to teach and evaluate critical thinking. *Journal of Nursing Education, 38*(1), 42–47.

Daley, B. J., & Torre, D. M. (2010). Concept maps in medical education: An analytical literature review. *Medical Education, 44*(5), 440–448.

Erickson, L. (2008). *Stirring the head, heart, and soul: Redefining curriculum, instruction, and concept-based learning.* Thousand Oaks, CA: Corwin Press.

Giddens, J. F. (2017). *Concepts for nursing practice* (2nd ed.). St. Louis, MO: Elsevier.

Giddens, J. F., Caputi, L., & Rodgers, B. (2015). *Mastering concept-based teaching: A guide for nursing educators.* St. Louis, MO: Elsevier.

Harrison, S., & Gibbons, C. (2013). Nursing student perceptions of concept maps: From theory to practice. *Nursing Education Perspectives, 34*(6), 395–399.

Ignatavicius, D. D., & Workman, M. L. (2016). *Medical-surgical nursing patient-centered collaborative care* (8th ed.). St. Louis, MO: Elsevier.

Kinchin, I. (2015). Concept mapping in university and professional education. *Knowledge Management & E-Learning, 7*(1), 1–5.

*King, M., & Shell, R. (2002). Teaching and evaluating critical thinking with concept maps. *Nurse Educator, 27*(5), 214–216.

Mammen, J. R. (2016). Computer-assisted concept mapping: visual aids for knowledge. *Journal of Nursing Education, 55*(7), 403–406.

*Novak, J. D. (2010). *Learning, creating, and using knowledge: Concept maps as facilitative tools in schools and corporations.* Mahwah, NJ: Lawrence Erlbaum.

*Novak, J. D., & Gowin, D. B. (1984). *Learning how to learn.* New York, NY: Cambridge University Press.

Oermann, M. H. (2017). *Teaching in nursing and role of the educator: The complete guide to best practice in teaching, evaluation and curriculum development* (2nd ed.). New York, NY: Springer Publishing.

Samawi, A., Miller, T., & Haras, M. S. (2014). Using high fidelity simulation and concept mapping to cultivate self confidence in nursing students. *Nursing Education Perspectives, 35*(6), 408–409.

*Schuster, P. (2000). Concept mapping: Reducing clinical care plan paperwork and increasing learning. *Nurse Educator, 25*(2), 76–81.

Schuster, P. (2016). *Concept mapping: A critical thinking approach to care planning* (4th ed.). Philadelphia, PA: FA Davis.

*Tanner, C. A. (2006). Thinking like a nurse: A research-based model of clinical judgment in nursing. *Journal of Nursing Education, 45*(6), 204–211.

---

*Indicates classic reference.

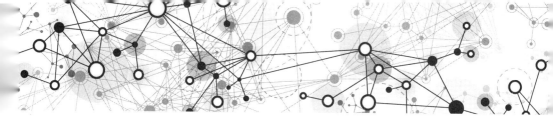

CHAPTER 9

Using Case Studies Effectively in a Concept-Based Curriculum

Donna Ignatavicius

CHAPTER LEARNING OUTCOMES

After studying this chapter, the reader will be better able to:

1. Review the origins of the nursing process and critical thinking in nursing.
2. Explain the relationship between clinical reasoning and clinical judgment.
3. Identify the four components of Tanner's Clinical Judgment Model.
4. Describe the purposes and use of case studies in the classroom or online to create clinical imagination in a concept-based curriculum (CBC).
5. Differentiate Single and Unfolding Case Studies to facilitate conceptual learning and clinical reasoning.
6. Explain the benefit and attributes of using Unfolding Case Studies in a CBC.
7. Explain the components of an Unfolding Case Study.
8. Describe the similarities and differences between the Unfolding and Continuing Case Study.

▶ Introduction to Case Studies

For a number of years, nursing education and clinical researchers have reported the lack of new graduates' ability to use critical thinking and clinical reasoning to provide safe, quality care in today's very complex healthcare environment (Benner, Stephen, Leonard, & Day, 2010; Del Bueno, 2005; Kavanagh & Szweda, 2017). Using case studies in a CBC can improve these skill sets and help students link classroom knowledge with clinical experience. This chapter begins with a discussion of clinical reasoning and clinical judgment as a basis for case studies to help students translate knowledge into practice, develop clinical reasoning, and promote conceptual learning in a concept-based curriculum (CBC).

▶ The Nursing Process and Critical Thinking

Nurses have used the *nursing process* as the basis for patient care since the first book on the topic was published by Yura and Walsh in 1967. At that time, the nursing process was a four-step problem-solving approach—assessing, planning, implementing, and evaluating—and preceded the work of the North America Nursing Diagnosis Association (now referred to as NANDA-I). This organization's work on developing and recognizing nursing diagnosis was consistent with the added nursing process step of Analysis. Alfaro-LeFevre (2017) relabeled this step as Diagnosis and defined it as "analyzing data to identify actual and potential health problems, risk factors, and strengths" (p. 8).

Although the work of NANDA-I has been useful in establishing the autonomy of nurses to make nursing diagnoses based on the interpretation of assessment data, it does not reflect the full scope of the current need for complex nursing thinking (Benner et al., 2010; Rischer, 2015). Another concern about nursing diagnoses is that nurses work collaboratively with patients, families, and members of the interprofessional team and therefore need to communicate effectively using a language that everyone understands. The work of the Quality and Safety Education for Nurses (QSEN) Institute also validated the need for nurses to learn how to communicate effectively for collaborative care using a common language (Cronewett, L., personal communication, 2009). The NANDA-I nursing diagnoses are not commonly used in the United States and Canada among nurses in clinical practice.

During the 1980s, a new term emerged in nursing education—*critical thinking*. Since then, many definitions of critical thinking have been reported in the general education and nursing literature. To measure critical thinking (also sometimes referred to as analytical thinking), various tests were developed for use on admission and at graduation to determine the growth of students during the program. Unfortunately, the results demonstrated that these tools were not sufficient to measure critical thinking in nursing because students either scored the same on both assessments or had decreased scores at graduation. Therefore, for over 30 years, there has been no clear and widely accepted definition and evaluation of critical thinking in nursing.

Clinical simulation literature focuses on critical thinking development. In their simulation study, Cazzell and Anderson (2016) equated critical thinking with the classic executive cognitive functions identified by Welsh (1991). These functions include:

- Problem solving
- Information processing
- Planning ahead
- Working memory
- Attention

Many nursing education researchers and experts have questioned the use of one type of thinking. For example, as a result of the most recent national study of nursing education, Benner et al. (2010) stated that nurses use multiple ways of thinking, including critical, scientific, creative, and criterial reasoning. Therefore, nursing students need to learn more than the nursing process and critical thinking to help them "think like a nurse" in today's complex practice arena.

Although the nursing process can be used with beginning students as a foundational tool, different types of thinking that are less linear and prescriptive are needed to ensure safe, high-quality care (Benner et al., 2010; Del Bueno, 2005; Rischer, 2015; Tanner, 2006). Currently most state Nurse Practice Acts include the term "nursing process." However, the National Council of State Boards of Nursing (NCSBN) 2016 NCLEX-RN® Detailed Test Plan defines nursing process as "a scientific clinical reasoning approach to client care which includes assessment, analysis, planning, implementation, and evaluation" (p. 5). This definition recognizes the movement away from the basic linear problem-solving approach and toward the more current terminology of clinical reasoning and clinical judgment, which are more in line with conceptual teaching and learning.

▶ Clinical Reasoning and Clinical Judgment

For more than a decade, the nursing education literature has shifted from an emphasis on the nursing process and critical thinking to focus more on the Professional Nursing and Health Care concepts of Clinical Reasoning and Clinical Judgment. Some experts use these terms synonymously, whereas others attempt to differentiate them. In either case, these skills better serve students for deep conceptual learning and thinking and are therefore the most appropriate to foster in a CBC.

For this book, Clinical Reasoning is a cognitive process that is more than the steps of the nursing process or critical thinking. In nursing practice, **Clinical Reasoning** is the process of thinking about a patient situation in a specific context while considering patient and family concerns (Benner et al., 2010; Tanner, 2006). **Clinical Judgment** is the conclusion or deduction about the patient's situation and the interventions used for decision making. This patient situation must be put into context to be patient-centered (Benner et al., 2010). Some organizations, such as the National League for Nursing (NLN), use the term *Nursing Judgment* rather than *Clinical Judgment.*

In their study of over 5000 new nursing graduates over a 5-year period, Kavanagh and Szweda (2017) found that novice nurses were not able to fully contextualize the patient experience when assessed on the Performance-Based Development System© (PBDS©). Although many could identify changes in patients' conditions and the concerns of both patients and families in the PBDS video vignettes, they were often not able to determine what actions or interventions to take and why.

These findings are consistent with the five rights of Clinical Reasoning identified by Levett-Jones, Hoffman, Dempsey, Jeong, and Noble (2010):

- Right patient
- Right time
- Right reason
- Right cues
- Right action

One contributing factor to the lack of ability to decide on appropriate action is the lack of connections that new graduates are able to make in a clinical situation. The need to make connections and recognize relationships has been described in previous chapters in this book (see Chapters 2 and 8).

In her meta-analysis, Tanner (2006) developed the well-known and highly respected model of Clinical Judgment, which includes four components: Noticing, Interpreting, Responding, and Reflecting. *Noticing* leads to accurate assessment and considers relationships, patient context, and background of the nurse. The Noticing component is affected by what the nurse brings to a patient situation, such as knowledge, bias, ethical perspective, and expectations. This is part of professional *relational practice* (Benner et al., 2010; Doane & Varcoe, 2015). *Interpreting* requires clinical reasoning to analyze what the patient's status is as a basis for whether to respond to the situation. *Responding* encompasses the actions that the nurse takes (or not) substantiated by current evidence. After the patient situation is managed, *reflecting* allows the nurse to think about his or her actions and determine the current status of the patient. Appropriate Clinical Judgment demonstrates clinical reasoning and accurate translation of nursing knowledge into practice. **TABLE 9-1** shows the relationship between the Nursing Process and Clinical Judgment. However, these models are not the same and do not require the same level of thinking.

The National Council of State Boards of Nursing (NCSBN) recently adopted a definition of clinical judgment as a basis for developing new formats for test items on the NCLEX®. Similar to other definitions, clinical judgment is a process in which the nurse determines and utilizes the best possible evidence-based solutions to ensure safe patient care. NCSBN recognizes five elements of clinical judgment which can be measured and correlated with Tanner's model as follows (Muntean et al., 2016):

- Cue recognition (Noticing)
- Hypothesis generation (Interpreting)
- Hypothesis evaluation (Interpreting)
- Taking action (Responding)
- Evaluating outcomes (Reflecting)

Test items that measure these elements of clinical judgment are being developed and tested over the next few years to best determine how to assess nursing graduates' clinical judgment and higher-order thinking.

TABLE 9-1 Relationship of the Nursing Process and Clinical Judgment

Clinical Judgment Model	Nursing Process
Noticing	Assessment
Interpreting	Analysis/Nursing Diagnosis
Responding	Planning
Responding	Implementation
Reflecting	Evaluation

▶ Translating Nursing Knowledge into Practice

Learning occurs in three domains—cognitive, psychomotor, and affective—representing the application of knowledge, skills, and attitudes that nurses need for safe, high-quality practice. Experienced nurses *integrate* clinical judgment, technical skill mastery, and ethical comportment based on patient context, which can rapidly change.

Benner et al. (2010) identified three professional apprenticeships that students need for professional practice, which include:

- *Cognitive:* Knowledge of science, theory, and principles needed for nursing practice
- *Practice:* Clinical reasoning, situated learning, and a sense of salience by doing
- *Ethical Comportment:* Ability to embody and enact good

Findings from her Carnegie Foundation Advancement for Teaching study (Benner et al., 2010) showed that students' integrative learning during their nursing program occurs primarily in the clinical setting or simulation, but not the classroom or online. In the clinical environment, the three apprenticeships are combined as students learn from caring for patients, sometimes referred to as experiential learning. Learning from a variety of specific patient situations is referred to as situated learning, also called situated cognition. **Situated learning** emphasizes that the student's knowledge is constructed within and linked to the activity, context, and culture in which it is learned.

Clinical nurse educators facilitate situating learning in the clinical environment through teaching by example and coaching students in the development of multiple skill sets. For example, they ask "what if" questions to promote clinical reasoning and anticipate changes in the patient's situation. They also help students set priorities for their patients while recognizing that priorities change as a basis for situated learning. By contrast, nurse educators in the classroom or online setting focus on acquiring knowledge rather than how to translate knowledge into clinical practice. No formal instruction on how to think, set priorities, develop rationales, or contextualize patient situations is typically provided in these learning environments.

> **Remember This . . .**
>
> *Clinical nurse educators facilitate situating learning in the clinical environment through teaching by example and coaching students in the development of these skill sets. For example, they ask "what if" questions to promote thinking and anticipate changes in the patient's situation.*

The result of the typically structured nursing curriculum is fragmentation and lack of deep understanding and thinking by students. In many programs, nurse educators in the classroom rely on lecture (which provides information or knowledge) and multiple PowerPoint slide presentations relaying disease pathophysiology, diagnostic tests, and medical treatments. Other than in the introductory courses, nursing care discussion is limited. Students may take notes and are often not questioned or coached to stimulate any type of thinking, reasoning, or judgment (Benner et al., 2010).

Boyer's Scholarship of Teaching calls for innovation in teaching/learning practices, including integrative pedagogies. The NLN's Core Competencies for the Academic Nurse Educator require that faculty facilitate learning and assist in learner development and socialization (www.nln.org/professional-development-programs /competencies-for-nursing-education/nurse-educator-core-competency). To meet the expected outcome of improving new graduate skills in Clinical Reasoning and Clinical Judgment, nurse educators need to use integrative teaching/learning strategies that connect the classroom with clinical patient situations and provide clinical imagination (Benner et al., 2010). **Clinical imagination** allows students in the classroom to practice or rehearse the clinical reasoning they need in practice through the use of real-world patient situations. One of the best strategies to create clinical imagination is case studies.

▶ Effective Use of Case Studies for Conceptual Learning and Clinical Reasoning

A **case study** is a student-centered learning activity that tells a story based on concepts that demonstrate application or translation of theory to practice. It usually consists of an actual or simulated clinical or healthcare scenario that involves a decision, problem, or issue. Regardless of purpose or type, be sure that clinical scenarios are realistic and reflect patient and family situations that students will likely encounter as professional nurses. Kavanagh and Szweda (2017) recommend that faculty get input from clinical agencies about typical issues and situations that commonly occur in these settings as a basis for case studies. If the nurse educator currently works in the clinical setting, actual patient situations and issues are readily accessible.

Case studies can vary in length and depth depending on their purpose. They may be called Single or Unfolding Case Studies, critical thinking exercises (CTEs), decision-making exercises, clinical reasoning cases, or clinical judgment challenges. Case studies may be assigned as homework or as a preclass activity. In this case, students write out or type their responses to the questions and may be required to bring the completed assignment to class as an Admit Ticket. If any student does not have an Admit Ticket, the nurse educator reminds the student of the assignment and requests that the student work on it outside the classroom until it is completed. Case studies also may be used in class, online, or during the clinical experience.

Regardless of learning environment, be sure that debriefing occurs to review the case study. During debriefing, the nurse educator clarifies misperceptions, highlights the most important concepts, identifies relationships, and summarizes the key points for the case study. Students need feedback so they can learn from their mistakes and refine their clinical reasoning skills.

Single Case Studies, Exercises, and Challenges

Herrman (2016) describes her frequent use of short CTEs in every class as a way to keep students engaged, apply concepts, and promote thinking. The routine use of these mini-cases is consistent with the classic THINK model of Scheffer and Rubenfeld (2000):

T = Total recall and memory (knowledge)

H = Habits of learning and thinking

EXHIBIT 9-1 Critical Thinking Exercises

- You are caring for an older adult diagnosed with new-onset cardiac dysrhythmias and advanced arthritis. What Health and Illness concepts will help you plan your care for this patient?
- A patient reports a pain level of 8 on a scale of 1 to 10 at 1 hour after receiving the prescribed analgesic. What action will you take to manage the pain and why?
- A nursing technician tells you that a postoperative patient's blood pressure decreased from 150/87 to 122/70 in 4 hours. What is your best action at this time?
- A patient tells you that she can no longer afford her diabetic medication and has decided to take half of the prescribed amount each day. How will you respond to her?

I = Inquiry and in-depth thinking (analytic thinking)

N = New ideas and creativity (creative thinking)

K = Knowing how one thinks and reflecting

Consider the CTEs about beginning concepts for a first-level nursing course in **EXHIBIT 9-1**. Unlike the NCLEX®-style test items discussed in Chapter 10, these brief scenarios each include one open-ended question rather than a list of potential answers. This technique allows each student to think about concepts in the classroom by presenting actual patient situations they may encounter in clinical practice. CTEs may be used to introduce concepts or reinforce them. Over time, students learn to think more quickly to answer the questions because they develop thinking as a habit.

Herrman (2016) also discusses the use of Quickie Case Studies, also called Single Case Studies, that are very brief vignettes and serve either to either start or end a class or function as a way to transition from one concept to another. Each case study is comprised of:

- Concept focus
- Decision making required by the student
- Patient/family context
- Supporting patient/family data

Be sure to be specific about patient context and supporting data to prevent overgeneralization by the students.

Some case studies are used to practice setting priorities and concept linkage. When used during class, they may be referred to as Interspersed Case Studies (Herrman, 2016). They are sometimes used before a test as a review for concepts being tested or at the end of class.

Decision-Making or Clinical Judgment Challenges are case studies used to help students "rehearse" for the real world, and may be utilized for pairs or small groups of learners. These scenarios tend to be a little longer than CTEs and more personal by adding identifying information such as name and age. More than one open-ended question is provided in these exercises, as shown in the basic example in **EXHIBIT 9-2**. This case study is appropriate to help students learn how to adapt care for children based on developmental stage.

EXHIBIT 9-2 Example of a Decision-Making Challenge: The Concept of Development

Demetri, a 13-month-old infant, was recently diagnosed with asthma due to his history of gastroesophageal reflux disease (GERD). He has a new prescription for three nebulizer treatments a day for the next week. His mother questions you about how she can give the treatments because Demetri is walking and always active. She is also concerned that the home day care provider may be too busy to give the treatments while caring for other infants and children.

1. Based on Demetri's developmental stage, what adaptation will the parents need to ensure that he successfully receives the medication needed to help control his asthma?
2. If Demetri does not like the mouthpiece for the treatment apparatus, what options are available? What are the advantages of each option?
3. How will you respond to the mother's concern about the day care provider's lack of time to administer the treatments?

Other Single Case Studies may be used to help students learn how to set priorities. Priority Setting is a professional nursing concept needed to ensure safe, high-quality care. In clinical settings, students are coached in establishing priorities of care, but minimal formal education in how to set these priorities is discussed or rehearsed in the classroom or online (Benner et al., 2010). Using case studies helps students to learn this concept and recognize that priorities frequently change as the patient situation changes.

As shown in the example in **EXHIBIT 9-3**, the mother has attempted breast feeding but the baby has not received adequate fluid. He is likely dehydrated, which explains

EXHIBIT 9-3 Clinical Judgment Challenge: The Concept of Priority Setting

A laboring woman (Carol) had an unexpected C-section early on a Friday morning because her cervix failed to achieve adequate dilation. She wanted to have a normal spontaneous vaginal delivery and expressed her disappointment at having an alternative delivery. After giving birth to a healthy 9-pound baby boy, the lactation specialist worked with her that day to assist her with breast feeding. Being an older mother, Carol stayed in the unit for another 2 days over the weekend. On the second hospital day, Carol and her husband reported that the baby "cries continuously no matter what we do." Both the nursing staff and pediatrician told the parents that "babies cry" and that they should not be concerned. When you assess mother-baby as the oncoming 7P-7A shift nurse, you note that only two diaper changes were documented during the last 20 hours. Carol is rocking the baby and expresses her frustration that he continues to cry.

1. What do you *notice* that is of concern in this patient situation? What are the Health and Illness concepts that need to be addressed in this clinical scenario?
2. What additional information do you need at this time for this mother-baby couplet to provide a complete assessment?
3. What is the priority for the care of this mother-baby couplet based on your *interpretation* of the information provided and why?

his continual crying. The lactation specialist may not be there over the weekend, and Carol has likely not had the support she needed to ensure success. She may not have taught about the importance of supplementing with bottle feeding and hydration.

Case studies also may be used in combination with other learning activities, such as clinical experiences or simulation. For example, Holland, Tiffany, Tilton, and Kleve (2017) restructured a second-semester junior community health course for prelicensure BSN students to help students learn the essential concepts of Care Coordination and Transitions of Care (CC/TC). Nursing students are not typically exposed to the continuum of care during their academic program, yet nurses in practice are responsible for ensuring seamless transitions of care from one healthcare agency/provider to another.

Following a community-based observational experience in which students attended support groups for patients with chronic physical or mental illness, each student prepared a written reflection guided by focused response items. The transitions-of-care clinical experience was designed through an electronic health records–based case study about a complex patient with multiple chronic diseases who is transitioning between care settings. As a result of this innovative approach to community health, the authors reported these study findings (Holland et al., 2017). The students were able to:

- Identify four key roles of the professional nurse in CC/TC, including educator, resource provider, care coordinator, and patient advocate.
- Value the patient and family experience during care coordination.
- Translate knowledge and skills that nurses need for CC/TC to practice.

Unfolding and Continuing Case Studies

A Single Case Study presents a patient/family/community situation for one care episode or point in time. An **Unfolding Case Study** evolves over time in a manner that is unpredictable to the learner as new elements (or phases of care) of the case are revealed during multiple patient encounters. The pedagogy of this learning tool is similar to Problem-Based Learning (PBL), an approach that has been used in academic health professions educational programs for more than a decade (Yuan, Williams, & Fan, 2008).

Marques (2017) reported the effective use of case studies for second-degree students to bridge the gap between pathophysiological concepts and clinical reasoning. Based on PBL, the author posted case-of-the-week (COW) exercises online to guide students in applying pathophysiological concepts using real-world scenarios. Although the COWs counted for only 20% of the final course grade, the students were very satisfied with these exercises and thought learning outcomes for the course were achieved.

Both Single and Unfolding Case Studies provide active learning for students, which is a required element of a CBC. These learning tools enable them to:

- Use clinical reasoning to make clinical judgments
- Analyze the supporting data and patient/family context
- Use decision-making approaches and skills
- Cope with ambiguities, or "what if?"

Kim et al. (2006) referred to Unfolding Case Studies as Teaching Cases. The authors identified five attributes of these teaching/learning tools:

- *Relevant:* Meets the level of the learners and allows learners to meet student learning outcomes (SLOs).

- *Realistic:* Information is disclosed over time; some supporting data are missing, requiring learners to make inferences and decisions before all information is available.
- *Engaging:* Allows groups of learners to explore multiple concepts and perspectives.
- *Challenging:* Provides complexity of concepts and thinking.
- *Instructional:* Directs learning and the interpretation of knowledge while allowing assessment of learning and thinking ability.

TABLE 9-2 presents a comparison between traditional teaching/learning and Unfolding Case Studies. As indicated in one of the attributes, using Unfolding Case Studies is ideal for collaboration in small groups of students when complex concepts are being explored. These tools replace a lecture; they should not be a part of or in addition to a lecture.

Remember This . . .

Using Unfolding Case Studies is ideal for collaboration in small groups of students when complex concepts are being explored. These tools replace a lecture; they should not be a part of or in addition to a lecture.

Yousey (2013) described a different approach to using Unfolding Case Studies for students enrolled in an online public health nursing course of an RN-to-BSN completion program. The author required students to collaboratively develop their own case studies based on the concepts of chronic illness. The assignment was scored using a grading rubric.

TABLE 9-2 Comparison of Traditional Teaching/Learning with Learning Through Unfolding Case Studies

Traditional Teaching/ Learning (Lecture)	Use of Unfolding Case Studies
Passive learning	Active learning
Faculty centered	Student centered and interaction between learners the nurse educator
Negates clinical reasoning skill development	Challenges learners to develop clinical reasoning
Creates learner boredom	Keeps learners engaged
Results in surface or superficial learning (memorizing)	Builds on existing knowledge (constructivism) and results in deep conceptual learning

Glendon and Ulrich (1997) introduced and identified seven areas for building an effective Unfolding Case Study:

- Purpose
- Patient context
- Biographical (supporting) data
- Content
- Focused questions
- Collaborative learning
- Reflective writing

As with for all learning activities, the development of Unfolding Case Studies is guided by SLOs for the concepts being learned. For example, consider these content SLOs about the concepts of Perfusion and Coping for patients experiencing trauma:

- Apply knowledge of pathophysiology and psychology to identify priority problems for the trauma patient experiencing impaired Perfusion and ineffective Coping.
- Prioritize whole-person care for the patient experiencing trauma.
- Plan referrals to members of the interprofessional healthcare team to help patients meet optimal clinical outcomes.

The purpose of an Unfolding Case Study to meet these SLOs would be centered on helping students contextualize the patient situation related to the concepts of Perfusion and Coping. Then the patient context, biographical (supporting) data, and content would be constructed to meet the purpose of the case study. Finally, focused thinking questions would be developed for each phase of the patient situation such that groups of students could learn collaboratively and reflect on their responses to the questions. **EXHIBIT 9-4** illustrates an example of an Unfolding Case Study that provides an opportunity for students to meet the previously mentioned SLOs.

EXHIBIT 9-4   Example of an Unfolding Case Study: Care of the Patient Experiencing Trauma

Phase 1: Critical Care

A 29-year-old woman, Cheryl, was admitted to the trauma unit following a motor vehicle accident as a front-seat passenger. She does not have any apparent brain, spinal cord, or internal organ injury. Her right leg sustained multiple compound fractures that are stabilized by an external fixator and extensive soft tissue damage, especially below her knee. Her right leg and foot are very swollen. She also has a right wrist fracture that is immobilized by a splint and multiple superficial lacerations and abrasions. When you first encounter Cheryl, she is crying and trying to talk with her parents, who are with her. When you introduce yourself, she tells you that the doctor told her that she might "lose her leg." She is also in severe pain and says she wishes she would have died in the accident.

1. What is your best response to Cheryl at this time?
2. What priority assessments will you need to perform and why?
3. What nursing interventions will you likely need to implement and why?
4. For what potential complications is Cheryl at risk and why?
5. What action will you take if she experiences any of these complications?

(continues)

EXHIBIT 9-4 Example of an Unfolding Case Study: Care of the Patient Experiencing Trauma (continued)

Phase 2: Acute Care

Two days after admission to the critical care unit, the vascular surgeon determined that Cheryl had adequate peripheral perfusion and was ready for a muscle flap graft followed by another surgery in 2 days to perform an open reduction, internal fixation of her tibia. After these two surgeries, Cheryl's pain remains uncontrolled with a pain intensity rating of no lower than 6 on a scale of 1 to 10 at any time. Her pain level at night is always higher than that in the daytime. One or both of her parents stay with her continuously and tell you that she has become very "emotional" about her situation.

6. What concepts are you concerned about at this time in Cheryl's care?
7. What priority assessments are needed postoperatively for Cheryl? Are they different from those in the first phase of care?
8. What additional subjective data do you need from Cheryl and her family at this time?
9. What referrals might be helpful for the patient to help her cope with the accident and why?

Phase 3: Rehabilitation Phase

After a 2-week stay in critical and acute care for four total surgeries, Cheryl was transferred to an acute rehabilitation unit on Saturday evening. As Cheryl's acute care nurse, you communicate her needs to the evening charge nurse of the rehabilitation unit, being sure to provide specific instructions in the plan of care about her surgical wound care, skin graft site care, pain management regimen, and mental/emotional support.

On Monday morning, Cheryl's parents report to the nurse manager of the rehabilitation unit that the weekend care for their daughter was less than satisfactory. Specific concerns about the lack of quality care included:

- Insufficient dressing supplies to follow the surgical wound care instructions provided by the hospital.
- Lack of knowledge by the nursing staff about how to redress a surgical wound with grafting.
- Inadequate pain management by refusing to give medication that was prescribed PRN for breakthrough pain. (The nurse stated that she was already getting OxyContin on a regular basis and could therefore not have additional medication.)
- Lack of knowledge by nursing staff on how to insert an intermittent urinary catheter for urinary retention; procedure took over an hour to locate the correct orifice for insertion.

10. If you were the nurse manager hearing these patient care concerns, how would you respond?
11. What might be the possible explanation for these issues, and how can they be prevented in the future?

BONUS QUESTIONS: What Health and Illness concepts is the nurse concerned with in this case study? What Professional Nursing concepts is the nurse concerned with in this case study? What Health Care Recipient concepts is the nurse concerned with in this case study?

Prior to working in groups to complete the case study in class, students would be reminded to review the concepts of Perfusion and Coping and read in their textbook about care of patients experiencing fractures. The nurse educator might begin class by asking if there were any questions from the assigned reading that needed clarifying. Then students could be randomly assigned to groups of four to discuss and complete the case.

The time to allot for this work depends on the complexity of the case and the number of care phases. Typically, most Unfolding Case Studies consists of three to four phases of care. If students do not read before class, they usually take longer to complete the case.

Similar to the Unfolding Case Study, the **Continuing Case Study** consists of more than one phase of care over minutes, hours, days, weeks, or months. However, rather than students completing the entire case study in one session, the phases or parts of the case are completed over time during a single class or over several classes during the term. The meta-concept of Perioperative Care would be an appropriate topic for a Continuing Case Study. The nurse educator could begin class with a discussion about preoperative care and then have students translate that knowledge for the case study on care of the patient having a total knee arthroplasty (TKA) (see **EXHIBIT 9-5**). Each student group would discuss, respond, and reflect on their answers to the focused thinking questions. Then the educator could present a video about the surgical procedure for a TKA and lead a class discussion about options for anesthesia and positioning as they might affect postoperative care. The next phase of care for the case (postoperative)

EXHIBIT 9-5 Portion of a Continuing Case Study: Care of the Perioperative Patient

Phase 1: Preoperative Care

A 65-year-old retired man, Marcus, is scheduled to have a total knee arthroplasty (TKA) in 3 months under general anesthesia. He has had multiple injections and arthroscopic surgeries for osteoarthritis in both knees and consequently walks with a limp as a result of his manufacturing job of 43 years. Marcus is 50 pounds overweight and has a history of hypertension and diabetes. His surgeon has recommended that he try to lose at least 10 pounds before surgery. He is married with no children and is anxious to "get this surgery over with." His current medications are:

Amlodipine 10 mg every morning for hypertension
HCTZ 25 mg every morning for hypertension
Ibuprofen 800 mg three times a day for osteoarthritis
Multivitamin 1 cap each day
Docusate Sodium (DOSS) 2 tablets every night

1. Why did the surgeon recommend that Marcus lose weight?
2. What medication(s) will Marcus need to discontinue prior to surgery and why?
3. What preoperative teaching will Marcus need?
4. Marcus tells you the surgeon told him he will have a regional nerve block and is not sure what to expect. How will you respond?
5. Given his history, for what complications is Marcus at risk and why?

could then be presented for students to discuss and complete. Finally, the rehabilitative care for the patient having a TKA could be presented as the third phase of care for groups of students to complete. During debriefing about the case, the educator could ask students to compare and contrast the care for a patient having a hip replaced.

▶ Chapter Key Points

- Using case studies in a CBC can improve clinical reasoning and clinical judgment skills and help students link classroom knowledge with clinical experience.
- Although the work of NANDA-I has been useful in establishing the autonomy of nurses to make nursing diagnoses based on the interpretation of assessment data, it does not reflect the full scope of the current need for complex nursing thinking.
- In nursing practice, clinical reasoning is the process of thinking about a patient situation in a specific context while considering patient and family concerns.
- Clinical judgment is the conclusion about the patient's situation and the interventions used for decision making. This patient situation must be put into context to be patient centered.
- In her meta-analysis, Tanner (2006) developed the well-known and highly respected model of clinical judgment, which includes four components: Noticing, Interpreting, Responding, and Reflecting.
- Clinical nurse educators usually teach by example and by coaching students in the development of these skill sets. For example, they tend to ask "what if" questions to promote thinking and anticipate changes in the patient's situation.
- Clinical imagination allows students in the classroom to practice or rehearse the clinical reasoning they need in practice through the use of real-world patient situations. One of the best strategies to create clinical imagination is case studies.
- A case study is a student-centered learning activity that tells a story based on concepts that demonstrate application or translation of theory to practice. It usually consists of an actual or simulated clinical scenario that involves a decision, problem, or issue.
- During case study debriefing, the nurse educator clarifies misperceptions, highlights the most important concepts, and summarizes the key points for the case study.
- An Unfolding Case Study evolves over time in a manner that is unpredictable to the learner as new elements (or phases of care) of the case are revealed during multiple patient encounters.
- Similar to the Unfolding Case Study, the Continuing Case Study consists of more than one phase of care over minutes, hours, days, weeks, or months. However, rather than students completing the case study in one session, the phases or parts of the case are completed over time.
- Similar to the Unfolding Case Study, the Continuing Case Study consists of more than one phase of care over minutes, hours, days, weeks, or months. However, rather than students completing the case study in one session, the phases or parts of the case are completed over time.

▶ Chapter References and Selected Bibliography

Alfaro-LeFevre, R. (2014). *Applying nursing process: The foundation for clinical reasoning* (8th ed.). Philadelphia, PA: Wolters Kluwer.

Alfaro-LeFevre, R. (2017). *Critical thinking, clinical reasoning, and clinical judgment: A practical approach* (6th ed.). St. Louis, MO: Elsevier.

Benner, P. (2012). Educating nurses: A call for radical transformation—how far have we come? *Journal of Nursing Education, 51*(4), 183–184.

Benner, P., Stephen, M., Leonard, V., & Day, L. (2010). *Educating nurses: A call for radical transformation.* San Francisco, CA: Jossey-Bass.

Billings, D. M., & Halstead, J. A. (2016). *Teaching in nursing: A guide for faculty* (5th ed.). St. St. Louis, MO: Elsevier.

*Boyer, E. L. (1990). *Scholarship reconsidered: Priorities of the professoriate.* San Francisco, CA: Jossey-Bass.

Cazzell, M., & Anderson, M. (2016). The impact of critical thinking on clinical judgment during simulation with senior nursing students. *Nursing Education Perspectives, 37*(2), 83–89.

Day, L. (2011). Using unfolding case studies in a subject-centered classroom. *Journal of Nursing Education, 50*(8), 447–452.

*Del Bueno, D. (2005). A crisis in critical thinking. *Nursing Education Perspectives, 26*(5), 278–282.

Doane, G. H., & Varcoe, C. (2015). *How to nurse: Relational inquiry with individuals and families in changing health and health care contexts.* Philadelphia, PA: Wolters Kluwer.

Dunne, D., & Brooks, K. (2004). *Teaching with cases.* Halifax, Nova Scotia: Society for Teaching and Learning in Higher Education.

*Glendon, K., & Ulrich, D. (1997). Unfolding case studies: An experiential learning model. *Nurse Educator, 22*(4), 15–18.

Herrman, J. W. (2016). *Creative teaching strategies for the nurse educator* (2nd ed.). Philadelphia, PA: F.A. Davis.

Holland, A. E., Tiffany, J., Tilton, K., & Kleve, M. (2017). Influence of a patient-centered care coordination clinical module on student learning: A multimethod study. *Journal of Nursing Education, 56*(1), 6–11.

Kavanagh, J. M., & Szweda, C. (2017). A crisis in competency: The strategic and ethical imperative to assessing new graduate nurses' clinical reasoning. *Nursing Education Perspectives, 38*(2), 57–62.

*Kim, S., Phillips, W. R., Pinksy, L., Brock, D., Phillips, K., & Keary, J. (2006). A conceptual framework for developing teaching cases: A review and synthesis of the literature across disciplines. *Medical Education, 40*(9), 867–876.

Levett-Jones, T., Hoffman, K., Dempsey J., Jeong, S. Y.-S., Noble, D., Norton, C. A., . . . Hickey, N. (2010). The "five rights" of clinical reasoning: an educational model to enhance nursing students' ability to identify and manage clinically "at-risk" patients. *Nursing Education Today, 30*(6), 515–520.

Marques, P. A. O. (2017). Nursing education based on "hybrid" problem-based learning: The impact of PBL-based clinical cases on a pathophysiology course. *Journal of Nursing Education, 56*(1), 60.

Muntean, W., Lindsay, M., Betts, J., Kim, D., Woo, A., & Dickison, P. (April, 2016). *Separating assessment of subject matter knowledge from assessment of higher-order cognitive constructs.* Paper presented at the American Educational Research Association Annual Meeting, Washington, D.C.

National Council of State Boards of Nursing (NCSBN). (2016). *2016 NCLEX-RN® detailed test plan.* Retrieved from www.ncsbn.org/2016_RN_DetTestPlan_Educator.pdf.

Popil, I. (2011). Promotion of critical thinking by case studies as teaching method. *Nurse Education Today, 31*(2), 204–207.

Reese, C. (2011). Unfolding case studies. *The Journal of Continuing Education in Nursing, 42*(8), 344–345.

Rischer, K. (2015). *Think like a nurse: Practical preparation for professional nursing practice* (2nd ed.). Bloomington, MN: Bethany Press.

*Scheffer, B. K., & Rubenfeld, M. G. (2000). A consensus statement on critical thinking in nursing. *Journal of Nursing Education, 39*(8), 352–359.

*Tanner, C. A. (2006). Thinking like a nurse: A research model of clinical judgement in nursing. *Journal of Nursing Education, 45*(6), 204–211.

Victor-Chmil, J. (2013). Critical thinking versus clinical reasoning versus clinical judgment: Differential diagnosis. *Nurse Educator, 38*(1), 34–36.

*Welsh, M. C. (1991). Rule-guided behavior and self-monitoring on the Tower of Hanoi disk-transfer task. *Cognitive Development, 6*(1), 59–76.

Yousey, Y. K. (2013). The use of unfolding case studies: Innovation in online undergraduate nursing education. *Journal of Nursing Education and Practice, 3*(4), 21–29.

Yuan, H., Williams, B., & Fan, L. (2008). A systematic review of selected evidence on developing nursing students' critical thinking though problem-based learning. *Nurse Education Today, 28*(6), 657–663.

*Yura, H., & Walsh, M. B. (1967). *The nursing process: Assessing, planning, implementing, and evaluating.* Washington, D.C.: Catholic University of America Press.

*Indicates classic reference.

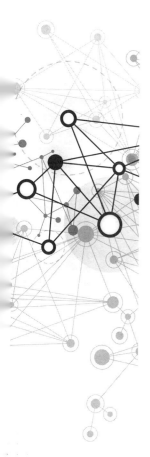

PART III

EVALUATION IN A NURSING CONCEPT-BASED CURRICULUM

CHAPTER 10 Evaluating Learning in the Concept-
Based Curriculum Classroom 185

CHAPTER 11 Evaluating Learning in the Concept-
Based Curriculum Clinical Setting 211

CHAPTER 12 Determining Systematic Methods
for Concept-Based Curriculum
Program Evaluation 233

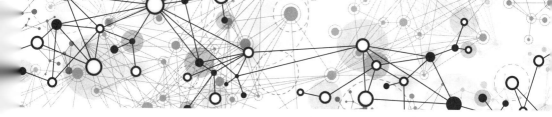

CHAPTER 10

Evaluating Learning in the Concept-Based Curriculum Classroom

Donna Ignatavicius

CHAPTER LEARNING OUTCOMES

After studying this chapter, the reader will be better able to:

1. Differentiate formative and summative methods for evaluating conceptual learning in nursing education.
2. Differentiate the purpose of norm-referenced and criterion-referenced evaluation methods.
3. Describe strategies for decreasing students' cognitive test anxiety to promote student success.
4. Explain the two major conceptual frameworks for the NCLEX® test plans.
5. Identify the components of a meaningful test blueprint to provide evidence of measurement validity.
6. Construct a cognitive test plan for a nursing program to emphasize higher-level conceptual thinking.
7. Distinguish the general principles and common formats for effective NCLEX®-style test item writing.
8. Explain the importance of establishing reliability of examinations.
9. Perform a test item analysis, including item difficulty and discrimination.
10. Describe the role of quizzes in evaluating conceptual learning.
11. Identify the role of papers and projects in evaluating conceptual learning.

▶ Introduction to Evaluation of Conceptual Learning in the Concept-Based Curriculum Classroom

In education, **evaluation** can be defined as the *process* of collecting and analyzing data gathered through one or more measurements to render a *judgment* about the subject of the evaluation (Keating, 2015; Oermann & Gaberson, 2017). Steps of this process are outlined in **BOX 10-1**. This chapter focuses on developing effective tools and methods to appropriately evaluate conceptual learning.

Two common terms are used in educational literature regarding how to determine if students have met course learning outcomes: *Assessment* and *Evaluation*. College, university, and school regional higher education accrediting bodies generally prefer the term *Assessment*. Many higher educational institutions have established Assessment departments or directors to ensure consistency across departments and programs to plan and enforce the institutional assessment plan.

In nursing programs, the term *Evaluation* is usually preferred to be congruent with the language of nursing accrediting bodies. This book uses the term *Evaluation* and recognizes that there are two types of evaluation: formative and summative (Billings & Halstead, 2016). **Formative evaluation** (sometimes referred to as assessment) occurs on an ongoing basis and provides opportunities for students to improve based on nurse educator feedback. Formative evaluation, then, is process-oriented, reflective, and diagnostic. **Summative evaluation** occurs at the end of a unit of study or course and assigns a final score or grade. By contrast to formative evaluation, summative evaluation is product-oriented, prescriptive, and judgmental.

Measurement tools or methods used to evaluate achievement of conceptual learning can be divided into two broad types based on how they are graded: criterion-referenced and norm-referenced. **Criterion-referenced evaluation** requires the learner to meet a predetermined standard or criteria; it is sometimes referred to as grading with an absolute scale. For example, the summative clinical evaluation tool used to measure

---

BOX 10-1 Steps of the Evaluation Process

1. Decide on the specific purpose(s) and faculty philosophy of evaluation.
2. Identify a timeframe for evaluation (formative vs. summative).
3. Establish standards for evaluation (e.g., norm-referenced or criterion-referenced; letter graded or pass/fail?).
4. Select the evaluator(s) (Faculty? Other students? Preceptor? Clients? Self?).
5. Select/develop an evaluation tool/method.
6. Collect and interpret results/data.
7. Use results to make decisions.
8. Evaluate the evaluation process for:
   - Technical accuracy
   - Effectiveness
   - Efficiency
   - Legal and ethical considerations

student clinical performance is a criterion-referenced tool. Students must meet all criteria to pass a clinical course or the clinical component of a course that has both theory and clinical requirements. Chapter 11 focuses on evaluating conceptual learning in the clinical learning environment.

Norm-referenced evaluation tools require the learner to successfully meet expectations, but scores vary and are compared with peer scores; it is sometimes referred to as grading with a relative scale. Using this method, students who perform better than other students receive better grades (Oermann & Gaberson, 2017). An example of a norm-referenced measurement tool is a unit examination.

Validity and Reliability Considerations

An effective evaluation tool requires evidence of measurement (or assessment) validity and reliability. For most evaluation methods and tools used to measure achievement of learning, the most important type of validity is *content-related evidence* of measurement validity. The purpose of content validation is to ensure that the nurse educator is measuring the content and related outcomes that the educator intended to measure.

Although there are several types of reliability, the most useful type to evaluate cognitive learning in the classroom or online is *internal consistency*. This type implies that if a tool is reliable, the same students would get the same scores if they were evaluated again using the same tool.

Learning Domain Considerations

As described briefly in Chapter 2 , learning can occur in one or more of three domains: *cognitive* (using and applying knowledge), *psychomotor* (performing skills as part of total care), and *affective* (appreciating and developing professional attitudes). Each domain has one or more taxonomies (classification systems) that help to show growth and progression in a variety of learning environments.

The development of evaluation methods depends on which learning domain is being measured. For instance, a scholarly paper would reflect learning in the cognitive domain. Reflective journaling would be effective for the affective domain. Skills demonstration in the clinical laboratory reflects learning in the psychomotor domain. In some education environments, such as clinical simulation or external clinical experiences, all three domains can be measured using a clinical performance tool as discussed in Chapter 11.

Other Considerations for Developing Evaluation Methods

The evaluation method also depends on the complexity of the content, the student learning outcomes (SLOs) being measured, and the purpose of the evaluation. For example, consider this SLO for a Doctor of Nursing Practice (DNP) course related to the concept of Systems-Based Practice: *Collaborate with community partners to design a plan to improve patient care outcomes in a local public health system.* The student's ability to meet this SLO using a summative approach cannot be measured using a single test item, quiz, or examination. The verb *Collaborate* indicates performance in working together with others to improve care. Additionally, the complexity of this SLO indicates the need for a student project rather than a test.

> **Remember This . . .**
>
> The evaluation method depends on the complexity of the content, the student learning outcomes (SLOs) being measured, and the purpose of the evaluation.

By contrast, this prelicensure nursing SLO focusing on the exemplar of Deep Vein Thrombosis for the concept of Clotting can easily be measured by one or more test items: *Prioritize nursing actions for the patient experiencing a deep vein thrombosis.* A sample test item to measure whether students met this SLO as part of the first adult health nursing course follows. The * indicates the correct answer.

A client is diagnosed with a lower extremity deep vein thrombosis. What is the nurse's **priority** *when teaching the unlicensed assistive personnel how to provide care for this client?*

    A.   *"Force fluids so that the clot will dissolve more quickly."*
    B.   *"Don't massage the affected leg to avoid dislodging the clot."**
    C.   *"Be sure to put anti-embolism stockings on both legs."*
    D.   *"Raise the bed at the knee to make the client more comfortable."*

▶ Examinations and Quizzes

Written or computerized examinations, usually referred to as tests, are norm-referenced measurement tools commonly used to evaluate cognitive application of concepts for scenarios in nursing education. Prelicensure nursing programs tend to use examinations more often than RN-to-BSN or advanced practice nursing programs. However, graduates from both prelicensure and clinical advanced practice programs must pass a high-stakes examination to become licensed or certified prior to beginning their practice.

Cognitive Test Anxiety

Many nursing students experience cognitive test anxiety (CTA), especially in prelicensure programs in which most of their theory course grade is derived from examination scores. Duty, Christian, Loftus, and Zappi (2016) correlated high CTA of nursing students with reduced academic performance. To help prepare students for the expectations of prelicensure nursing programs and decrease anxiety, targeted strategies and courses have been developed and successfully implemented. For example, Walker (2016) implemented a Nursing Success Boot Camp focused on student test-taking strategies, critical thinking, and clinical reasoning. Latham, Singh, Lim, Nguyen, and Tara (2016) developed a special course for first-generation and minority nursing students that created a sense of community, decreased anxiety, and student success. Some nursing programs also have Student Success Coaches or Retention Coordinators who work with students throughout the program to help them improve academic performance and reduce CTA.

Quinn and Peters (2017) conducted an integrative literature review on ways to decrease student anxiety before and during an examination. Strategies for CTA reduction were divided into two categories: environmental adjustments and student behavioral modifications. Examples of *environmental adjustments* include having students use lemon oil on their hands (to smell) during the test, pet therapy, and music therapy (especially soothing or classical music). The author has had students use pretest stretching and other exercises in the classroom prior to taking an examination. Exercise increases endorphin levels to improve mood, relieve stress, and reduce anxiety. *Student behavioral modifications* include biofeedback, meditation, mindfulness, and progressive muscle relaxation.

Although these approaches are helpful before taking a test, students also have CTA after a test, especially if they fail. One method that can allay anxiety is to provide a test review for all students as soon as possible either in class or online. Students deserve to know what the correct answers are and evaluate where they made their errors. Some faculty do not provide this group review for fear of controversy and confrontation by students. However, the nurse educator needs to know how to manage the classroom or online environment and conduct a professional and respectful test review. The author has found that providing an opportunity for learning through collaborative testing decreases controversy and reduces CTA. Chapter 5 describes this learning activity in detail.

After the group test review, the role of the nurse educator is to identify students at high risk for course failure and intervene as early as possible to plan strategies for student success. One tool to help students identify their trends in testing is found in **EXHIBIT 10-1**. Wiles (2015) described another useful tool for test analysis that also included major areas on the NCLEX®, such as pharmacology, psychosocial integrity, physiological integrity, and nursing process. This tool helps prelicensure students identify specific content areas in which they need improvement.

With both types of tools, students review their test individually with the nurse educator to determine what problems in testing they demonstrated. For example, a student may lack confidence and frequently change his or her answers. Another student may miss key words or not comprehend certain vocabulary. After this review, the nurse educator and/or success coach (if available) can advise the student on ways to improve for future tests.

NCLEX®-Style Tests

To simplify grading of examinations, most nurse educators use objective-formatted items rather than short-answer or essay-type questions when possible. This chapter focuses on objective-type items because both the NCLEX® and nursing certification examinations for specialty advanced practice incorporate these items. Essay-type questions may be useful for higher-level thinking, but require a grading rubric to minimize subjectivity. Because most graduate programs in nursing are not conceptually based, the discussion of testing is limited to prelicensure testing. However, the same principles apply in all types of programs.

Currently the NCLEX®, a computerized adaptive test (CAT), is available in all 50 U.S. states, U.S. territories, and Canada. Graduates who pass the NCLEX® demonstrate *minimal safety* and are therefore eligible to be licensed in their state, province, or territory to practice nursing. The graduate who qualifies to take the NCLEX-RN® has between 75 and 265 test items to complete in 6 hours. The NCLEX-PN® has between 85 and 205 test items to take in 5 hours.

EXHIBIT 10-1 School of Nursing and Health Sciences Individual Test Analysis

Semester: _Spr '17_   Date: _____   Test #: _____   # Items on the Test: _____

Questions Missed							
#	Q #	Subject	Misread Question	Misunderstood Question	Read into the Question	Missed Important Keyword in Question	Did Not Remember/ Recognize Subject Matter
1							
2							
3							
4							
5							
6							
7							
8							
9							
10							
11							
12							
13							
14							
15							
16							
17							
18							
19							
20							
21							
22							
Summary...							

Correct: _____   # Missed: _____   Final Score: _____

Did Not Understand Subject Material	Did Not Recognize Rationale for Correct Answer	Guessed Wrong	Changed Answer	Marked Scantron Incorrectly	Did Not Read All Responses Carefully	Used Incorrect Rationale for Selecting Response

Nurse educators teaching in prelicensure nursing programs typically use NCLEX®-style tests to evaluate conceptual learning and clinical judgment. Advantages of using this type of test include:

- Allows students preparing to take the NCLEX-RN® or NCLEX-PN® an opportunity to practice similarly constructed test items
- Provides a measurement of student learning and clinical reasoning as a summative evaluation method
- Provides feedback for nurse educators regarding effectiveness of the learning and the need for remediation
- Consists of objective-type formatted items, which simplifies grading
- Can be statistically analyzed to determine the quality of the test

NCLEX® Test Plans

The National Council of State Boards of Nursing (NCSBN) provides several versions of the most recent test plans for both the NCLEX-RN® and NCLEX-PN® (www.ncsbn.org). The most useful version of the plan for nurse educators is the Detailed Test Plan – Item Writer/Item Reviewer/Nurse Educator Version. For the NCLEX-RN®, the test plan is dated 2016; for the NCLEX-PN®, the test plan is dated 2017. Every 3 years, the NCSBN conducts a survey of nurses who have been practicing for a year. Prior to the most recent NCLEX-PN® test plan, nurses were surveyed after 6 months in practice. The survey asks nurses to identify what knowledge (cognitive learning domain), skills (psychomotor learning domain), and attitudes (affective learning domain) they must have to function as a safe competent nurse. Survey data are analyzed and compiled into Nursing Activity Statements, which are included throughout the NCLEX® test plans by category.

Based on these statements from the practice analysis and expert opinion of the NCLEX® Examination Committee and members of various state boards of nursing, specific competencies are outlined in the detailed test plans as a basis for test items. Nurse educators can apply as item writers to develop test items for both licensure examinations through their state board of nursing or other local regulatory body. Each item is aligned with a competency and reviewed by nurse educator item reviewers. The final versions of the items are then assessed as part of future licensure examinations through the standardized psychometric steps required to establish validity and reliability. For that reason, 15 of the NCLEX-RN® items and 25 of the NCLEX-PN® items for graduates do not count as part of their score to determine passing or failing the examination because they are being pretested.

The NCLEX-RN® and NCLEX-PN® test plans have a similar structure based on major concepts and sub-concepts rather than medical diagnosis. Both plans identify a list of Integrated Processes (IP), which include:

- Nursing process (for RN)/Clinical Problem-Solving Approach (for PN)
- Caring
- Teaching and Learning
- Communication and Documentation
- Culture and Spirituality

Each of these IPs is defined and is consistent with the scope of practice for the RN and LPN/LVN (see www.ncsbn.org). The Nursing Process is defined as a scientific

EXHIBIT 10-2 Example of NCLEX®-Style Test Item That Assesses Caring

A nursing assistant states that the client's blood pressure decreased from 142/88 to 104/60 over the past 2 hours. What is the nurse's **best** response?

   A. "That can't be right; there's no reason why the blood pressure would be so low."
   B. "Take it again just to make sure you got the correct reading."
   C. "Thank you for telling me; I'll go check on the client now."
   D. "I think these machines aren't giving us accurate readings."

Correct response: C

Rationale: The correct response demonstrates respect and trust between the nurse and nursing assistant. Mutual respect and trust are consistent with the definition for Caring provided in the NCLEX® test plans.

clinical reasoning approach to care. Culture and Spirituality was added as an IP to the most recent NCLEX® test plans. Each item in the test bank for the licensure examinations is aligned with one of the IPs. Interestingly, Caring is an affective or "soft" concept measured as part of the licensure examinations. A sample test item that evaluates caring is cited in **EXHIBIT 10-2**.

In addition to identifying the five IPs, the test plans are organized by four major Client Needs Categories (CNC). Two of the four are subdivided into conceptual categories for a total of eight total categories (see www.ncsbn.org):

- Safe and Effective Care Environment
  - Management of Care (for RN)/Coordinated Care (for PN)
  - Safety and Infection Control
- Health Promotion and Maintenance
- Psychosocial Integrity
- Physiological Integrity
  - Basic Care and Comfort
  - Pharmacological and Parenteral Therapies (for RN)/Pharmacological Therapies (for PN)
  - Reduction of Risk Potential
  - Physiological Adaptation

As the name implies, Safe and Effective Care Environment focuses on safe practices. Examples of topics within this category include prioritization; assignment, delegation and supervision; case management; security plans; and home safety. Consider this multiple-choice item to measure the student's ability to apply the concept of Delegation. The * indicates the correct response.

Which task or activity is appropriate for the nurse to delegate to the nursing assistant?

   A. A gastrostomy tube feeding
   B. Stage I pressure injury care*
   C. Urinary catheterization
   D. Intravenous site care

Health Promotion and Maintenance includes healthy perinatal care, lifespan development (from newborn through older adulthood), health screenings, health teaching, and immunizations. Psychosocial Integrity focuses on topics such as therapeutic communication, cultural awareness, suicide risk, abuse/neglect, and substance use disorder. Physiological Integrity is the largest Client Needs Category and includes concepts such as:

- Mobility/Immobility
- Nutrition
- Elimination
- Dosage calculation
- Medication administration
- Laboratory tests
- Medical emergencies
- Fluid and electrolyte imbalance

Both NCLEX® test plans outline percentage ranges for each CNC to represent how much of the examination is dedicated to each category. For example, Psychosocial Integrity is 9% to 15% of the NCLEX-PN® (see www.ncsbn.org). Most items for both licensure examinations focus on Safe and Effective Care Environment and Physiological Integrity.

Cognitive Levels of NCLEX®-Style Test Items

The concept of **Cognition** is "the complex integration of mental processes and intellectual function for the purposes of reasoning, learning, and memory" (Ignatavicius, Workman, & Rebar, 2018, p. 16). From his classic research, Bloom (1956) developed a cognitive taxonomy to describe the levels of cognition that learners demonstrate. NCLEX® test items are based on the *revised* Bloom's cognitive taxonomy developed by Anderson and Krathwohl (2001). **TABLE 10-1** compares Bloom's original six cognitive (thinking) levels with those of Anderson and Krathwohl. The major difference is that the *revised* Bloom's levels are verbs or gerunds rather than nouns. The other change was that the highest level in Bloom's levels is evaluation; the highest level in the *revised* Bloom's taxonomy is creating.

EXHIBIT 10-3 presents examples of multiple-choice items for Remembering and Applying cognitive levels to show the difference in the thinking required to answer each question. Note in the first item (A. Remembering) that the student is required only to regurgitate the memorized normal value of serum potassium. In the second item (B. Applying), the student has to determine the most appropriate nursing intervention based on an accurate interpretation of the serum potassium value. According to the NCLEX-RN® and NCLEX-PN® test plans, the majority of the licensure examination items are at the Applying and higher levels and present clinical scenarios that require more complex thinking.

Although there are six cognitive levels in the revised Bloom's taxonomy, they can be divided into two broad categories: not critical thinking/clinical reasoning (Remembering and Understanding) and critical thinking/clinical reasoning (Applying and higher). Although this simplified approach may seem unconventional, it serves as a way to determine items that require (or not) the ability of the student to make appropriate clinical judgments using critical thinking and clinical reasoning. **EXHIBIT 10-4** provides a useful tool to determine whether an NCLEX®-style test item is at the Applying or higher level.

TABLE 10-1 Comparison of the Original Bloom's Cognitive Taxonomy with the Revised Bloom's Taxonomy (from Lowest to Highest Level)

Original Bloom	Description of Level for Evaluation of Learning	Revised Bloom
Knowledge	Lowest cognitive level in which learner regurgitates memorized knowledge of concept; no understanding of concept.	Remembering
Comprehension	Learner demonstrates understanding and recalls knowledge of one concept.	Understanding
Application	Learner uses knowledge in new situations; requires recall of two or more concepts or principles.	Applying
Analysis	Learner is required to break down the situation and identify key concepts to answer the question.	Analyzing
Synthesis	Learner is required to put concepts together with information to create a question.	Evaluating
Evaluation	Learner makes judgment about the situation to derive an answer.	Creating

Using these two broad categories, nursing faculty can determine when to introduce higher-level items into the program and how to show progression of more complex thinking. For example, consider this cognitive plan for testing in an associate-degree nursing program that has four nursing semesters:

	Semester 1	Semester 2	Semester 3	Semester 4
Remembering/ Understanding (not critical thinking/clinical reasoning)	50%	30%	15%	0%
Applying and higher (critical thinking/clinical reasoning)	50%	70%	85%	100%
Total	100%	100%	100%	100%

EXHIBIT 10-3 Examples of Multiple-Choice Test Items at Two Different Cognitive Levels

A. Remembering

A client is preparing to have a serum potassium level drawn. What is the normal value of serum potassium?

A. 4.5 – 6.0 mg/dL
B. 4.0 – 5.5 mg/dL
C. 3.5 – 4.5 mg/dL
D. 2.0 – 3.0 mg/dL

Correct response: C

SLO = State the normal value of serum potassium as part of the concept of Fluid and Electrolyte Balance.

B. Applying

*A client is receiving an IV of 5%D/0.45%NS with 40 mEq of potassium added. The nurse notes that the most recent serum potassium level is 5.2 mg/dL. What is the nurse's **priority** action?*

A. Inform the primary healthcare provider.
B. Assess the client for any changes in condition.
C. Document the serum potassium level.
D. Stop the intravenous fluid immediately.

Correct response: D

SLO = Apply knowledge of the concept of Fluid and Electrolyte Balance to determine priority nursing interventions.

This program's cognitive plan shows progression across the curriculum. By having 100% of the test items at a higher thinking level by the end of the program, the student should be prepared to successfully answer the questions on the NCLEX®. Remember, though, that if a test needs to consist of 85% Applying items, the corresponding SLOs have to be at that level.

Evidence of Measurement Validity

To establish content-related evidence of measurement validity, create a blueprint (also known as a test plan) before developing a test. *Avoid the pitfall of developing the blueprint after giving the examination, which is not best practice.* A test blueprint illustrates how student learning outcomes (SLOs) and concepts align with the test items. It also demonstrates congruency of the test with the NCLEX® test plan (see **EXHIBIT 10-5**).

Remember This . . .

Avoid the pitfall of developing the blueprint after administering the examination, which is not best practice.

Examinations and Quizzes **197**

EXHIBIT 10-4 How to Determine if a Nursing Test Item Is Written at the Applying Level or Above

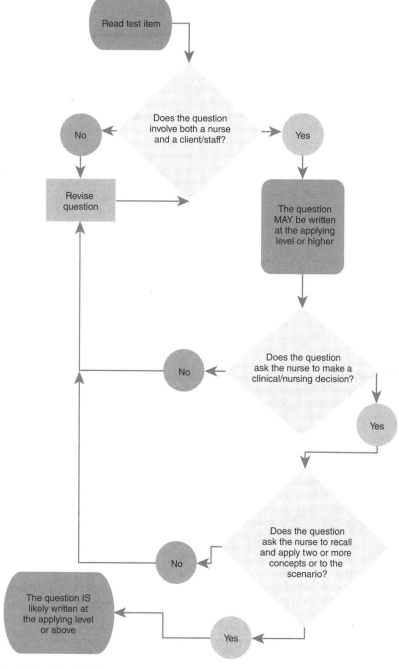

Read test item

Does the question involve both a nurse and a client/staff?

No

Yes

Revise question

The question MAY be written at the applying level or higher

Does the question ask the nurse to make a clinical/nursing decision?

No

Yes

Does the question ask the nurse to recall and apply two or more concepts or to the scenario?

No

Yes

The question IS likely written at the applying level or above

Courtesy of Donna Ignatavicius and Lee Henderson

EXHIBIT 10-5 Portion of a Sample Test Blueprint Form to Demonstrate Measurement Validity

Item #	SLO#	Cognitive Level	Concept	Integrated Process	Client Needs Category
1	3	Understanding	Cognition	Caring	Psychosocial Integrity
2	7	Applying	Elimination	Nursing Process	Physiological Integrity
3	5	Applying	Mood and Affect	Communication and Documentation	Safe and Effective Environment

The most important part of the test blueprint for faculty-created tests is the alignment of each test item with a content-level SLO and concept. The cognitive level of the SLO must match the cognitive level of the test item. For example, the Applying level test item in Exhibit 10-3 does not align with the SLO for the Remembering item, even though both questions are about Fluid and Electrolyte Balance related to potassium. It would be unfair for the nurse educator to provide a low cognitive level SLO such as "state the normal value of serum potassium," and then require the student in a test item to prioritize care for the client who has a high potassium level.

Another column of the test blueprint is for identifying the Health (or Health and Illness), Professional Nursing and Health Care, or Health Care Recipient concept being evaluated. For example, both test items in Exhibit 10-3 relate to the concept of Fluid and Electrolyte Balance.

The remaining components of the blueprint are the NCLEX® IP and Client Needs Category. Both test questions in Exhibit 10-3 relate to the IP of the Nursing Process and the Client Needs Category of Physiological Integrity. If the nurse educator desires to identify the sub-category within the broader one for these test items, both are aligned with Physiological Adaptation.

Test blueprints are guidelines and, therefore, many nurse educators share them with students to help them prepare for the test. Other educators are concerned that sharing the blueprint will "give away the test." However, no specific information about the type of test item or clinical scenario is provided. Nurse educators share the student learning outcomes and should therefore use the blueprint as a type of study guide for students in preparing for the test.

Types of NCLEX® Item Formats

Examples of all of the NCLEX® item formats are included in the NCLEX® test plans. All items can be broadly divided into selected response and constructed response questions. **Selected response test items** provide choices from which the test taker must choose to get the correct answer, also referred to as multiple-choice items. **Constructed response test items** require the test taker to either manipulate information provided in the question or create an answer.

Currently there are two types of selected response test items on the NCLEX®: single response and multiple response. A **single-response item** consists of a stem and four choices; only one choice is the best response or answer. Examples of this type of test item may be found in Exhibit 10-3.

A **multiple-response item** consists of a stem (clinical scenario) and five to seven choices; two or more choices are the best response or answer. This item is also called a Select All That Apply (SATA) question and is graded as either correct or incorrect; no partial credit is given. These items often test the following content areas:

F = Risk *F*actors

A = *A*ssessment Findings

C = Potential *C*omplications

T = Nursing *T*reatments (interventions)

An example of a SATA item that measures the students' understanding and application of the concept of Cognition is:

Which assessment findings will the nurse expect when caring for a client with delirium? **Select all that apply.**

    A.   Acute confusion
    B.   Restlessness
    C.   Wandering
    D.   Forgetfulness
    E.   Agitation

    Correct response: A, B, D, E

SATA test items are considered to be the most difficult type of item, and, as a result, students typically do not like them. However, because they are difficult and higher-level questions, graduates who pass the NCLEX in 75 items report that SATA items comprise over half of the licensure examination. For that reason, some programs develop a progression plan to gradually increase this type of item.

Currently there are four types of constructed response test items on the NCLEX®, but they are less commonly seen on the examination when compared to the number of SATA questions:

- Fill-in-the-blank (completion)
- Drag and drop/Rank order/Ordered response
- Hot spot
- Exhibit

Fill-in-the-blank items require a numeric calculation, such as drug dosage, IV calculation, intake and output, and drainage. *Drag and drop/Rank order/ordered response* items ask the test taker to rearrange steps of a procedure or prioritize care interventions. *Hot spot* test items provide the test taker with a graphic on which to indicate the correct answer by an "X" or a mouse click; for example, to show where the nurse places a stethoscope to listen to breath sounds in the base of the left lung. *Exhibit items* require the test taker to open the exhibit, which is usually parts of the medical record, to obtain additional information to best answer the question. Laboratory data, vital signs, primary healthcare provider prescriptions, and the medication administration record may be accessed.

Any item format can include graphic or audio options. For example, consider this single-response, multiple-choice item that measures the student's understanding and application of the concept of gas exchange:

*A client reports difficulty breathing after walking to the bathroom. The nurse hears these breath sounds. What is the nurse's **best** action?*

- A. *Document the assessment findings in the health record.*
- B. *Begin oxygen via nasal cannula at 2 Liters/minute.*
- C. *Tell the client to take more time when walking.*
- D. *Keep the head of the bed in semi-Fowler's position.*

This test item requires the test taker to listen to recorded breath sounds to answer the question. Other items list graphics or pictures as choices rather than phrases or sentences. This option is useful when asking about equipment to use or demonstrating how to draw up parenteral medications.

In the item presented previously, the wrong choices, also called **distractors**, are viable and relate to the client's problem. When writing distractors, be sure that each choice is distinct and discrete. Do not include the same terminology in multiple choices.

General Principles of NCLEX®-Style Test Writing

Because the NCLEX® is a timed test within a set number of hours, students should have an equitable amount of time for unit and final examinations during the program, or 1.5 minutes per item. The average unit examination is typically 40 to 50 items; the typical number of unit examinations per semester is four and a comprehensive final, which is approximately twice as long as each unit examination.

Once the test blueprint is developed, item writing can begin. Because most items on the NCLEX® are at the Applying or higher level, each item should consist of a short scenario in which there is interaction between a nurse and a patient/client or a nurse and a staff member. The test item asks what the nurse will do in each situation. Demographic or patient variables should not be included unless they are needed to answer the question. The client's medical diagnosis is also not included unless needed to answer the test item. For example, consider this test item. The * indicates the correct responses.

*A client is on seizure and aspiration precautions. What emergency equipment will the nurse have at the bedside? **Select all that apply.***

- A. *Padded tongue blade*
- B. *Suction apparatus**
- C. *Oxygen setup**
- D. *Vest restraint*
- E. *Artificial airway**

The SLO for this item could be: Plan appropriate interventions for clients on seizure and aspiration precautions to promote *oxygenation*. (NOTE: Oxygenation is the concept being tested.) In this item, the medical diagnosis is not necessary to answer the question.

However, the following test item stem needs the medical diagnosis to arrive at the correct response. The * indicates the correct response.

*The nurse is teaching a new diabetic client about foot care. Which statement by the client indicates a need for **further** teaching?*

    A.   *"I will wash and dry my feet every day."*
    B.   *"I will use lotion every day to prevent dryness."*
    C.   *"It's OK to walk barefooted this summer."**
    D.   *"I will inspect my feet carefully every day."*

The SLO for this test item is: Evaluate the effectiveness of health teaching about impaired *perfusion* associated with diabetes. (NOTE: Perfusion is the concept being tested; diabetes is the exemplar.)

When writing an NCLEX-style item, avoid the pitfall of using negative words such as "not," "except," and "but." Negative items make the test taker select the best *wrong* answer, which can be very confusing to the student. However, in the previous item, the student must select the wrong response by the client. This is an acceptable way to write a negative item without using negative terms. The test taker is determining how to evaluate the effectiveness of teaching.

Remember This . . .

When writing an NCLEX-style item, avoid the pitfall of using negative words such as "not," "except," and "but." Negative items make the test taker select the best wrong answer, which can be very confusing to the student.

For all NCLEX®-style test items, use "a client" and "the nurse" as frequent terms in each test item. Other current language includes:

"The client reports" (rather than "complains")

"Primary healthcare provider" (rather than "physician")

"Prescribe" or "prescription" (rather than "orders" or "order")

The nurse "will" (rather than the nurse "should")

Additionally, key words such as "first," "best," and "next" are all bolded in the item stem.

Another consideration for writing test items is to be aware that unintentional cultural bias is common. For example, nurse educators often refer to the nurse as "she." Foods that are locally or regionally limited are sometimes used in test questions and should be avoided. For example, "pop" is commonly used in the Midwest to describe a carbonated beverage. Terms used in other parts of the country and Canada include "soda," "coke," and "soft drink." International students often have difficulty interpreting the meaning of these terms. Avoid regional foods, such as "fatback," "scrapple," and "hoghead cheese." Recognize that English as a second language/English-language learners (ESL/ELL) students may have never had hot dogs, bologna, or cold cuts.

Also avoid idioms and metaphors that would only be understood by students whose primary language is English. For example, consider these phrases:

- Motherhood and apple pie
- Totally stressed out
- Cold turkey

These phrases are difficult for ESL/ELL students to understand, and therefore they may not correctly answer questions that include this language.

Another concern about vocabulary is reading level. Nonmedical words with multiple syllables are not used when a shorter word is available. Students have high CTA and may not recall the definitions of more difficult lay terms. Avoid using words such as "concurrently," "unequivocal," and "spontaneously." The National Council of Boards of Nursing uses a team of cultural experts to ensure that the NCLEX® is culturally sensitive and educationally appropriate.

Evidence of Test Reliability

A basic principle of research and measurement is that if reliability is not established, then validity could be threatened. The most important evidence of reliability for an NCLEX®-style unit or comprehensive examination is internal consistency because it is not practical to repeat the examination for test-retest reliability (McDonald, 2014). The Kuder-Richardson (KR)-20 is a commonly used reliability coefficient because test items in nursing education are often scored as either right or wrong. The KR-20 is based on the proportion of correct responses and the standard deviation of the score distribution. The potential numeric range for KR-20 is 0 (no reliability) to 1.00 (perfect). When scoring is dichotomous, the alpha coefficient is the most appropriate indicator of internal consistency (McDonald, 2014).

No measurement is perfect; all tools contain error. Although measurement error cannot be avoided, the purpose of writing a good test is to decrease the error and increase test reliability and confidence in the scores. Therefore, when interpreting the KR-20 of a test, keep in mind that these factors can affect the reliability coefficient:

- *Length of test*: If the test is too short, the KR-20 will be low. Be sure your examinations are at least 40 to 50 items.
- *Difficulty of test items*: If the test is too easy or too difficult, the KR-20 will be low. Be sure that the difficulty level represents a range of levels. (See discussion of item difficulty in the next section.)
- *Test item discrimination*: The greater the test item discrimination values, the higher the KR-20 will be; conversely, low item discrimination can result in a low KR-20 value. Be sure to write items that discriminate well. (See discussion of item discrimination later in the next section.)
- *Size and homogeneity of the test group*: A small class size will result in a lower KR-20 than a larger class because the range and distribution of scores is narrow. As the class becomes more homogeneous and those students who cannot meet academic standards fail or leave a program, the KR-20 may also decrease. A large heterogeneous test group usually yields a higher reliability coefficient.

Test Item Difficulty

Item analysis is the best way for the nurse educator to determine the fairness of the test and improve the quality of selected test items that may be used on potential future examinations (McDonald, 2014). It is also an opportunity to address poorly written items and provide allowances on the *current* test for students. Item difficulty affects test reliability and is calculated using a Scantron® machine (paper and pencil testing), computerized software program, or the testing component of a learning management system. If needed, item difficulty can easily be calculated by hand. Each of these methods provides the nurse educator with information about how many students selected each choice in a multiple-choice item. For example, consider this item. The * indicates the correct response.

A	B	C	D
35*	8	7	0

In this item for a class of 50 test takers, 35 students selected the correct response. Test item difficulty is defined as the percent of students who got the item correct or 35/50 = 70%. This item was not too easy or too difficult. When reported as a p level, the percent is changed to a decimal, such that for this item, p = 0.70.

Although differences in opinion exist regarding the desired item difficulty range for a test, consider that nursing tests should not represent the "normal curve." There is nothing "normal" about failing an examination if the score is below 80. In nursing education, the score required to pass a course is higher than for other departments or colleges. If items are consistently *below* 80%, no one in the class will pass the test. Some testing experts have called for writing test items that are between a p value of 0.60 and 0.90 (McDonald, 2014).

Another controversial discussion is about mastery items. Is it ever appropriate for the nurse educator to want all test takers to get an item correct? In nursing and health care, failing to take the best action may result in a complication or even death. The author and others advocate mastery test items if they are designated as such *before* giving the test and do not comprise more than 10% to 15% of the total test score. Consider this mastery item. The * indicates the correct response:

*The nurse is preparing to give metoprolol XL 25 mg to an adult client. What is the **most important** assessment for the nurse to obtain?*

    A.   *Temperature*
    B.   *Oxygen saturation*
    C.   *Apical pulse**
    D.   *Pain level*

To answer this item correctly, the student needs to know what the drug is and its action. All of these vital signs are important, but apical pulse is the most important assessment because beta blockers can cause bradycardia. Failing to note this dysrhythmia could compromise the client's safety.

Test Item Discrimination

As mentioned earlier, test item discrimination affects test reliability more than any other factor. Therefore, it is important that items discriminate between those who know (high test scorers) and can clinically reason and those who cannot (low test scorers). Two statistical tests may be used to determine item discrimination, although some software or web-based programs do not provide both types. These types are point biserial index and item discrimination ratio, or index.

If a test item is easy or mastery, low or no discrimination is expected because nearly all students answered the item correctly; there is little or no difference in test performance for high and low scorers. Therefore, the author recommends that test item discrimination be most closely analyzed for items that less than 50% of the class answered incorrectly. The preferred discrimination statistic is the point biserial index (PBI), also called a point biserial coefficient (PBS). Although several scales delineate PBI range, good test items are those above 0.30; weak or poor items are below 0.10. The mean PBI value correlates with the correct answer. A high PBI indicates a good test item that discriminates well between high and low achievers. A low PBI for the correct answer reflects that the test item did not discriminate well. Wrong answers should have low PBI values. High values for the incorrect choices indicate that more high achievers selected the wrong answer, which means that those choices need revision.

Consider the item statistics in **EXHIBIT 10-6**, Item A. The PBI for the correct answer A is high, reflecting very good discrimination although only 45% of the students got the item correct. All of the distractors have low PBI values indicating that low scorers selected these choices, which is the desired outcome. In Item B, 37% of test takers chose the correct response, but the PBI is very low, indicating that the item discriminated poorly. In this case, the nurse educator can decide (if consistent with program policy) to nullify the item for this test. **Nullifying** means that all choices are acceptable because the test item was poorly constructed. The test takers who chose A do *not* receive extra credit but are given credit for the test item like the rest of the class.

The second method for evaluating test item discrimination is the item discrimination ratio (IDR) or index. For this statistic, the software or web-based program compares the highest scorers (usually upper 27% of test takers) and the lowest scorers (usually lower 27% of test takers) to determine item difficulty for each of these two

EXHIBIT 10-6 Examples of Item Analysis Statistics

A. Example of Good Test Item Discrimination (No need for revision.)		
p value	**PBI value**	
A = 0.45	0.43	CORRECT
B = 0.35	−0.02	
C = 0.06	−0.13	
D = 0.14	0.05	

(continues)

EXHIBIT 10-6 Examples of Item Analysis Statistics (continued)

B. Example of Poor Test Item Discrimination (Item needs revision and should be nullified.)

p value	PBI value	
A = 0.37	0.09	CORRECT
B = 0.35	0.21	
C = 0.15	−0.13	
D = 0.13	0.05	

sub-groups. The expected result is that the many more students in the upper group should answer the items correctly, compared to the lower group. To calculate the actual IDR, subtract the lower group value from the upper group value. For example, for a test item in which 85% of the upper group answered correctly and only 37% of the lower group answered correctly, the IDR is 85% – 37% = 48%, or 0.48. The desired IDR value is a difference of 25% or 0.25. In this case, the item discriminated well because the IDR met the desired value.

However, consider these values:

Upper group = 24% (0.24)

Lower group = 62% (0.62)

The difference in this situation is a negative 38% or –0.38. This value indicates that the item discriminated poorly; it should be nullified now and revised for future tests.

Commercial Standardized Testing

Many prelicensure RN and LPN/LVN programs use standardized testing products sold by companies such as Kaplan, Assessment Technologies Institute (ATI), and Elsevier (HESI). Each company offers a comprehensive array of tests that can be used throughout a nursing program to compare the program's nursing students' performance with national norms. Although the scoring is standardized, the content being tested is not.

Some programs use standardized tests as a high stakes evaluations, despite the National League for Nursing's (NLN's) recommendation *not* to use high stakes testing. Students are given the opportunity to take several practice versions of the test during a course followed by the proctored examination that counts as a grade or score at the end of the course. Faculty require remediation if the student does not meet the recommended cut score on the test. In some programs, the student cannot progress to the next course without passing the proctored examination. In lieu of the high stakes use of these examinations, some programs count the examinations as a percentage of the course grade. Considerations for using commercial standardized testing products include:

- Be selective in how and when tests are used.
- Select the products that best meet your program's needs and curriculum.
- Collect and analyze data from tests to help make program/curriculum changes.

Keep in mind that commercial testing is based on the traditional curricular model, which is content saturated. *No test at the time of this writing is based on concepts and conceptual learning.* Currently there is lack of evidence that commercial standardized testing products are beneficial in increasing student program success or predicting NCLEX® first-time pass rates (Sosa & Sethares, 2015).

Quizzes

Quizzes are short measurement tools used most often for formative evaluation. They usually test at the Remembering level to determine if the students gained the knowledge needed to use in more complex situations. Quizzes may be assigned as a preclass activity as an Admit Ticket, in-class or online activity, or at the end of the class as an Exit Ticket. Students may take quizzes individually, in pairs, or as small groups, depending upon the purpose of their use.

Multiple item formats may be used on a quiz. Each item should meet a student learning outcome as discussed earlier in this chapter. Examples of test item types that are appropriate to assess the Remembering level include:

- *True-false items*: The student is asked to determine if the statement is true or false. For example: *The normal urinary output is at least 30 mL/hour.*
- *Correction true-false items*: The student is asked to determine if the statement is true or false and then correct the false statements. For example: *The normal urinary output is at least 50 mL/h.* The student would need to change the value to the correct number of 30.
- *Matching items*: The student is asked to match a term in one column with its counterpart, often a definition, value, or purpose. For example, a list of drug names could be in one column and a list of their common usage could be in the other column. The student would need to match the drug with its therapeutic purpose.
- *Completion items*: Completion items on a quiz are usually not the same format as on an NCLEX®-style test. Often the test taker has to fill in the blank with a word or several words. For example: *The client who has a serum calcium level of 8.3 mg/dL has _____.* The desired answer is hypocalcemia.
- *Short-answer items*: Instead of requiring the test taker to supply one or more missing words in a sentence, the item is presented as a question. For example: *What assessment findings are common for the client having left-sided heart failure?* Another question that guides the test taker more specifically is *What are four common pregnancy-induced complications?*

▶ Papers and Projects

Similar to all evaluation methods or assignments, papers and projects have a variety of purposes and should relate to the learning outcomes of the course. These types of assignments are typically used more in postlicensure nursing programs than in prelicensure programs. Among prelicensure programs, BSN programs usually require more papers and projects than other types of nursing programs.

Papers may measure learning in the cognitive and/or affective domain. Papers in the cognitive domain are usually assigned as an individual evaluation method and are usually referred to as scholarly papers. Papers that measure affective learning are discussed in Chapter 11. These assignments vary in length, depending on their purpose, and are graded using a grading rubric. In a concept-based curriculum, papers tend to measure conceptual learning that focuses on professional nursing and health care. For example, the nurse educator may assign a scholarly paper requiring the student to research a state legislative bill that would affect the scope of practice for the LPN. This assignment would be appropriate to measure learning about the concept of Health Care Law. The student might be required to analyze the bill and present a strong argument as an opinion paper supported by well-respected sources in favor of or in opposition to the bill.

Projects are often developed by student pairs or larger groups. For instance, students may be required to select a concept that they were introduced to earlier in the curriculum and create a poster that demonstrates how the concept is applied in a specific context, such as for mother-baby content. The student may be permitted to select the concept or be limited to a selection presented by the nurse educator. Examples of concepts that would be appropriate for this activity could include Ethics, Sexuality, Culture, Health Promotion, and Patient Education.

A current trend in writing is to achieve mastery learning. For a paper or project, the nurse educator may assign that selected parts or steps of the assignment be submitted for formative evaluation and feedback. In this way, all students have the opportunity to improve and correct any misconceptions such that the final product reflects excellence.

Regardless of the purpose of the paper or project, these assignments should be scored by the nurse educator using a grading rubric anonymously (Oermann & Gaberson, 2017). In addition, students may critique each other's work using the rubric. Other recommendations about written assignments include (Oermann & Gaberson, 2017):

- Provide clear instructions and expectations for the paper or project.
- Be sure that the assignment is meaningful to the adult learner.
- Avoid requiring too many assignments in any one course; reading and tests count as assignments.
- Place most of the assignment grading weight on content and organization rather than style or grammar.
- Read papers at least twice in random order.
- Have a nurse educator peer evaluate any assignment in which the grading is difficult or uncertain.

▶ Chapter Key Points

- In education, evaluation can be defined as the *process* of collecting and analyzing data gathered through one or more measurements to render a *judgment* about the subject of the evaluation.
- Formative evaluation (sometimes referred to as assessment) occurs on an ongoing basis and provides opportunities for students to improve based on nurse

educator feedback. Formative evaluation, then, is process-oriented, reflective, and diagnostic.

- Summative evaluation occurs at the end of a unit of study or course and assigns a final score or grade. By contrast to formative evaluation, summative evaluation is product-oriented, prescriptive, and judgmental.

- Criterion-referenced evaluation requires the learner to meet a predetermined standard or criteria; it is sometimes referred to as grading with an absolute scale.

- Norm-referenced evaluation tools require the learner to successfully meet expectations, but scores vary and are compared with peer scores; it is sometimes referred to as grading with a relative scale. Using this method, students who perform better than other students receive better grades.

- Many nursing students experience cognitive test anxiety, especially in prelicensure programs in which most of their theory course grade is derived from examination scores. Duty et al. (2016) correlated high cognitive test anxiety with reduced academic performance.

- Written or computerized examinations, often referred to as tests, are commonly used to evaluate application of concepts for scenarios in nursing education.

- The National Council of State Boards of Nursing (NCSBN) provides several versions of the most recent test plans for both the NCLEX-RN® and NCLEX-PN®. (www.ncsbn.org). The most useful version of the plan for nurse educators is the Detailed Test Plan – Item Writer/Item Reviewer/Nurse Educator Version.

- The NCLEX-RN® and NCLEX-PN® test plans have a similar structure based on major concepts and sub-concepts rather than medical diagnosis.

- NCLEX® test items are based on the revised Bloom's cognitive taxonomy developed by Anderson and Krathwohl (2001) (see Table 10-1).

- According to the NCLEX-RN® and NCLEX-PN® test plans, the majority of the licensure examinations consists of questions at the Applying and higher levels that present clinical scenarios that require more complex thinking.

- To establish measurement validity, create a blueprint (also known as a test plan) before developing a test.

- The most important part of the test blueprint for faculty-created tests is the alignment of each test item with a content-level student learning objective and concept.

- In addition to identifying the five Integrated Processes, the NCLEX® test plans are organized by four major Client Needs Categories.

- Selected response test items provide choices from which the test taker must choose to get the correct answer, also referred to as multiple-choice items.

- Constructed response test items require the test taker to either manipulate information provided in the question or create an answer.

- When writing an NCLEX-style item, avoid the pitfall of using negative words such as "not," "except," and "but." Negative items make the test taker select the best *wrong* answer, which can be very confusing to the student.

- The Kuder-Richardson (KR)-20 is a commonly used reliability coefficient because test items in nursing education are often scored as either right or wrong.

- Test item difficulty is defined as the percent of test takers who got the item correct; when the value is presented as a decimal, it is called the p level.

- Point biserial index and item discrimination index, or ratio, compares performance between high and low test scorers.

- Quizzes are short measurement tools used most often for formative evaluation. They usually test at the Remembering level to determine if the students gained the knowledge needed to use in more complex situations.
- *Some prelicensure nursing programs use standardized tests as high stakes evaluations, despite the National League for Nursing's recommendation *not* to use high stakes testing; these tests are not based on concepts or conceptual learning.
- Similar to all evaluation methods or assignments, papers and projects have a variety of purposes and should relate to the learning outcomes of the course.
- Use a grading rubric for written assignments such as papers and projects.

▶ Chapter References and Selected Bibliography

*Anderson, L. W., & Krathwohl, D. R. (2001). *A taxonomy for learning, teaching and assessing: A revision of Bloom's educational objectives.* San Francisco, CA: Jossey-Bass.

Billings, D. M., & Halstead, J. A. (2016). *Teaching in nursing: A guide for faculty* (5th ed.). St. Louis, MO: Elsevier.

*Bloom, B. S. (1956). *Taxonomy of educational objectives: Handbook 1.* New York, NY: David McKay Company.

Duty, S. M., Christian, L., Loftus, J., & Zappi, V. (2016). Is cognitive test-taking anxiety associated with academic performance among nursing students? *Nurse Educator, 41*(2), 70–74.

Ignatavicius, D. D., Workman, M. L., & Rebar, C. R. (2018). *Medical-surgical nursing: Concepts for interprofessional care.* St. Louis, MO: Elsevier.

Keating, S. B. (2015). *Curriculum development and evaluation in nursing.* New York, NY: Springer Publishing.

Latham, C. L., Singh, H., Lim, C., Nguyen, E., & Tara, S. (2016). Transition program to promote incoming nursing student success in higher education. *Nurse Educator, 41*(6), 319–323.

McDonald, M. (2014). *The nurse educator's guide to assessing learning outcomes* (3rd ed.). Sudbury, MA: Jones & Bartlett Learning.

Oermann, M. H., & Gaberson, K. B. (2017). *Evaluation and testing in nursing education* (5th ed.). New York, NY: Springer Publishing.

Quinn, B. L., & Peters, A. (2017). Strategies to reduce nursing student test anxiety: A literature review. *Journal of Nursing Education, 56*(3), 145–151.

Sosa, M.-E., & Sethares, K. A. (2015). An integrative review of the use and outcomes of HESI testing in baccalaureate nursing programs. *Nursing Education Perspectives, 36*(4), 237–243.

Walker, L. P. (2016). A bridge to success: A nursing student success strategies improvement course. *Journal of Nursing Education, 55*(8), 450–453.

Wiles, L. L. (2015). "Why can't I pass these exams? Providing individualized feedback for nursing students. *Journal of Nursing Education, 54*(3 Suppl.), S55–S58.

*Indicates classic reference.

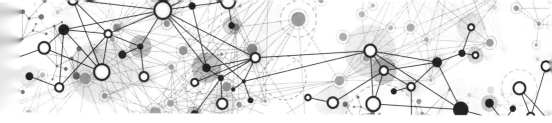

CHAPTER 11

Evaluating Learning in the Concept-Based Curriculum Clinical Setting

Donna Ignatavicius

CHAPTER LEARNING OUTCOMES

After studying this chapter, the reader will be better able to:

1. Identify three ways to ensure fairness and minimize subjectivity in clinical evaluation.
2. Describe how to provide evidence of measurement validity and reliability when using a clinical evaluation tool to measure achievement of student learning outcomes.
3. Explain the purpose and format for a weekly or daily formative evaluation tool to evaluate conceptual learning.
4. Explain the purpose of a summative clinical evaluation tool at the end of a course.
5. Identify the use of standardized patient methodology, clinical simulation, and the objective structured clinical examination as part of the clinical evaluation process to measure conceptual learning.
6. Differentiate ways to evaluate selected focused conceptual learning activities, such as reflection papers and data mining.

▶ Introduction to Evaluation of Learning in the Concept-Based Curriculum Clinical Setting

When compared to evaluation of learning for theory assignments, clinical evaluation is much more subjective. The desired outcome for the nurse educator is to be fair in clinical evaluation and minimize subjectivity. Oermann and Gaberson (2017) suggest that ensuring fairness requires the nurse educator to:

- Create a supportive clinical learning experience for all students.
- Develop clinical evaluation tools (CETs) that are based on preestablished criteria or student learning outcomes (SLOs).
- Identify his or her own values, biases, and beliefs that could affect the process of evaluation.

Creating a supportive clinical learning environment is especially important to help allay student anxiety. Students in the clinical setting often fear that they will accidentally harm the patient, be unprepared for an often-complex and changing clinical setting, and/or not have the knowledge to provide needed patient care. The nurse educator needs to create an atmosphere of learner-centeredness in partnership with the student.

Although the nursing literature indicates that many programs provide a CBC, few articles have been published about evaluating students in this type of curriculum. As discussed in Chapter 6, learning in a CBC clinical setting is different from that in the traditional nursing curriculum. Clinical experiences for students in the CBC clinical environment are categorized as either direct care activities (DCAs) or focused learning activities (FLAs). Each type of clinical activity is graded differently: DCAs are typically graded as satisfactory/pass or unsatisfactory/fail and are criterion-referenced; FLAs are usually scored using a grading rubric and can either be criterion- or norm-referenced.

In addition to clinical experiences in external community-based settings, in-house laboratory skills demonstrations and simulations provide an opportunity for students to meet specific outcomes in a safe environment using varying types of mannequins as patients. These experiences are typically used for learning, but they may also be used as a summative clinical evaluation, sometimes called the Objective Structured Clinical Examination (OSCE). Most nurse educators also usually require clinical paperwork assignments that are evaluated using a grading rubric. This chapter focuses on how to develop and use these clinical evaluative tools in a CBC. Recall that clinical experiences reflect knowledge, skills, and attitudes (KSAs) in the cognitive (thinking), psychomotor (doing), and affective (feeling) learning domains.

▶ Validity and Reliability Considerations

Clinical evaluation methods are measurement tools and thus need evidence of validity and reliability. For example, *content-related evidence of measurement validity* is established by correlating the course SLOs with the tool. An example is provided later in Exhibit 11-2. The most important type of reliability to establish when using a clinical evaluation tool to measure student performance is interrater reliability. Interrater reliability is essential when multiple raters use the same tool for the same purpose with the same class of students.

Various methods may be used to establish *interrater reliability*. Ideally a group of clinical educators would observe the same clinical situation in which a student provides nursing care and rate the student independently. Then the raters would compare their scores to achieve the goal of at least 90% agreement. However, it is often difficult to get a group of clinical educators together, especially when many may be part-time. As an alternative method, have students videotape themselves performing a psychomotor skill or providing patient care in the simulation laboratory. Then each clinical educator can view the recording independently by a certain date to determine the percent of agreement. If the expected 90% agreement is not achieved the first time, plan time to discuss the reasons why the ratings differ. In most cases, the wording of the competency is not clear and changing a few words can make the expectation better understood by both the educator and students.

▶ Direct Care Activities

As for any curriculum, appropriate clinical experiences are selected to provide the opportunity for students to achieve course learning outcomes in a CBC. DCAs can be planned for either in-house laboratory simulation or external community-based settings. For all DCAs, the nurse educator selects weekly conceptual activities with corresponding clinical SLOs as discussed in Chapter 6. These SLOs should correlate with classroom or online didactic learning. Providing ongoing feedback to students on their performance in meeting the SLOs is essential in the clinical learning environment. This feedback is called *formative evaluation*.

Formative Evaluation of Direct Care Activities in the Community-Based Clinical Setting

Weekly or daily evaluation is formative and provides ongoing instructor feedback for the student in the external community-based clinical setting. As discussed in Chapter 1, most prelicensure and RN-to-BSN nursing programs use the six major competency areas of the Quality and Safety Education for Nurses (QSEN) Institute plus professionalism and other meta-concepts or themes to organize their curricula. These themes are also typically used as part of the clinical evaluation process (Lewis, Stephens, & Ciak, 2016). Certain behaviors for each theme are expected; these behaviors may also be referred to as *competencies*. **Competencies** are the KSAs that make up a person's role. They are context-specific and show demonstration of abilities and skills (behaviors) in a variety of situations. Consider these examples of weekly clinical expectations (SLOs) for students as they relate to QSEN as part of the formative evaluation process.

- Identifies patient using two qualifying identifiers (Safety and Quality).
- Explains all procedures thoroughly to patients before performing them (Patient-Centered Care).
- Consistently uses proper hand hygiene (Evidence-Based Practice).
- Demonstrates professional behavior at all times (Professionalism).

■ Communicates appropriately in a timely manner with members of the nursing team (Teamwork and Collaboration).
■ Documents appropriately and timely using correct medical terminology (Informatics).

Each of these student behaviors is expected on every clinical day in both simulation and community-based settings throughout the course.

In addition to these ongoing behaviors, the nurse educator needs to specify weekly expectations regarding concept application to promote deep learning. For instance, if students are introduced to the concept of Oxygenation in the first nursing theory course, they may be required to "Perform a focused assessment of the patient's oxygenation status" in the clinical setting. DCAs that would help them meet this learning outcome might include physical assessment, such as:

■ Performing a focused respiratory assessment on an assigned patient.
■ Performing a focused cardiac assessment on an assigned patient.

Another DCA to help meet this SLO is to assess the oxygen saturation of the patient using pulse oximetry. The patient's laboratory values also may be assessed, including complete blood count, hemoglobin, hematocrit, and arterial blood gases (if available). Diagnostic tests such as pulmonary function studies also may be available to review.

The nurse educator lists these SLOs on the weekly assessment form as part of the clinical formative evaluation. **EXHIBIT 11-1** illustrates a portion of this formative assessment for a clinical day/week. Note that the ongoing SLOs related to QSEN stay the same each week, but the weekly SLOs would change depending on the concept(s) being studied. The nurse educator may decide that if a student did not have an opportunity to meet one or more SLOs, or if the student achieved an unsatisfactory rating, then he or she may be given a second chance to meet the expectations to achieve mastery.

Each behavior or competency is scored as satisfactory (S), needs improvement (NI), or unsatisfactory (U). If there is not opportunity to meet the competency, an NO (no opportunity) is assigned. This scoring system is easier to use than a numeric rating scale of 1 to 3, 1 to 4, or 1 to 5, which is sometimes used for summative evaluation and discussed later in this chapter.

Other concepts lend themselves to formative evaluation of DCAs. For example, consider the concept of Cognition. Students might be assigned to clients in an assisted living facility or community-based geriatric clinic where they could assess cognitive status and plan interventions for older clients with a potential for or actual impaired Cognition. DCAs related to this concept and its primary exemplars of Delirium, Dementia, and Depression might include:

■ Conduct a Short-Form Depression Inventory for the assigned client.
■ Perform a focused neurological and mental status assessment on the assigned client.
■ Plan nursing interventions for the client with impaired cognition.
■ Plan referral to interprofessional health care team members as needed to manage care for the client with impaired cognition.

For the child-bearing client, many concepts apply. One of the most important concepts to ensure the safety and well-being of both mother and baby is Patient Education. The nurse educator may assign students to a prenatal clinic, nurse midwife, or obstetrics and gynecology office to assist with scheduled check-ups and health

EXHIBIT 11-1 Sample Portion of a Weekly Clinical Formative Evaluation Tool

Student Name: _____ Date: _____
Week #: _____

Ongoing Student Learning Outcomes	S/NI/U/NO
Identifies patient using two qualifying identifiers (Safety and Quality).	
Explains all procedures thoroughly to patients before performing them (Patient-Centered Care).	
Consistently uses proper hand hygiene (Evidence-Based Practice).	
Demonstrates professional behavior at all times (Professionalism).	
Communicates appropriately in a timely manner with members of the nursing team (Teamwork and Collaboration).	
Documents appropriately and timely using correct medical terminology (Informatics).	
Weekly Student Learning Outcomes for Concept of Oxygenation	
Performs a focused respiratory assessment on assigned patient and document findings.	
Performs a focused cardiac assessment on assigned patient and document findings.	
Assesses laboratory tests to determine oxygenation status, including complete blood count, hemoglobin, hematocrit, and arterial blood gases, if performed.	
Assesses pulse oximetry for oxygen saturation level.	
Reviews diagnostic tests, if any, that assess the patient's oxygenation status.	

Key: S (Satisfactory), NI (Needs Improvement), U (Unsatisfactory), NO (No Opportunity).

teaching. As part of DCAs, the student needs to plan specific patient education for the pregnant woman, taking into consideration factors such as:

- Developmental age of the pregnant woman
- Cultural and spiritual factors influencing patient education and care
- Third-party payer source
- Readiness to learn
- Educational level/reading ability

The SLO for the concept of Patient Education in this context may be stated as: "Applies knowledge of developmental, cultural, educational, and financial factors to provide appropriate Patient Education for the pregnant woman." For example, the author's students were assigned to work with a midwife whose primary clientele were Amish women in a rural farmland area. When pregnant, they incorporated integrative therapies into their prenatal care and would not be examined in the presence of their husbands. To provide whole-person, culturally appropriate care, the students learned that the midwife had to understand and incorporate the values and practices of this population to be accepted as their primary healthcare provider.

Summative Evaluation of Direct Care Activities in the Community-Based Clinical Setting

Tools used for summative evaluation in the clinical learning environment vary in format and length. However, all of them determine by the end of a course whether the student has been successful or not in completing course requirements. *The summative clinical evaluation tool (CET) should not be used as the weekly formative tool.* Formative and summative evaluation are not the same, as discussed in Chapter 10 (Billings & Halstead, 2016).

The summative clinical evaluation tool varies by program. However, all summative CETs should be based on course SLOs, which provide content-related evidence of measurement validity. Consider the CET for an Adult Health course in **EXHIBIT 11-2**. Specific competencies or behaviors are delineated that demonstrate achievement of each course SLO for this Adult Health course. The rating scale has two levels, met (M) and unmet (U). All competencies are expected to be met by the end of the course to pass. If any competency is not met, the student fails the course. This method simplifies scoring and is most fair for the students. Some programs select certain behaviors to label as "critical" and are the only competencies that must be met by the student. However, if the behavior is important enough to be listed on a CET and indicates meeting the course SLO, then all behaviors should be met, rather than just a subset.

Some nurse educators add a third rating column for "Exceeds expectations." This level may be helpful for encouraging high-achieving students to perform, but their grade remains as a Pass.

Remember This . . .

The summative clinical evaluation tool varies by program. However, all summative clinical evaluation tool should be based on course student learning objectives, which provides content-related evidence of measurement validity.

EXHIBIT 11-2 Summative Clinical Evaluation Tool for Adult Health Course

NUR # 220
ADULT HEALTH I
CLINICAL EVALUATION TOOL

Scoring of Clinical Evaluation Tool

This form will be completed at Midterm and at the end of the semester for a Final clinical grade. Each student behavior will be assessed using an "M" (Met) or "NM" (Not Met) at Midterm. For the Final grade, each student behavior will be assessed using the same choices. Students must receive an "M" for *all* behaviors to pass the clinical component of the course by **the completion of the clinical experience**. The clinical instructor and student should write comments at the end of the tool.

Course Learning Outcomes (CLOs)

CLO 1: Utilize the nursing process and critical thinking to make clinical judgments in collaboration with adult patients with common health problems to meet optimal outcomes. (Clinical Judgment)

	M	NM
Perform focused assessments and interpret relevant data.		
Provide care that is adequate, applicable, and prioritized to include patient education and discharge planning.		
Perform psychomotor skills according to predetermined standards.		
Implement interventions that are based on available evidence and best practices.		
Manage care for 1 or 2 patients in an inpatient adult health setting.		

CLO 2: Communicate effectively with the patient and members of the healthcare team to ensure patient safety and quality care. (Teamwork & Collaboration, Safety and Quality Improvement)

	M	NM
Seek information from members of the interprofessional health care team to collect data and ensure adherence to the patient's collaborative plan of care.		

(continues)

EXHIBIT 11-2 Summative Clinical Evaluation Tool for Adult Health Course (continued)

	M	NM
Coordinate care for patients to create a culture of safety.		
Consistently communicate with the patient and family in a facilitative manner.		
Provide for safety, comfort, and well-being of patient.		
Use computer programs (e.g., electronic medical record, medical databases) to skillfully access patient data and current research, and communicate essential information as needed.		
Coordinate continuing care with the patient, family, case manager/discharge planner, and other healthcare team members as needed.		
Seek internal and community resources to assist in health teaching to meet the patient's and/or family's learning needs.		

CLO 3: Document care appropriately and accurately using the electronic patient record and/or other medical record format. (Communication)

	M	NM
Document care consistent with protocols of the facility and best practices.		
Integrate cultural and spiritual assessment data into the patient's collaborative plan of care.		
Ensure that documentation is clear, concise, complete, relevant, and accurate.		
Promptly respond to and document/report changes in a patient's condition.		

CLO 4: Prioritize and organize care for two patients in a general medical-surgical healthcare setting. (Management of Care)

	M	NM
Provide nursing care in a safe and competent manner.		

EXHIBIT 11-2 Summative Clinical Evaluation Tool for Adult Health Course (continued)

	M	NM
Provide care that respects and is sensitive to the patients' preferences.		
Assume responsibility for clinical assignment as directed.		
Organize care to ensure that patient receives medication and treatments as scheduled.		
Use time management principles to organize care for two patients.		
Begin to use principles of delegation and supervision to coordinate care with other staff members and nursing students.		

CLO 5: Adapt patient care as needed based on the adult's age, culture, and developmental stage. (Patient-Centered Care)

	M	NM
Provide care that is consistent with best practices based on developmental stage and changes of aging.		
Communicate patient's preferences, values, and needs to other relevant healthcare providers.		

CLO 6: Use information technology to locate and validate evidence for planning and implementing patient care for adults in a variety of medical-surgical nursing settings. (Informatics/Technology)

	M	NM
Apply knowledge of best, current evidence when planning and giving care.		
Research relevant resources to determine best practice for patients' current condition and needs.		
Maintain security and confidentiality of all patient and family information.		

(continues)

EXHIBIT 11-2 Summative Clinical Evaluation Tool for Adult Health Course (continued)

CLO 7: Apply legal, ethical, and professional standards in clinical nursing practice. (Professionalism)

	M	NM
Consistently evaluate self and performance identifying areas needing improvement.		
Seek learning opportunities to gain new knowledge and clinical experiences.		
Apply professional, legal, and ethical standards of care in practice.		
Respect the patient's rights and responsibilities and maintains client confidentiality.		
Serve as a role model for professional nursing behavior.		
Use quality improvement data to alter own practice.		

Midterm Progress

FACULTY COMMENTS:

STUDENT COMMENTS:

Faculty Signature/Date_____

Student Signature/Date_____

Final Grade

FACULTY COMMENTS:

STUDENT COMMENTS:

Faculty Signature/Date_____

Student Signature/Date_____

Other rating scales are more complicated and vary from one program to another. Some programs continue to use scales developed and published more than 20 years ago. However, their validity and reliability are not clearly evident. For example, consider this 4-level rating scale:

4 = Above expectations

3 = Meets expectations

2 = Below expectations

1 = Does not meet expectations

As stated, the nurse educator has no specific criteria for determining the student's rating. However, some programs have developed more detailed criteria to qualify and quantify student performance. **BOX 11-1** illustrates an example of specific criteria for the 1 to 4 rating scale as listed previously. Note that terminology such as "minimum," "occasional," and "moderate" are not defined and would be very subjective for the nurse educator in evaluating the student.

BOX 11-1 Sample Criteria for a Clinical Evaluation Tool That Uses a Numeric Rating Scale

A "4" means the student functions above expectations:

- Demonstrates all the criteria in "3" below.
- Functions consistently with minimum guidance in the clinical setting.
- Is self-directed in learning.

A "3" means the student functions meets expectations:

- Functions satisfactorily with moderate guidance in the clinical setting.
- Demonstrates appropriate knowledge and integrates knowledge with skills and attitudes among interprofessional team members.
- Needs occasional prompting for engaging in self-direction in learning.
- Prepares for all clinical learning experiences.
- Performs care safely.
- Identifies own learning needs and seeks appropriate assistance.

A "2" means the student functions below expectations:

- Functions safely with moderate to extensive amount of guidance in the clinical situation.
- Demonstrates adequate knowledge and requires *moderate* assistance in integrating knowledge with skills.
- Requires some direction in recognizing and utilizing learning opportunities.

A "1" means the student does not meet expectations:

- Requires *intense* guidance for the performance of activities at a safe level.
- Has difficulty providing nursing care.
- Demonstrates gaps in necessary knowledge
- Requires frequent or almost constant assistance in integrating knowledge and skills.
- Has limited insight into own behavior.
- Is unable to identify own learning needs and neglects to seek appropriate assistance.

A small number of programs use more specific percentages or numbers of cues to better quantify these criteria. For example, a 4 might mean that the student requires only 1 or 2 cues or provides safe quality care 100% of the time. Being able to accurately use these numeric values would mean that the nurse educator has to supervise each student 100% of the time or count cues for each student. Most clinical educators have group sizes of 6 to 10 nursing students, making it impossible to do this type of supervision.

Oermann and Gaberson (2017) list multiple issues with numeric rating scales, including personal bias, leniency error (scoring all students at the high end of the rating scale), severity error (scoring all students at the low end of the scale), and halo effect (making judgments based on the general impression of the student). Another issue that the author has noted is the tendency of some faculty to convert the total numeric score to a letter grade. This conversion most often occurs in programs in which letter grading rather than a pass/fail system is used. *Avoid this pitfall if possible because there is no evidence that any particular numeric value is equivalent to specific letter grades.* In this case, a quantitative, objective approach is applied to a qualitative, subjective process which is not a "good fit" or best practice.

▶ Standardized Patient Methodology

Standardized patients (SPs) are actors and actresses who portray a patient with a variety of signs and symptoms and have been used in health care education for many years. Each SP is coached to represent a specific scenario to help the students learn important concepts. For instance, in prelicensure and RN-to-BSN programs, SPs may be used to help students learn interviewing skills when taking a nursing history. Some programs have used SP methodology to learn and evaluate the concepts of Therapeutic Communication and Patient-Centered Care (Webster, 2013).

In graduate nursing education, SPs are often used to help students transition to their new role in which the risk for error is high (Ballman, Garritano, & Beery, 2016). Examples of the purpose of SPs for nurse practitioner programs include to:

- Improve cultural competence and communication skills
- Improve interprofessional interactions
- Assess the use of clinical practice guidelines for a particular health problem
- Increase student confidence
- Increase competence in assessment skills

Regardless of type of program, several challenges are posed by using SP methodology, including development of case scenarios, intensive coaching of actors or actresses, coordinating learning experiences, and evaluating student performance. SPs may be used for either formative or summative evaluation. In some programs, the SP provides feedback for the student, especially when interpersonal skills and bedside manner are being assessed. However, this method is not appropriate when students are being evaluated on whether they used the appropriate clinical practice guidelines for a particular health problem or made the correct differential medical diagnosis. In this case, a subject matter expert, usually a nurse practitioner preceptor or nurse educator, evaluates student performance using predetermined criteria (Ballman et al., 2016).

▶ Clinical Simulation

Over the last decade, the use of simulation in the laboratory setting has dramatically increased in nursing education (**FIGURE 11-1**). In some prelicensure nursing programs, high-fidelity simulation (HFS) is used as a substitute for external clinical experience in community-based settings as much as 50% of the time. The allowed amount of clinical time that can be used for clinical simulation is determined by each state board or provincial regulatory body. The major advantage of clinical simulation is that the health care situation can be controlled and can focus on specific concepts to be learned and evaluated to improve clinical reasoning and judgment. Most HFS studies, however, have focused on student satisfaction rather than evaluation of learning.

A quasi-experimental study by Curl, Smith, Chisholm, McGee, and Das (2016) compared the effectiveness of integrated simulation and clinical experiences (50% simulation and 50% external clinical) with the traditional clinical experience for AD nursing students in three Texas community colleges. Achievement of SLOs in the two student groups was measured by multiple methods, including:

- Health Education Systems Incorporated (HESI) exit examination scores
- HESI specialty examination scores
- Clinical performance evaluations by nurse educators

The results of these outcome measures showed that students performed better on HESI examinations in the group that had 50% integrated simulation. Students in both groups met the clinical SLOs.

Professional Nursing concepts may be embedded in HFS experiences, including Ethics and Communication. For example, Krautscheid (2017) reported embedding microethical dilemmas to extend ethics education beyond the cognitive learning domain. Common dilemmas such as breaching patient confidentiality, poor infection control practices, and unsafe medication practices were selected for inclusion. As a result of this integration of affective learning in simulation, students reported increased confidence and empowerment to advocate for patients as needed. They also learned how to best communicate their concerns about these ethical issues.

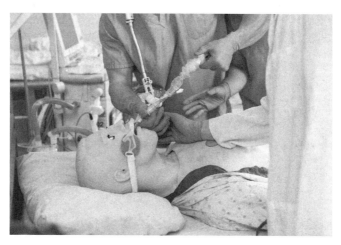

FIGURE 11-1 Nursing students participating in a high-fidelity laboratory simulation
© Tyler Olson/Shutterstock

Prebriefing is an important component of a simulation experience to help students notice various aspects of the clinical situation, anticipate the patient's needs, and focus on the conceptual knowledge needed for making timely and appropriate clinical decisions (Page-Cutrara, 2014). Simulation scenarios may be low-fidelity, mid-fidelity, or high-fidelity; they may include role playing or computer-based simulation. Nursing programs often calculate 1 contact hour of simulation to be equal to 1 or 2 hours of traditional community-based experience. Following the simulation, structured debriefing that is facilitated by the simulation coordinator or clinical nurse educator is crucial to provide an opportunity for students to reflect and build on previous conceptual learning and thinking (Dreifuerst, 2012).

Like formative and summative evaluations in community-based clinical settings, evaluating student performance in a simulated experience can result in educator bias and subjectivity. In most programs, simulation is assessed as a formative experience so students can learn from participating in the experience and debriefing with the nurse educator.

Over the past few years, several tools have been developed for evaluating the effectiveness of simulation and student performance. Although none of these tools are universally used, some examples of evaluation tools reported in the literature include:

- Lasater Clinical Judgment Rubric (LCJR) (Lasater, 2007)
- Creighton Competency Evaluation Instrument (C-CEI) (Todd, Hawkins, Hercinger, Matz, & Tracy, 2014)
- Quality and Safety Education for Nurses (QSEN) Rubric (Luetke & Benbenek, 2012)

More study is needed to determine the best tool for evaluating student performance.

▶ Objective Structured Clinical Evaluation

The objective structured clinical evaluation (or examination) (OSCE) has been used in healthcare education for many years, but has only more recently been applied in nursing education. An OSCE is a method used to evaluate students to determine if they are ready for practice. They have been used primarily in advanced practice RN programs for assessing competency of students preparing to graduate. An OSCE provides a high-fidelity simulation or SP situation to evaluate student performance in the cognitive, psychomotor, and affective learning domains (Benbenek et al., 2016). Performance checklists that consist of predetermined competencies or criteria are used by faculty to evaluate student performance. Concepts such as Communication, Patient-Centered Care, and Evidence-Based Practice are evaluated as part of the OSCE. At this time, only a few prelicensure nursing programs are beginning to use the OSCE as part of evaluating students' readiness for practice. However, Benner, Stephen, Leonard, and Day (2010) in the Carnegie Foundation study of nursing education recommended testing of clinical skills for prelicensure nursing students before graduation.

▶ Focused Learning Activities

As discussed in Chapter 6, a focused learning activity (FLA) is an assignment completed in the clinical or laboratory setting that is associated with or supports achievement of one or more clinical competencies and applies concept(s) for deep learning. FLAs may be accomplished individually, in pairs, or in small groups working collaboratively and are scored using a grading rubric. Ways to evaluate selected FLA examples are provided in this section.

> ### Remember This . . .
>
> Focused learning activities may be accomplished individually, in pairs, or in small groups working collaboratively and are scored using a grading rubric.

To assist the nurse educator, the QSEN website's (www.qsen.org) Teaching Strategies section is an outstanding resource for focused learning activities and how they can be evaluated. These strategies are open source ideas and can be used without permission of the educator who submitted them.

Reflection Papers

FLAs may focus on Professional Nursing and Health Care concepts, Health/Health and Illness concepts, or Health Care Recipient concepts. Concepts within the Professional Nursing and Health Care category are often difficult for students to learn and for the nurse educator to evaluate. One popular assignment to meet this goal is the reflection paper. As a clinical assignment, this paper is usually short (1 to 3 pages). The purpose of the clinical reflection paper is to help reinforce conceptual learning, focus on the student's personal feelings and experiences, and synthesize conceptual knowledge with applied experiences. This assignment should relate to a course SLO.

Grading rubrics are generally norm-referenced, but expectations vary depending on the purpose of the assignment and the nurse educator's personal philosophy about assignment expectations. An example of a grading rubric for a reflection paper is presented in **TABLE 11-1**. Note that the majority of the grade is on the content of the reflection paper rather than grammar, spelling, or organization.

From her literature review, Elliott (2017) found that the evaluation of learning in a CBC has been limited. In her recent study, the author reviewed 75 student FLAs in which students from two colleges wrote short reflection papers about the theme of Professional Values. The focus of the study was to evaluate overall student conceptual learning rather than determine individual learning and was based on Essential VIII of the American Association of Colleges of Nursing (AACN's) *The Essentials of Baccalaureate Education for Professional Nursing Practice*. The competency states that the BSN student should "reflect on one's own beliefs and values as they relate to professional practice" (AACN, 2008, p. 29). Two core concepts emerged from the study's framework analysis methodology: Appreciation for Professional Values and Disillusionment with Unprofessional Behaviors. Three themes were evident as part of Appreciation for Professional Values:

- Focus on the relationship with the patient
- Focus on the healthcare team
- Focus on the self

TABLE 11-1 Sample Grading Rubric for Clinical Reflection Paper*

Criteria	Excellent (4 points)	Acceptable (3 points)	Minimally Acceptable (2 points)	Unacceptable (1 point)
Depth and content of reflection (points × 2 for 50% of grade)	Paper demonstrates an in-depth reflection on and understanding of selected concepts presented in the course. Viewpoints and interpretations are insightful and well supported. Clear, detailed examples are provided.	Paper demonstrates a general reflection on and beginning understanding of selected concepts presented in the course. Viewpoints and interpretations are supported. Appropriate examples are provided, as applicable.	Paper demonstrates a minimal reflection on and understanding of selected concepts presented in the course. Viewpoints and interpretations are unsupported or supported with flawed arguments. Examples are not provided or are irrelevant to the assignment.	Paper demonstrates a lack of reflection on or understanding of selected concepts presented in the course. Viewpoints and interpretations are missing, inappropriate, and/or unsupported. Examples are not provided.
Structure and organization (25% of the grade)	Writing is clear, concise, and well organized, with excellent sentence/paragraph construction. Thoughts are expressed in a coherent and logical manner. There are no more than two spelling and grammatical errors per page of the paper.	Writing is mostly clear, concise, and well organized, with good sentence/paragraph construction. Thoughts are expressed in a coherent and logical manner. There are no more than three spelling, grammar, or syntax errors per page of the paper.	Writing is unclear and/or disorganized. Thoughts are not expressed in a logical manner. There are more than four spelling or grammatical errors per page of the paper.	Writing is unclear and disorganized. Thoughts ramble and make little sense. There are numerous spelling and grammatical errors throughout the paper.
Evidence and practice (25% of the grade)	Paper shows strong evidence of synthesis of ideas presented and insights gained. The implications of these insights for the student's clinical practice are thoroughly detailed.	Paper shows some evidence of synthesis of ideas presented and insights gained. The implications of these insights for the student's clinical practice are presented.	Paper shows little evidence of synthesis of ideas presented and insights gained. Few implications of these insights for the student's clinical practice are presented.	Paper shows no evidence of synthesis of ideas presented and insights gained. No implications for the student's clinical practice are presented.

*Possible score of 4 to 16 points for paper

Three themes were evident as part of Disillusionment with Unprofessional Behaviors:

- Negativity toward to patient
- Negativity toward the healthcare team
- Negativity toward the self

These findings inform the nurse educator about the need to help students learn how to cope with negative nurses and demonstrate professional values and behaviors. **BOX 11-2** provides specific examples of sub-concepts that were identified in the Elliott study for each core concept.

Clinical Paper Assignments

In addition to reflection papers, conceptual learning can be measured using other clinical paper assignments. Examples of these assignments include journaling, evidence-based practice papers, and case studies.

Journaling provides an opportunity for students to share and reflect on their clinical experiences. Journal entries may be structured or semi-structured such that the nurse educator assigns the concept for reflection. For example, the students may be asked to share a clinical experience and provide an example of how they demonstrated patient-centeredness with a focus on the concept of Culture. Journal entries may or may not be graded, but could be part of a student portfolio. The nurse educator should provide feedback for the student to assist them with the process of journaling as needed.

BOX 11-2 Examples of Core Concepts Derived from Elliott's Study on the Competency of Professional Values

Appreciation for Professional Values

- Advocacy
- Caring
- Collegial relationships
- High standards
- Leadership
- Lifelong learning
- Making a difference
- Professional autonomy
- Respect

Disillusionment with Unprofessional Behaviors

- Disrespect for patients
- Disrespectful communication
- Inadequate communication
- Inattentiveness
- Lack of compassion
- Making students feel unwelcome

Data from Elliott, A. M. (2017). Professional values competency evaluation for students enrolled in a concept-based curriculum. *Journal of Nursing Education, 56*(1), 12–21.

Evidence-based assignments can help students learn to critically think to determine best practice. These assignments may require students to select a clinical practice, procedure, or policy that they observed or performed at the clinical site and compare it to evidence in the literature to determine if it is best practice. For example, the author had students in a long-term care setting in which tympanic thermometers were used. After a thorough literature search, the students found that this type of thermometer should not be used for older adults due to inaccuracies in that population.

A more complex assignment is an activity and evaluation related to using the Beers Criteria to prevent medication-related problems older adults. This assignment available on the QSEN website helps measure learning about the concepts of Safety and Development. Students are asked to complete a form similar to the abbreviated one in **EXHIBIT 11-3**, and then post their findings on a blog or journal. The students are evaluated by the clinical nurse educator using a grading rubric. The clinical SLO for the week that correlates with the FLA regarding the concept of Safety might be: "Evaluate an older adult's medications to determine if they are safe based on the revised Beer's Criteria and make recommendations for change as needed."

Case studies may also be used as FLAs. They can be assigned to individuals, pairs, or groups in the clinical setting while other students are performing direct care activities. Case studies should focus on selected concepts and pose thinking questions to promote effective deep learning. Chapter 9 is devoted to developing and evaluating several types of case studies.

Data Mining Assignments

Data mining assignments are appropriate when the student is in a healthcare agency and has access to a medical record, either paper or electronic. This FLA focuses on one or more specific concepts and requires the student or group of students to find client data that relate the concepts being studied. The value of this assignment is to help students discover conceptual knowledge. For example, consider the concept of Nutrition. Students may be asked to retrieve and document the following data about their assigned patient, as available:

- Medical diagnosis
- Age and gender
- Prescribed and over-the-counter medications
- Current weight
- Trend in gaining or losing weight over the past 3 months
- Body mass index (BMI)
- Hemoglobin and hematocrit
- Serum iron level or iron-binding capacity value
- Serum protein panel
- Serum prealbumin
- Status of skin, hair, and mucous membranes
- Special diet, if prescribed
- Daily caloric intake for 3 days

All of these indicators of nutritional status can then be interpreted to determine if the patient has adequate nutrition to meet current needs. If not, students may be asked to plan and implement collaborative interventions to promote or improve their patient's nutritional status.

EXHIBIT 11-3 Beers Criteria Assignment

I.   *During the clinical day*, select an older adult patient for whom you are caring who is taking at least eight medications. Medications include routinely scheduled, as needed (PRN), over-the-counter medications, and supplements. List all current medications with dose, route, frequency, and indications for use.

Medication Name	Dose	Route	Frequency	Indications for This Patient's Use
Routine medications				
PRN medications				
Over-the-counter medications				
Herbal medications				
Mineral and vitamin supplements				

II. *After the clinical day*, evaluate the patient's medications by using the article, "American Geriatrics Society 2015 updated Beers Criteria for potentially inappropriate medication use in older adults," at the website www.guideline.gov/content.aspx?id=49933, using all five tables for the evaluation.

   A.   Table. 2015 American Geriatrics Society (AGS) Beers Criteria for Potentially Inappropriate Medication Use in Older Adults
   B.   Table. 2015 AGS Beers Criteria for Potentially Inappropriate Medication Use in Older Adults Due to Drug-Disease or Drug-Syndrome Interactions That May Exacerbate the Disease or Syndrome
   C.   Table. 2015 AGS Beers Criteria for Potentially Inappropriate Medications to Be Used with Caution in Older Adults
   D.   Table. 2015 AGS Beers Criteria for Potentially Clinically Important Non-Anti-infective Drug–Drug Interactions That Should Be Avoided in Older Adults
   E.   Table. 2015 AGS Beers Criteria for Non-Anti-Infective Medications That Should Be Avoided or Have Their Dosage Reduced with Varying Levels of Kidney Function in Older Adults

(continues)

EXHIBIT 11-3 Beers Criteria Assignment (continued)

Med of Concern	Rationale	Recommendation	Quality of Evidence (high, moderate, low)	Strength of Evidence (strong, weak, insufficient)	Safety Issues	Toxicity	Drug Interactions?	Fall Risk?	Other Concerns

Modified from Saidleman, V. QSEN Beers Criteria Teaching Strategy. Accessed from www.qsen.org/using-beers-criteriato-prevent-medication-related-problems-in-older-adults

Compare and Contrast Assignments

Some FLAs allow students to compare and contrast patients that students are assigned to or additional patients, clients, or residents, depending on setting. For example, for the data mining FLA described in the previous section, the students may be asked to collect nutrition data for three different patients and then compare and contrast their nutritional status. Questions that might be posed to the students by the clinical nurse educator could include:

- Compare and contrast the nutritional status of the three patients. How are they similar and how are they different?
- How does each patient's medical diagnosis affect his or her nutritional status?
- How might medications that the patients are taking affect their nutritional status?
- What other factors, such as age, might affect each patient's nutritional status and why?
- Are there any factors that are common to all three patients that may contribute to their nutritional status?

This FLA would be done during the clinical experience in pairs or groups. The clinical nurse educator would facilitate learning by working with the group during their data mining and discussion to apply the concept of Nutrition for patient care. Then the assignment could be graded.

Graphic Organizers

Graphic organizers, as discussed elsewhere in this text, are effective methods for evaluating concepts and meaningful learning. The most common tool as part of clinical learning and evaluation is concept mapping, which is described in detail in Chapter 8.

▶ Chapter Key Points

- Each type of clinical experience is graded differently: direct DCAs are graded as satisfactory/pass or unsatisfactory/fail and are criterion-referenced; FLAs are scored using a grading rubric and can either be criterion- or norm-referenced.
- Clinical evaluation methods are measurement tools and, as such, need evidence of validity and reliability.
- Competencies are the knowledge, skills, and attitudes that make up a person's job. They are context-specific and show demonstration of abilities and skills (behaviors) in a variety of situations.
- In addition to ongoing performance behaviors, the nurse educator needs to specify weekly expectations regarding concept application to promote deep learning.
- Tools used for summative evaluation in the clinical learning environment vary in format and length. However, all of them determine by the end of a course whether the student has been successful or not in completing clinical course requirements.
- Standardized patients are actors and actresses who portray a patient with a variety of signs and symptoms and have been used in healthcare education for many years. Each standardized patient is coached to represent a specific scenario to help the students learn important concepts.
- Like formative and summative evaluations in community-based clinical settings, evaluating student performance in a simulated experience can result in educator bias and subjectivity. In most programs, simulation is evaluated as a formative experience so students can learn from debriefing.

- Grading rubrics are generally norm-referenced, but expectations vary depending on the purpose of the assignment and the nurse educator's personal philosophy about assignment expectations.
- The purpose of the clinical reflection paper is to help reinforce conceptual learning, focus on the student's personal feelings and experiences, and synthesize conceptual knowledge with applied experiences. It is typically scored using a grading rubric.
- In addition to reflection papers, conceptual learning can be measured using other clinical paper assignments. Examples of these assignments include journaling, evidence-based practice papers, and case studies.

▶ Chapter References and Selected Bibliography

American Association of Colleges of Nursing (AACN). (2008). *The essentials of baccalaureate education for professional nursing practice.* Washington, DC: Author.

Ballman, K., Garritano, N., & Beery, T. (2016). Broadening the reach of standardized patients in nurse practitioner education to include the distance learner. *Teaching and Learning in Nursing, 41*(5), 230–233.

Benbenek M., Dierich, M., Wyman, J., Avery, M., Juve, C., & Miller, J. (2016). Development and implementation of a capstone objective structured clinical examination in nurse practitioner and nurse-midwifery programs. *Nurse Educator, 41*(6), 288–293.

Benner, P., Stephen, M., Leonard, V., & Day, L. (2010). *Educating nurses: A call for radical transformation.* San Francisco, CA: Jossey-Bass.

Billings, D. M., & Halstead, J. A. (2016). *Teaching in nursing: A guide for faculty* (5th ed.). St. Louis, MO: Elsevier.

Curl, E. D., Smith, S., Chisholm, L. A., McGee, L. A., & Das, K. (2016). Effectiveness of integrated simulation and clinical experiences compared to traditional clinical experiences for nursing students. *Nursing Education Perspectives, 37*(2), 72–77.

Dreifuerst, K. T. (2012). Using debriefing for meaningful learning to foster development of clinical reasoning in simulation. *Journal of Nursing Education, 51*(6), 323–333.

Elliott, A. M. (2017). Professional values competency evaluation for students enrolled in a concept-based curriculum. *Journal of Nursing Education, 56*(1), 12–21.

Keating, S. B. (2015). *Curriculum development and evaluation in nursing.* New York, NY: Springer Publishing.

Krautscheid, L. C. (2017). Embedding microethical dilemmas in high-fidelity simulation scenarios: Preparing nursing students for ethical practice. *Journal of Nursing Edcuation, 56*(1), 55–58.

Lasater, K. (2007). Clinical judgment development: Using simulation to create an assessment rubric. *Journal of Nursing Education, 46*(11), 496–503.

Lewis, D. Y., Stephens, K. P., & Ciak, A. D. (2016). QSEN: Curriculum integration and bridging the gap to practice. *Nursing Education Perspectives, 37*(2), 97–100.

Luetke, R., & Benbenek, M. (2012). Simulation evaluation: A comparison of two simulation evaluation rubrics. Presented at the 2012 QSEN National Forum, Tucson, AZ, May 31.

Oermann, M. H., & Gaberson, K. B. (2017). *Evaluation and testing in nursing education* (5th ed.). New York, NY: Springer Publishing.

Page-Cutrara, K. (2014). Use of pre-briefing in nursing simulation: A review of the literature. *Journal of Nursing Education, 53*(3), 136–141.

Todd, M., Hawkins, K., Hercinger, M., Matz, J., & Tracy, M. (2014). Creighton Competency Evaluation Instrument. Creighton University School of Nursing. Retrieved from www.creighton.edu/nursing/simulation/.

Webster, D. (2013). Promoting therapeutic communication and patient-centered care using standardized patients. *Journal of Nursing Education, 52*(11), 645–648.

*Indicates classic reference.

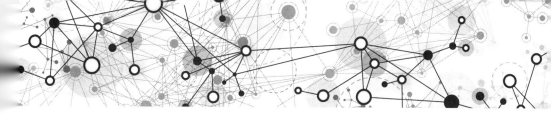

CHAPTER 12

Determining Systematic Methods for Concept-Based Curriculum Program Evaluation

Donna Ignatavicius

▶ Introduction to Program Evaluation

Program evaluation is a continuous assessment and analysis of the components of a nursing program or department to provide data for faculty as a basis for informed program decisions about the ability to meet program outcomes. A secondary purpose for program evaluation is the requirement of state boards of nursing, provincial nursing regulatory bodies, and nursing accrediting organizations for programs to demonstrate compliance with established standards by each organization.

Faculty are responsible for developing the systematic plan for evaluation (SPE) that consists of the process, data, analysis, and plans for revision or change based on that analysis. In other words, the SPE serves as a tool to document the program's continuous quality improvement process (**FIGURE 12-1**). Some programs assign program evaluation responsibility to an assessment or evaluation committee, but all faculty need to participate in systematic evaluation. This chapter describes the most important components of the program evaluation process, with the emphasis on how to evaluate the effectiveness of a concept-based curriculum (CBC).

▶ Commonly Used Program Evaluation Models

Accrediting bodies and regulatory agencies do not typically prescribe the evaluation model or framework to use for program evaluation. That decision is up to each program faculty. Several models have been used as frameworks for quality improvement and educational programs over the past 30 to 40 years, including those published by Donabedian, Piskurich, and Stufflebeam.

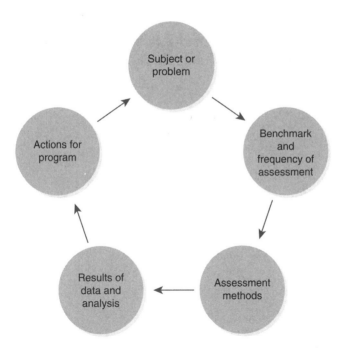

FIGURE 12-1 Continuous Quality Improvement Process for Nursing Program Evaluation

The classic Donabedian (1989) framework of "structure, process, and outcome" has been used for many years for quality assurance/improvement activities in healthcare organizations. *Structure* refers to the resources and fixed elements in an organization; *process* is defined as actions taken to deliver healthcare services. *Outcomes* have become more important over the past few decades because in health care they are the measurable results of client care that are attributed to the structure and processes of care. Higher education programs, including nursing, have focused more on outcomes to demonstrate quality.

Piskurich (1993) developed five criteria around the structure, process, and outcome framework and applied them to the assessment of educational programs. The five criteria are:

- Sufficiency of the structure
- Usability of the process
- Currency of the process
- Compliance with both the structure and process
- Effectiveness of the outcomes in harmony with the structure and process

The third model for approaching program evaluation is the CIPP model posited by Stufflebeam (2000). The CIPP model—context, input, process, and product—uses an accountability approach in program evaluation and quality. This model is most commonly used in nursing education and has been promoted by Singh (2004), Kalb (2009), and others as an effective program evaluation approach.

Escallier and Fullerton (2012) reported their experience in developing and implementing a program evaluation plan for their school of nursing (SON). The faculty combined use of the Piskurich framework with the CIPP model. The authors shared the lessons that were learned from this experience, which included:

- The need for the SON to develop a new standing faculty committee to focus on program evaluation and outcomes.
- The need for all faculty to be fully engaged in the program evaluation process on an ongoing basis.
- The need for all faculty to be responsive to changes that need to be implemented.

These findings are consistent with the need for the continuous quality improvement process in nursing education programs.

▶ The Systematic Plan for Program Evaluation

Determining the key components of the systematic plan for evaluation (SPE) (sometimes referred to as the systematic evaluation plan [SEP]) for the program or department is somewhat dependent on specific state or provincial regulations. This decision is also influenced by which nursing organization, if any, accredits the nursing program. For example, the Accreditation Commission for Education in Nursing (ACEN) 2017 Standards for Accreditation no longer require that programs include every standard and criterion in their SPE (www.acenursing.org). They also no longer require that new graduate and employer satisfaction data be collected, aggregated, trended, and analyzed. Both the National League for Nursing Commission for Nursing Education Accreditation (CNEA) (www.nln.org/accreditation-services) and the Commission on Collegiate Nursing Education (CCNE) (www.aacn.nche.edu/ccne) do require that satisfaction data be collected and analyzed from stakeholders, including alumni and employers.

Most nursing programs require measurement of three components: program outcomes, curricular outcomes, and faculty outcomes. Some programs also include every element and criteria of the accreditation standards, including physical, fiscal, and learning resources; policies; and mission and governance.

> ### Remember This . . .
>
> *Determining the key components of the systematic plan for evaluation (SPE) (sometimes referred to as the systematic evaluation plan [SEP]) for the program or department is somewhat dependent on specific state or provincial regulations. This decision is also influenced by which nursing organization, if any, accredits the nursing program.*

The format of the SPE is often tabular and typically consists of all or most of these areas:

- Component being measured
- Expected outcome, or expected level achievement (ELA)
- Method of measurement
- Frequency and date of measurement
- Person or committee responsible for data collection and analysis
- Actual outcome, or data
- Data analysis
- Plan of action
- Follow-up to plan

The expected outcome, or ELA, states a benchmark or level that the program deems as most appropriate to measure the component. The ELA should be specific and measurable. For example, consider this ELA: *90% of faculty state they are satisfied with available learning resources as evidenced by rating a 3 (agree) or 4 (strongly agree) on the annual faculty survey.* As stated, this expectation is clearly specific and measurable. The method of assessment is a faculty survey and the frequency of measurement is annually. Many programs use a program evaluation calendar to keep track of when all of the components are measured.

The person or committee responsible keeps everyone accountable of what is expected when. This responsibility needs to be divided among faculty and nursing administration and not just a designated Assessment or Program Evaluation Committee. Actual data are aggregated, trended, and analyzed by comparing the actual outcome or data with the ELA. If the outcome was met at the specified level, the plan would likely be to continue to monitor the data. However, if the outcome was *not* met, the faculty are obligated to develop and implement a plan of action to reach the intended level of achievement. When the measurement occurs the next time, the effectiveness of the action plan can be determined.

Program Outcomes

All accrediting and regulatory bodies require that the achievement of program outcomes be measured. Regional college, university, and school accrediting organizations also require that programs and departments track these outcome data to inform decision making. The three outcomes that all nursing programs in the United States usually track are:

- Program completion rates
- Employment rates
- Certification or licensure first-time pass rates

For both prelicensure and graduate programs in nursing, program completion data are essential to track by student cohort, program location, and program option. Although some variance exists, as a general rule, program completion is calculated as 150% of the length of the full-time or part-time nursing program. For example, if an associate degree (AD) full-time program in nursing is four semesters once a student is admitted, the student's program completion rate would be based on six semesters (150% of the full-time program). Additionally, if that program offered both a generic and an LPN-to-RN program option, both options would need to be reported separately and then combined.

A program's completion rate should be compared to national trends or whatever is reasonable for the specific program. For instance, AD programs desire a student completion rate of at least 70%, which reflects the national average. However, in an urban college where there might be a high population of international and/or educationally disadvantaged students, that number might be set at a lower expected outcome.

Consider the data for program completion listed in **EXHIBIT 12-1**. Note that the completion rates for all students consistently meet the expected outcome of 70%.

EXHIBIT 12-1　Portion of a Systematic Plan for Evaluation for Program Completion

Component Being Evaluated	Expected Level of Achievement (ELA)/Benchmark	Data and Analysis	Plan of Action
Program completion rate for generic AD nursing students	70% of the generic AD nursing students admitted to the program will complete the program in six semesters.	2013 = 85%; ELA met. 2014 = 87%; ELA met. 2015 = 83%; ELA met.	2013 = Continue to monitor. 2014 = Continue to monitor. 2015 = Continue to monitor.
Program completion rate for LPN-to-RN nursing students	70% of the LPN-to-RN nursing students admitted to the program will complete the program in four semesters.	2013 = 62%; ELA not met. 2014 = 66%; ELA not met. 2015 = 55%; ELA not met.	2013 = Continue to monitor. 2014 = Change admission criteria to include preadmission test. 2015 = Preadmission test not predictive of program completion; continue to monitor.

However, the completion rates for the LPN-to-RN cohorts are consistently below 70%, but the faculty made minimal plans for ways to improve the rate of program completion for this group. This process was not effective for improving this program outcome.

Employment rates are also required to be tracked for program graduates within 6 to 12 months of graduation. Graduates of prelicensure programs seek employment as LPNs or RNs for the first time, but most postlicensure graduates are already employed as nurses. Instead, for RN-to-BSN graduates, a program outcome might include: *75% of graduates will obtain a new position or be promoted, obtain a pay raise, or be more involved in agency or unit activities.*

Nursing program pass rates for the NCLEX® or advanced practice registered nurses certification examinations should reflect national trends. For example, the current national NCLEX® first-time pass rates are between 80% and 85%. Nursing accrediting bodies usually require or recommend a pass rate of at least 80%. However, some states require higher expectations.

Programs beginning a CBC should compare program outcomes data of the graduates of the new curriculum with the data for graduates from the traditional curricular model. Outcomes related to the CBC are discussed later in this chapter.

Curricular Outcomes

A major component of the SPE is measuring curricular student learning outcomes (SLOs) for a CBC. Measuring learner achievement of SLOs may be direct or indirect. **Direct measurement of learning**, the preferred and most meaningful approach, requires students to demonstrate performance or SLO achievement using a specific evaluation method. Examples are tests, projects, portfolios, and clinical performance. **Indirect measurement of learning** requires students to provide their perception or opinion about how well they think they performed or achieved the SLOs. Examples are course surveys, program exit surveys, and alumni satisfaction surveys.

End-of-Program Student Learning Outcomes

As discussed earlier in this book, SLOs are developed at three tiers in a nursing program. The end-of-program SLOs, sometimes called program learning outcomes (PLOs), are broad statements that incorporate the organizing framework of the curriculum and reflect national trends and standards or competencies for a program's new graduates. For example, consider these new graduate SLOs for a BSN program:

- Provide safe, evidence-based nursing care for patients and families in a variety of health inpatient and community care settings.
- Collaborate with the interprofessional healthcare team using informatics and technology to facilitate communication and improve care.
- Utilize leadership and management of care principles within the legal and ethical framework of the generalist nursing role.

As mentioned in Chapter 1, these competencies are measured at the end of the program and could include *direct* evaluation methods such as:

- Performance on a standardized comprehensive examination that predicts NCLEX® performance and conceptual learning (for pre-RN licensure BSN options)

- Portfolio containing graded assignments (known as "artifacts") that demonstrate end-of-program SLO achievement and conceptual learning
- End-of-program objective structured clinical examination (OSCE) to measure clinical performance and conceptual learning

These measurement tools are administered near the end of the last nursing course in most programs.

As described in Chapter 4, the most commonly used standardized tests used in prelicensure programs are:

- HESI® Comprehensive Exam (Available through Elsevier)
- Kaplan Readiness Test (Available through Kaplan)
- ATI™ Predictor Exam (Available through Assessment Technologies Institute)

Although some programs use these tests as "high stakes," that is not their intended purpose. Most programs require a more appropriate use of these tests to demonstrate that students have met the end-of-program SLOs. The faculty set a desired level or expected outcome, also known as an expected level of achievement (ELA) or benchmark, that specifies how many students taking the test will obtain the recommended score on the test. For example, consider this ELA: *85% of graduating students will score 850 or above on the HESI Comprehensive Exam after two attempts.* Students who do not achieve an 850 on the first attempt as the actual outcome remediate in their low scoring areas then retake the examination. There is no penalty for not achieving the 850 score on the second try, but students need to study those areas where performance was low in preparation for the NCLEX®.

These tests are also useful to inform faculty about the quality of their CBC. For the previously mentioned ELA, if less than 85% of students achieve the desired HESI score, the faculty need to analyze the data to determine what curricular concepts might need improvement. For example, if a program determines that graduating students over the past several classes score low in Basic Care and Comfort, Teamwork and Collaboration, and Management of Care, the faculty of the program needs to consider strengthening that conceptual content in the curriculum. In this way, the data inform faculty decision making and provide evidence for curricular revision.

Another direct measurement method is the portfolio. A **portfolio** is a purposeful collection of materials, sometimes called artifacts, that communicates personal and professional development, self-assessment, and self-reflection skills. The portfolio is also used as a direct measurement of end-of-program SLOs and may be graded or reviewed for mastery in paper or digital format.

The least utilized direct method for measuring learner achievement of end-of-program SLOs in prelicensure nursing programs is the Objective Structured Clinical Examination (OSCE). However, this method is used more often in advanced practice nursing programs and in other health profession educational programs, including medicine and anesthesia.

A recent study by Kavanaugh and Szweda (2017) supports the need for more testing of students' clinical performance before they graduate from their nursing programs. The authors found that new graduates employed at a large Midwestern academic health system in the United States were unprepared and often overwhelmed intellectually, emotionally, and physically. To address this challenge, the institution implemented a new graduate residency program based on quantifiable analysis of the preparation-to-practice gap. The Performance-Based Development System (PBDS©), a web-based competency assessment tool, was used to identify new graduate clinical judgment ability using a series of video vignettes and narrative clinical case scenarios in medical-surgical nursing. The major components of the PBDS© system are listed in **BOX 12-1**.

The researchers found that over a 5-year period (2011–2015) of assessing more than 5,000 new graduates from 140 nursing programs in 21 states that only 20% to 24% (depending on the year) of new graduates had acceptable clinical judgment skills. Just over 75% of the new graduates were able to identify an urgency or problem in clinical situations, but less than 50% were able to demonstrate how to manage the urgency or problem. There was no difference in performance between AD and BN degree graduates.

As a result of these alarming statistics, the authors recommended that nursing program curricular revisions include performance evaluation, including OSCEs, to ensure that graduates can critically think, especially when planning and implementing how to manage a patient problem. Clinical or nursing judgment is an essential meta-concept in a CBC and is often not effectively measured. The authors also suggested that pedagogies, such as realistic case studies, be developed in nursing education that keep students "focused on the patient experience" (p. 61) and connect the classroom and clinical learning. These pedagogies may be created more effectively through partnering with clinical agencies to ensure a competent workforce.

Indirect methods for measuring student achievement of end-of-program SLOs include exit and/or new graduate surveys conducted at 6 to 12 months after graduation. As part of these surveys, the SLOs should be included so graduates can indicate how strongly they think they have met them or not. Most surveys use a rating scale similar to the one in **EXHIBIT 12-2**. Data from these surveys are aggregated, trended, and analyzed by cohort, program option, and program location.

Course Student Learning Outcomes

Course SLOs also may be measured using direct and indirect methods. Many nursing programs at all levels use comprehensive final examinations as a *direct* approach to course evaluation. Others may use standardized proficiency tests produced by the companies described earlier in this chapter; some may use these tests to determine student progression. However, as discussed in Chapter 4, high-stakes testing is not recommended by major nursing education organizations.

BOX 12-1 Major Components of the PBDS© Competency Assessment

Problem/urgency identification focus:

- Problems/risk identification
- Relative priority—urgency
- Justification for actions

Problem management focus:

- Identification of independent nursing actions
- Communication of essential information to the primary healthcare provider
- Anticipation of appropriate medical orders/prescriptions
- Justification of actions

EXHIBIT 12-2 Sample of Part of a New Graduate Survey Tool

I was prepared by my nursing program to meet these End-of-Program Student Learning Outcomes	1 Strongly Disagree	2 Disagree	3 Agree	4 Strongly Agree
Provide safe, evidence-based nursing care for patients and families in a variety of health inpatient and community care settings.				
Collaborate with the interprofessional healthcare team using informatics and technology to facilitate communication and improve care.				
Utilize leadership and management of care principles within the legal and ethical framework of the generalist nursing role.				

Clinical course SLOs are most often measured using the summative clinical evaluation tool (CET). A nursing program may set an ELA for the percentage of students who will successfully meet the performance criteria (also called competencies) outlined on a clinical CET as a way to determine student achievement of course outcomes. For example, consider this ELA: *95% of students will successfully meet all CET competencies.* If the actual data showed that less than 95% were successful, the faculty would need to trend the data to determine where the students had difficulty to develop a plan for improvement. Exhibit 11-2 in Chapter 11 illustrates an example of a summative clinical evaluation course.

One or more clinical performance examinations or OSCEs also may be used to measure achievement of course SLOs. Meaningful evaluations would serve to assess critical thinking, deep learning, and clinical judgment skills. As discussed earlier, research shows that new graduates need improvement in these skill sets to meet the complex needs of today's patients.

Some course SLOs are best measured directly by projects or papers. For example, consider these two course SLOs for a Community and Global Health course:

- *Conduct a health assessment of a community or vulnerable population.*
- *Develop a plan to improve the health of a selected vulnerable population based on a needs assessment.*

These SLOs would not be best met using a test or CET. Rather, a community health project (a direct measure) might be the most appropriate measurement to ensure that students achieved these SLOs.

Most programs ask students to complete course surveys about their satisfaction with the course, instructor, and program resources. Course surveys are *indirect* measures for program evaluation. However, students often provide very useful information that helps faculty revise or alter their course for the next group. An ELA for an SPE might be: *85% of students rate a 3 (agree) or 4 (strongly agree) that they have met the course SLOs.* Again, if the students do not meet the expected level or outcomes, the faculty need to respond by developing and implementing a plan for improvement.

Remember This . . .

Most programs ask students to complete course surveys about their satisfaction with the course, instructor, and program resources. Course surveys are indirect measures for program evaluation.

Faculty Outcomes

In a CBC, nurse educators need to learn how to teach conceptually in all learning environments. Therefore, most nursing programs develop expected faculty outcomes related to credentialing, clinical expertise, and scholarship. Credentialing and clinical expertise are dictated by regional higher institutional accrediting organizations, state or provincial nursing regulatory bodies, and/or nursing accreditation groups. Scholarship is usually determined by the college, university, school, or program.

The transition from a traditional to a conceptual learning paradigm requires faculty development and curricular expertise. Therefore, scholarship activities to promote professional growth and development of faculty is particularly important for a successful CBC. Nursing programs either develop their own definitions of scholarship, use the educational institution's definition, or adopt Boyer's classic four aspects of scholarship (1990). These aspects include:

- Scholarship of Discovery: Searching for new knowledge, often demonstrated through research.
- Scholarship of Integration: Bringing knowledge together from various disciplines, often demonstrated through research, publications, and presentations.
- Scholarship of Application (Practice): Finding ways that new knowledge can help promote practice, often through certifications and recognition as a master practitioner or expert.
- Scholarship of Teaching: Using innovative practices in teaching/learning, often demonstrated through presentations and publications.

For a CBC, the most important model is the Scholarship of Teaching. Effective teaching and learning in a CBC requires an innovative approach to help students achieve deep learning, critical thinking, and clinical reasoning. Examples of ELAs for faculty outcomes related to credentialing, clinical expertise, and scholarship might include:

- 100% of full-time faculty have a graduate degree in nursing or above.
- 100% of all faculty will demonstrate clinical expertise consistent with the content of the course(s) in which they teach.
- 100% of all full-time faculty will demonstrate evidence of at least one Scholarship of Teaching activity related to conceptual teaching and learning.
- 100% of all faculty will participate in at least two scholarship activities each academic year.
- 30% of full-time faculty will earn their Certified Nurse Educator™ credential in AY17-18.

▶ Evaluating Concept-Based Curriculum Outcomes

For several years after the CBC movement began in 2004 at the University of New Mexico, NCLEX-RN® pass rates of that program markedly decreased (Giddens & Horton, 2010). A few other programs reported slightly lower pass rates, but no trend in licensure pass rate decline has occurred as a result of moving from the traditional curriculum model to the CBC model. A descriptive survey reported in a white paper by Sportsman (2013) found that 30% of respondents indicated that graduates' NCLEX® pass rates increased after CBC implementation, 42% had no change in pass rates, and only 5% had decreased NCLEX® pass rates.

Some faculty continue to be reluctant to pursue conceptual learning in a CBC because they fear a potential decrease in the NCLEX® pass rates. Patterson, Crager, Farmer, Epps, and Schuessler (2016) reported their experience with their CBC and found that based on three BSN graduating classes since new curriculum implementation, program outcomes stayed the same or improved. In particular, the authors found that their NCLEX-RN® pass rates were the same, at 91%, before and after CBC implementation. New graduate satisfaction with the program also stayed the same at between 87% and 97%. Additional findings included that:

- Student critical thinking scores trended upward since CBC implementation.
- Unsolicited nursing staff and formal feedback from clinical settings indicated that students exhibited better critical thinking skills at the bedside since CBC implementation.

Lewis (2014) reported that program outcomes improved as a result of CBC implementation in a small diploma nursing program in North Carolina. Findings included that:

- Program completion rate increased by 4% (statistically significant)
- Employer satisfaction increased by 1.7% (not statistically significant)
- NCLEX® pass rates increased by 1% (not statistically significant)

As expected from these data, student retention and on-time graduation rates also increased.

Harrison (2016) found a significant increase in NCLEX® pass rates as a result of changing from a traditional model to a CBC in an AD in nursing program. The researcher also found an increase in students' critical thinking scores when compared to those for students in the traditional curriculum.

Another faculty (and administrative) concern about the change from a traditional model to a CBC model is "curricular drift." Curricular drift occurs over time, often only a few months or years, when faculty begin to revert to old familiar ways of teaching and content. This phenomenon can be the result of one or more factors. First, some faculty may not have "bought in" to the new curriculum and therefore did not change their content or teaching/learning practices. In other cases, faculty may not have understood how to teach concepts and therefore continued with the traditional medical model. The second factor is faculty turnover that may result in new faculty who may or not be formally educated in nursing education. Third, new faculty may not be adequately oriented and mentored so that they gain the knowledge and skills needed to be effective in a CBC.

To prevent these types of problems, nursing accreditation and regulatory bodies dictate the need for faculty to regularly review the curriculum for currency, integrity, and rigor. This element is met in most programs several ways:

- Each nurse educator develops a report or synopsis that summarizes, reflects, and evaluates his or her course.
- Many programs have extended annual or bi-annual meetings or retreats in which all faculty participate to review and evaluate the strengths and identify the areas of improvement for the curriculum.

When transitioning to a CBC, this review and evaluation are even more critical due to nature and scope of the change. Patterson et al. (2016) reported concerns about curricular drift and the continued use of the medical model by some faculty after the CBC model was implemented in their BSN program. They also noted that instead of complex concepts being expanded with new knowledge in each new context as the program progresses, the same content was repeated.

The new curriculum consisted of:

- Four Health Care of the Client courses (HCC1 through HCC4)
- Four Professional Nursing Concepts courses (PC1 through PC4)
- Four Clinical Practice courses (CP1 through CP4)
- Seven support courses, such as Evidence-Based Practice and Pathopharmacology

To address the identified problems, the faculty used a conceptual grid to assess and improve their new curriculum. The conceptual grid aligned courses for each of four semesters both vertically and horizontally. Faculty formed vertical and horizontal committees to ensure that everyone was engaged and actively pursuing best practices in conceptual teaching and learning. The vertical committees were organized by course across the four semesters (e.g., faculty teaching in PC1, 2, 3, and 4 comprised the Professional Nursing Concepts courses vertical committee). Horizontal committees were organized by semester across the three types of concepts courses (e.g., faculty teaching in HCC1, PC1, and CP1 made up a horizontal committee). Therefore, each faculty served on more than one committee and was aware of what all other nurse educators were teaching and evaluating. Faculty teaching in the support courses were placed on one or more of the committees depending on where they were placed in the curriculum and which concept course was most supported. For instance, Health Assessment and Pathopharmacology 1 and 2 were aligned with the first-semester courses where they were taught.

More studies are needed to determine the outcomes of conceptual teaching and learning in nursing. Increasing numbers of dissertations are being published to add to the body of knowledge needed to develop the most effective concept-based programs such that students will be competent in critical thinking and clinical judgment to provide safe, high-quality care.

▶ Chapter Key Points

- Program evaluation is a continuous assessment and analysis of the components of a nursing program or department to provide data for faculty as a basis for informed program decisions about the ability to meet program outcomes.
- Several models have been used as frameworks for quality improvement and educational programs over the past 30 to 40 years, including those published by Donabedian, Piskurich, and Stufflebeam. Stufflebeam's CIPP model is more commonly used for nursing program evaluation.
- The SPE typically consist of these components: program outcomes, curricular outcomes, and faculty outcomes.
- The three program outcomes that all nursing programs in the United States usually track are program completion rates, employment rates, and certification or licensure first-time pass rates.
- The expected outcomes, or ELAs, are benchmarks or levels that the program deems most appropriate to measure the component.
- Measuring learner achievement of SLOs may be direct or indirect. Direct measurement of learning, the preferred approach, requires students to demonstrate performance or SLO achievement using a specific evaluation method.
- Indirect measurement of learning requires students to provide their perception or opinion about how well they think they performed or achieved the SLOs.
- A portfolio is a purposeful collection of materials, sometimes called artifacts, that communicates personal and professional development, self-assessment, and self-reflection skills.
- The portfolio is also used as a direct measurement of end-of-program SLOs and may be graded or reviewed for mastery in paper or digital format.
- The least utilized direct method for measuring learner achievement of end-of-program SLOs in prelicensure nursing programs is the Objective Structured Clinical Examination (OSCE).
- *Indirect* methods for measuring student achievement of end-of-program SLOs include exit and/or new graduate surveys conducted at 6 to 12 months after graduation.
- Many nursing programs at all levels use comprehensive final examinations as a *direct* approach to course evaluation; others may use standardized proficiency tests. Some course SLOs are best measured directly by projects or papers.
- Clinical course SLOs are most often measured using the summative clinical evaluation tool.
- Most nursing programs develop expected faculty outcomes related to credentialing, clinical expertise, and scholarship.
- Nursing programs either develop their own definitions of scholarship, use the educational institution's definition, or adopt Boyer's classic four aspects of scholarship (1990); for a CBC, the most important model is the Scholarship of Teaching.

- No trend in NCLEX® pass rate decline has occurred as a result of moving from the traditional curriculum model to the CBC model. In most programs, the pass rate has stayed the same or increased.
- Some data show that program completion rates, employer satisfaction rates, alumni satisfaction rates, and critical thinking scores have remained the same or increased as a result of CBC implementation.

▶ Chapter References and Selected Bibliography

Billings, D. M., & Halstead, J. A. (2016). *Teaching in nursing: A guide for faculty* (5th ed.). St. Louis, MO: Elsevier.

*Boyer, E. (1990). *Scholarship reconsidered: Priorities for the professoriate.* Princeton, NJ: The Carnegie Foundation for the Advancement of Teaching.

*Donabedian, A. (1989). Institutional and professional responsibilities in quality assurance. *Quality Assurance in Health Care, 1*(1), 3–11.

Escallier, L. A., & Fullerton, J. T. (2012). An innovation in design of a nursing evaluation protocol. *Nurse Educator, 37*(5), 187–191.

*Gard, C., Flannigan, P., & Cluskey, M. (2004). Program evaluation: An ongoing systematic process. *Nursing Education Perspectives, 25*(4), 176–179.

Giddens, J., & Horton, N. (2010). Report card: An evaluation of a concept-based curriculum. *Nursing Education Perspectives, 31*(6), 372–377.

Harrison, C. V. (2016). *Evaluating the outcomes of a concept-based curriculum in an associate degree in nursing program.* (Doctoral dissertation). Retrieved from http://mospace.umsystem.edu/xmlui/bitstream/handle/10355/48987/HarrisonEvaOutCon.pdf?sequence=1.

Kalb, K. (2009). The three Cs model: The context, content, and conduct of nursing education. *Nursing Education Perspectives, 30*(3), 176–180.

Kavanaugh, J. M., & Szweda, C. (2017). A crisis in competency: The strategic and ethical imperative to assessing new graduate nurses' clinical reasoning. *Nursing Education Perspectives, 38*(2), 57–62.

Keating, S. B. (2015). *Curriculum development and evaluation in nursing.* New York, NY: Springer Publishing.

Lewis, L. S. (2014). Outcomes of a concept-based curriculum. *Teaching and Learning in Nursing, 9*(2), 75–79.

Oermann, M. H., & Gaberson, K. B. (2017). *Evaluation and testing in nursing education* (5th ed.). New York, NY: Springer Publishing.

Patterson, L. D., Crager, J. M., Farmer, A., Epps C. D., & Schuessler, J. B. (2016). A strategy to ensure faculty engagement when assessing a concept-based curriculum. *Journal of Nursing Education, 55*(8), 467–470.

*Piskurich, G. (1993). *Self-directed learning: A practical guide to design, development and implementation.* San Francisco, CA: Jossey-Bass.

*Singh, M. D. (2004). Evaluation framework for nursing education programs: Application of the CIPP model. *International Journal of Nursing Education Scholarship, 1*, Article 13.

Sportsman, S. (2013). *Concept-based curricula in nursing: Perceptions of the trend.* St. Louis, MO: Elsevier.

*Stufflebeam, D. L. (2000). The CIPP model for evaluation. In D. L. Stufflebeam, G. F. Madaus, & T. Kellaghan (Eds). *Evaluation models* (2nd ed.). Boston, MA: Kluwer Academic Publishers.

*Indicates classic reference.

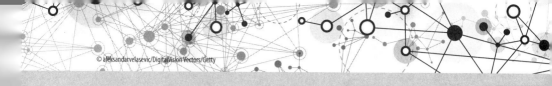

Appendix A

Lesson Plan/Student Study Guide

▶ NUR 320: Adult Health Nursing I

Topic	Student Learning Outcomes	Related Course SLOs	Learning Activities	Evaluation Methods
Osteoarthritis	1. Recall the anatomy and physiology of the musculoskeletal system, including the synovial joints. 2. Explain the pathophysiology of osteoarthritis (OA) and risk factors for its development. 3. Apply knowledge of pathophysiology to identify typical assessment findings for the patient with OA. 4. Use nursing judgment to plan safe, evidence-based care for patients with OA.	1, 2	*Before class:* ■ Review musculoskeletal system with focus on joints. ■ Read content in Ignatavicius and Workman (2015) on osteoarthritis. *During class:* ■ Lecture and discussion ■ NCLEX® practice questions ■ Case study in small groups *After class:* ■ Review notes and come to class with questions.	■ Unit examination questions on Exam #2

(continues)

Topic	Student Learning Outcomes	Related Course SLOs	Learning Activities	Evaluation Methods
	5. Apply knowledge of pharmacology to delineate nursing implications for administering drug therapy used for patients with OA.			
	6. Determine which healthcare team members to collaborate with to manage pain and promote mobility and activities of daily living for the patient with OA.			
	7. Provide health teaching for the patient and family to manage pain and promote mobility for patients with OA.			

▶ Reference

Ignatavicius, D. D., & Workman, M. L. (2015). *Medical-surgical nursing: Patient-centered collaborative care* (8th ed.). St. Louis: Elsevier.

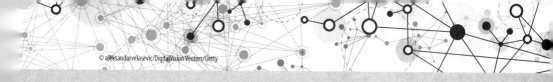

Appendix B

Concept Presentation: Mobility

Topic	Description
Definition of Mobility	The ability of an individual to perform purposeful physical movement of the body. When a person is able to move, he or she is usually able to perform activities of daily living (ADLs), such as eating, dressing, and walking. This ability depends primarily on the function of the central and peripheral nervous system and the musculoskeletal system.
Scope or Categories of Mobility	The scope of mobility can be described as a continuum of a person's ability to move, with high-level (normal) mobility on one end of the continuum and total immobility on the other end. Many patients have varying degrees of impaired or altered physical mobility.
Common Risk Factors for Impaired or Altered Mobility	Patients who have dysfunction of the musculoskeletal or nervous system are most at risk for impaired mobility or immobility. For example, a patient with a fractured hip is not able to walk due to pain and hip joint instability until the hip is surgically repaired and healed. Patients who have severe brain or spinal cord injuries have impaired mobility or total immobility due to lack of neuronal communication or damaged nerve tissues that enable body movement. Any person who is bedridden or on prolonged bedrest is at risk for immobility issues regardless of health problem or medical diagnosis.
Physiological Consequences of Impaired or Altered Mobility	<ul><li>Pressure injuries</li><li>Disuse osteoporosis</li><li>Constipation</li><li>Weight loss or gain</li><li>Muscle atrophy</li><li>Atelectasis/hypostatic pneumonia</li><li>Venous thromboembolism (VTE) (e.g., deep venous thrombosis [DVT] and pulmonary embolus)</li><li>Urinary system calculi</li><li>Depression</li><li>Changes in sleep-wake cycle</li><li>Sensory deprivation</li></ul>

(continues)

Topic	Description
Assessment of Mobility Status	The mobility level of the patient is high (or good) if he or she can move purposely to walk with an erect posture and coordinated gait and perform ADLs without assistance. Several functional assessment tools are available to measure the level at which a patient can perform ADLs. Assessment of muscle strength and joint range of motion (ROM) also can be measured using a scale of 0–5, with 5 being normal and 0 indicating no muscle contractility.
Collaborative Interventions to Prevent Impaired or Altered Mobility	■ Teach patients to do active ROM exercises every 2 hours. Assess and manage pain to promote more comfortable movement. ■ Teach patients to perform "heel pump" activities and drink adequate fluids to help prevent VTE, such as DVT. ■ In collaboration with the occupational therapist, evaluate the patient's need for assistive devices to promote ADL independence, such as a plate guard or splint; encourage self-care. ■ Evaluate the patient's need for ambulatory aids, such as a cane or walker; encourage ambulation; collaborate with the physical therapist if needed.
Interventions for Patients with Impaired or Altered Mobility	■ Perform passive ROM exercises for patients who are immobile or have severe impaired mobility. ■ Turn and reposition the patient every 1–2 hours; assess for skin redness and intactness. ■ Keep the patient's skin clean and dry; use pressure-relieving or pressure-reducing devices as indicated. ■ In collaboration with the registered dietitian, teach the patient and family the need for adequate nutrition, including high-fiber and protein-rich foods to promote elimination and slow muscle loss. ■ Teach the patient to eat high-calcium foods to help prevent bone loss; avoid excessive high-calorie foods to prevent obesity. ■ Encourage deep breathing and coughing exercises; teach the patient how and when to use incentive spirometry. ■ Teach the patient and family the need for adequate hydration to prevent renal calculi (stones) and constipation. ■ Teach the patient and family to report signs and symptoms of complications of immobility, such as pressure injuries, swollen, reddened lower leg, and excessive respiratory secretions. ■ Collaborate with the physical therapist to ambulate the patient with mobility aids (e.g., walker, cane), if needed.
Interrelated Concepts	Functional Ability, Comfort, Sensory Perception

Appendix C

Concept Presentation: Clinical Judgment

Topic	Description
Definition of Clinical Judgment	The conclusion or deduction about the patient's situation and the interventions used for decision making. Clinical reasoning is the process used to reach a clinical judgment.
Scope or Categories of Clinical Judgment	In her classic systematic review, Tanner (2006) concluded that *sound* clinical judgment is influenced by how well the nurse knows the patient's typical response pattern and the situational context or culture of the nursing care unit. *Poor* clinical judgment can result in Failure to Rescue situations in which patients are harmed. Failure to Rescue occurs when beginning or subtle patient signs and symptoms are not noticed or accurately interpreted and, therefore, action to improve the patient's condition is not implemented (Garvey, 2015).
Attributes and Theoretical Links for Clinical Judgment	Tanner (2006) describes four components of clinical judgment: ■ Noticing ■ Interpreting ■ Responding ■ Reflecting Each of these processes requires clinical reasoning to ensure that the most appropriate clinical decision is made in a timely manner.
Examples of Context for Clinical Judgment in Nursing and Health Care	The Joint Commission's National Patient Safety Goals specify that each healthcare organization must establish criteria for patients, families, or staff to call for additional assistance in response to an actual or perceived change in the patient's condition. Most acute care hospitals have a Rapid Response Team who respond to these patient changes.
Interrelated Concepts	Safety, Quality Improvement, Professionalism

▶ References

Garvey, P. K. (2015). Failure to rescue: The nurse's impact. *MEDSURG Nursing, 24*(3), 145–149.

*Tanner, C. A. (2006). Thinking like a nurse: A research-based model of clinical judgment in nursing. *Journal of Nursing Education, 45*(6), 204–211.

*Indicates classic reference.

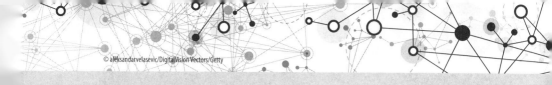

Appendix D

Example of Lesson Plan for Concept Introduction: Gas Exchange

Concept	Student Learning Outcomes	Related Course SLOs	Learning Activities/ Assessment	Evaluation Methods
Gas Exchange	1. Define the concept of gas exchange. 2. Briefly explain the process of ventilation and diffusion. 3. Describe the scope of gas exchange. 4. Assess risk factors for impaired gas exchange. 5. Describe the possible physiological consequences of impaired gas exchange. 6. Explain how to assess a patient's gas exchange status.	1, 2, 4	*Before Class:* ■ Complete gas exchange worksheet and bring to class. (NOTE: May use as an Admit Ticket.) (#1) ■ Review respiratory system with focus on ventilation and diffusion of gases. (#2) *During Class:* ■ Have students pair and draw the scope of gas exchange. Then do Pair Activity to discuss where patients would be on the gas exchange continuum. (#3) ■ NCLEX® practice items (#4) ■ In-class discussion (#5) ■ Video on respiratory assessment (#6) ■ Case study (#7 & #8)	■ Worksheet worth a possible 1 point ■ Unit examination questions on Exam #3

(continues)

Concept	Student Learning Outcomes	Related Course SLOs	Learning Activities/ Assessment	Evaluation Methods
	7. Identify collaborative interventions to promote gas exchange and prevent inadequate gas exchange. 8. Identify collaborative interventions to manage patients with inadequate gas change.		*After Class:* ■ Review notes; apply knowledge of gas exchange in clinical experience this week as directed.	

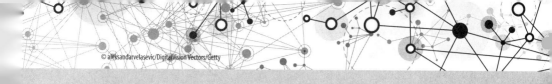

Appendix E

Lesson Plan/Student Study Guide for Exemplar

▶ NUR 320: Nursing Concepts I

Exemplar	Student Learning Outcomes	Related Course SLOs	Learning Activities/ Assessment	Evaluation Methods
Gas Exchange: Chronic Obstructive Pulmonary Disease (COPD)	1. Recall the introduction to gas exchange, including anatomy and physiology. 2. Explain the pathophysiology of COPD as it affects gas exchange, including risk factors. 3. Outline the role of the nurse in caring for patients with COPD having diagnostic testing to measure gas exchange. 4. Apply knowledge of pathophysiology to document assessment findings for the patient with COPD to determine the status of gas exchange.	1, 2, 5	*Before class:* ■ Complete gas exchange worksheet and bring to class. (NOTE: May use as an Admit Ticket.) ■ Review respiratory system with focus on ventilation and diffusion of gases. ■ Read COPD section in Ignatavicius and Workman (2015). ■ Review chapter on end-of-life in Ignatavicius and Workman (2015).	■ Worksheet worth a possible 1 point ■ Unit examination questions on Exam #1 ■ Discussion forum due prior to next class; 3 points possible (see rubric)

(continues)

5. Use nursing judgment to plan safe, evidence-based care to promote gas exchange in the patient with COPD.
6. Apply knowledge of pharmacology to delineate nursing implications for administering drug therapy used to promote gas exchange in the patient with COPD.
7. Collaborate with the healthcare team for care coordination to improve gas exchange in the patient with COPD.
8. Apply knowledge of pathophysiology to reduce potentially life-threatening complications of COPD that affect gas exchange and perfusion.
9. Provide health teaching for the patient and family to manage transitions in care, including smoking cessation if applicable, to promote gas exchange.
10. Explain the professional role of the nurse in assisting patients and families with end-of-life and palliative care for patients with COPD.

During class:
- Have students pair and draw graphics to demonstrate what happens in the pathophysiology of COPD. Be prepared to explain the graphics in class. (#2)
- i-Clicker questions (#3)
- Unfolding case study in small groups (#4–#6, #9)
- Create drug cards for assigned selected prototype bronchodilators.
- NCLEX® Practice Test Items (#6 and #7)
- 3Rs (Recognize, Respond, and Rescue) activity on cor pulmonale in small groups. (#8)

After class:
- Online discussion forum about ethics and end-of-life care. (#10)

▶ Reference

Ignatavicius, D. D., & Workman, M. L. (2015). *Medical-surgical nursing: Patient-centered collaborative care* (8th ed.). St. Louis: Elsevier.

Glossary

A

Academic-practice liaison (APL): A faculty member who assists in educating leadership and clinical staff in the healthcare agency and advocates for adequate clinical units to meet the students' needs each semester or other term.

Affective domain: A hierarchical learning domain that involves developing attitudes, values, and beliefs.

Asynchronous online learning: An event in the online setting in which a group of students are engaged in learning at different times.

B

Backward design: A three-stage pedagogical approach that includes developing desired student learning outcomes and program outcomes; determining evaluation strategies; and determining course content, student expectations, and teaching/learning strategies.

Blended online learning: A hybrid or mix of face-to-face instruction and online learning.

Blog: A web page run by an individual or group that is written in informal or conversational style.

C

Case study: Written simulated learning activity in which a clinical or healthcare situation is followed by thinking questions for students to answer; it is a student-centered learning activity that tells a story based on concepts that demonstrate application or translation of theory to practice.

Chat room: An online area where learners can communicate often about a particular topic.

Clinical coordinator: A nurse educator who arranges all clinical experiences and makes rounds in each agency to ensure students have the opportunity to meet outcomes related to conceptual learning.

Clinical imagination: A learning environment that allows students in the classroom to practice or rehearse the clinical reasoning they need in practice through the use of "real-world" patient situations.

Clinical judgment: The conclusion or deduction about the patient's situation and the interventions used for decision making.

Clinical reasoning: The process of thinking about a patient situation in a specific context while considering patient and family concerns.

Cognition: "The complex integration of mental processes and intellectual function for the purposes of reasoning, learning, and memory" (Ignatavicius, Workman, & Rebar, 2018, p. 16).

Cognitive domain: A hierarchical learning domain that describes the levels of cognition (thinking) in one's brain.

Cognitive presence: The process of building knowledge throughout an online course.

Collaborative Testing: A learning strategy in which students work together in pairs or groups to answer test questions.

Competencies: The knowledge, skills, and attitudes (KSAs) that make up a person's role.

Computer-assisted concept mapping (CACM): Use of computer software to develop an individualized concept map for a variety of electronic devices, including the iPad.

Concepts: Classifications/categories of information (knowledge) that can be ideas or mental images; they are not objects or things, and can be flexible and dynamic.

Concept-based curriculum (CBC): A curriculum designed by organizing specific content around identified program concepts.

Concept-based teaching: An innovative approach that ensures meaningful learning to help students apply patterns of knowing across a variety of contexts.

Concept map (CM): A graphic organizer learning tool that is used to develop clinical judgment.

Concept mapping: An innovative approach in healthcare education that creates meaningful learning as students are better able to organize knowledge, create connections, and develop clinical judgment skills that ultimately improve patient safety and quality care.

Concept presentation: An introduction that provides an in-depth analysis of a concept.

Conceptual learning: Learning process that is student-centered and requires active engagement.

Constructed response test items: Test items that require the test taker to either manipulate information provided in the question or create an answer.

Constructivism: A learning theory that is similar to Malcolm Knowles' classic adult learning theory and posits that new knowledge is best understood if it can be connected to previous knowledge or experiences and previous knowledge and experiences influence the understanding and interpretation of new knowledge.

Continuing case study: A case study that consists of more than one phase of care over minutes, hours, days, weeks, or months; the parts of the case are completed over time rather than students completing the case study in one educational session.

Criterion-referenced evaluation: Evaluation that requires the learner to meet a predetermined standard or criteria; it is sometimes referred to as grading with an absolute scale.

Curriculum: The formal and informal structure and process in which a learner gains the knowledge, skills, attitudes, and abilities to meet established educational outcomes.

D

Debriefing: An important part of learning during which the educator clarifies, highlights, summarizes, and updates class content at various points during class and other learning environments.

Decision-making trees: A learning and thinking tool that allows the user to determine the best decision to make based on answers to a series of questions.

Deep learning: Long-term learning that results when new neuronal connections are created or expanded in the brain during each meaningful teaching/learning experience.

Degree plan: A plan of study that results in receiving a college degree.

Direct care activities: Clinical learning activities in which students provide total or focused patient care to *achieve* one or more competencies related to applying Health and/or Professional Nursing concepts.

Direct measurement of learning: The preferred and most meaningful way to measure learning because students have to demonstrate performance or student learning outcome achievement using a specific evaluation method.

Discussion boards: An online activity that provides a "threaded" forum in which students and the educator can engage asynchronously.

Distractors: The wrong choices in a test item; they should be viable and feasible.

E

English language learners (ELL): Students who learn English as a second (or third or fourth) language.

Evaluation: The *process* of collecting and analyzing data gathered through one or more measurements to render a *judgment* about the subject of the evaluation.

Exemplars: Specific content topics that relate to and represent identified concepts.

F

Flipped classroom: A model in which lecture and homework are reversed; that is, the lecture occurs *before* class and homework that engages students in active learning is done in the classroom.

Focused learning activities: Activities and assignments that promote learning in the laboratory or external clinical setting; they *support* achievement of one or more clinical competencies related to applying concepts for deep understanding.

Formative evaluation (sometimes referred to as assessment): Evaluation that occurs on an ongoing basis and provides opportunities for students to improve based on nurse educator feedback; it is process-oriented, reflective, and diagnostic.

G

Gaming: A learning activity that is an excellent method for assessing student knowledge (but not how to apply or translate knowledge).

Graphic organizers: A group of learning tools in which concepts are presented visually to show relationships, which are particularly helpful for visual learners.

Group rooms: An online area that gives groups of students places to store files that are exclusive to their work, but are not necessary for the rest of the class to access.

H

Hybrid online learning: Another term for blended online learning (see above definition).

I

Indirect measurement of learning: A way to measure learning that requires students to provide their perception or opinion about how well they think they performed or achieved student learning outcomes.

Interprofessional education (IPE): Process that allows students from two or more health professions to learn together during the same learning activity or in the same setting and promotes team building.

L

Learning Management System (LMS): A type of software or application that is used to structure and manage an online course.

Lecture: A one-way teaching experience in which the instructor talks and the students are expected to listen and learn.

Lesson plan: A guide for faculty as they prepare for class, and a study guide for students to delineate learning expectations and assessments.

Let's Discuss: A learning activity in which the instructor initiates discussion of a topic or statement with the entire class or with student pairs or groups.

Linking words: One or more words on a concept map that provide the meaning of the *relationships* between two or more concepts.

M

Macroconcepts: Broad concepts that provide a way to link sub-concepts.

Microconcepts: Specific concepts that provide disciplinary depth for understanding and deep learning.

Mission: A broad statement about the institution's, department's, or program's goal or purpose.

Multiple-response test item: A test item that consists of a stem (clinical scenario) and five to seven choices; two or more choices are the best response or answer. On the NCLEX® examination, these items are called Select All That Apply (SATA).

N

Norm-referenced evaluation: Evaluation that requires the learner to successfully meet expectations, but scores vary and are compared with peer scores; it is sometimes referred to as grading with a relative scale.

Nullifying: A process in which all choices of a test item are accepted because the test item was poorly constructed.

O

Objective Structured Clinical Examination (OSCE): A process in which a high-fidelity simulation or standardized patient situation is used to evaluate student performance in the cognitive, psychomotor, and affective learning domains.

Online course: A course that is delivered via the Internet using a learning management system.

Online presence: The mechanism by which the nurse educator establishes first contact with learners in an online learning environment.

Organizing curriculum framework: A plan that identifies the major underpinnings, themes, or core concepts that organize a program's curriculum; also may be called an organizational framework or conceptual framework.

P

Pedagogies: Teaching/learning activities and strategies.

Philosophy: A set of beliefs and their related concepts that flows from the mission; it drives a program's curriculum.

Plan of study: A plan that outlines the sequence of courses needed for a student to graduate from a program; may also be called a program of study (POS).

Portfolio: A purposeful collection of materials, sometimes called artifacts, that communicates personal and professional development, self-assessment, and self-reflection skills.

Program evaluation: A continuous assessment and analysis of the components of a nursing program or department to provide data for faculty as a basis for informed program decisions about the ability to meet program outcomes.

Proposition: The building blocks of knowledge in a concept map that are formed when two or more concepts are connected with linking words and lines to establish meaning.

Psychomotor domain: A hierarchical learning domain that involves the development of technical skills, including competencies associated with informatics and technology.

R

Reflection: A learning tool that may be utilized as an assignment in the classroom, laboratory, simulation, or clinical environment to promote self-awareness about the benefit of a learning activity and the impact of the activity on the student to help develop professionalism.

S

Scrambled classroom: A model in which learning is facilitated by mixing engaging collaborative student activities with multiple short periods (5 to 10 minutes each); the instructor clarifies, updates, and prioritizes class content.

Selected response test item: A test item that provides choices from which the test taker must choose to get the correct answer; also referred to as a multiple-choice item.

Send a Problem (sometimes called Pass a Problem): A learning activity in which students individually, in pairs, or in groups of 3 or 4 develop test questions or case studies to share with other students.

Single-response test item: A test item that consists of a stem and four choices; only one choice is the best response or answer.

Situated learning: Learning that emphasizes that a student's knowledge is constructed within and linked to the activity, context, and culture in which it is learned.

Socratic questioning: A technique that nurse educators can use to stimulate thinking and deep conceptual learning in the classroom, laboratory, and simulation.

Social presence: Perceived presence and salience that increases inter-learner and learner-facilitator (educator) interactions, which in turn, enriches the educational process.

Structured Controversy: A learning and thinking activity used when exploring controversial issues or ethical dilemmas; students debate each side of the issue for 1 minute each.

Student learning outcomes (SLOs): The desired expectations regarding knowledge, skills, and attitudes that students are expected to achieve during an educational program.

Summative evaluation: Occurs at the end of a unit of study or course and assigns a final score or grade; it is product-oriented, prescriptive, and judgmental.

Superficial learning: Short-term learning in which knowledge is fragmented, disorganized, and compartmentalized.

Synchronous online learning: An event in the online setting in which a group of students are engaged in learning at the same time.

T

Taxonomy: Classification system.

Teaching presence: The elements of instruction that make up an online course, including the course syllabus.

Test Item Checks: Practice test items that are used for learning or formative assessment of learning during face-to-face or online courses.

Think-Pair-Share: A learning activity in which the instructor presents a topic or statement to the class but each student first writes his or her own response on paper or a mobile device within a 2- to 3-minute timeframe. After this time elapses, students in each pair share and compare their answers for another 2 to 3 minutes.

U

Unfolding Case Study: A case study that evolves over time in a manner that is unpredictable to the learner as new elements (or phases of care) of the case are revealed during multiple patient encounters.

V

Venn diagrams: Graphic organizers that use two or more circles to show comparisons between and among concepts.

W

"What If . . . ?": A learning activity that provides an opportunity for students to critically think and then decide on the action they would take. This question could be asked for the entire class to consider or used as a pair discussion either in the classroom or online.

Wikis: A collaborative effort created by different members of an online course that gives students opportunities to collectively share notes or study tips, or creatively present work.

Index

A

academic-practice liaison (APL), 99
Accreditation Commission for Education in
        Nursing (ACEN), 235
adult health nursing I, 247–248
advanced nursing practice programs
    length of, 16
    and organizing curriculum framework,
        9–10
affective domain, 65–67, 70–71, 187
Appreciation for Professional Values, 225
artifacts, 239
assessment. *See* formative evaluation
assimilation theory, 148
asynchronous online learning, 126
attendance, LMS and, 134

B

backward design, 10
blended or hybrid course, 126–127
blogs, LMS and, 134
Bloom's taxonomy, 194–196
Boyer's model of scholarship
    Scholarship of Application (Practice), 242
    Scholarship of Discovery, 242
    Scholarship of Integration, 242
    Scholarship of Teaching, 242

C

calendar feature, LMS and, 134
caring, 193
case studies
    description of, 83
case studies, concept-based curriculum and,
        167–180
    clinical judgment, 169–170
    clinical reasoning, 169–170
        effective usage of, 172–180

conceptual learning and clinical
        reasoning, effective usage of,
        172–180
    single case studies, exercises, and
        challenges, 172–175
    unfolding and continuing case studies,
        175–180
    critical thinking, 168–169
    description of, 172
    introduction, 167–168
    nursing process, 168–169
    transformation, knowledge into practice,
        171–172
CBC. *See* concept-based curriculum
chat room, LMS and, 134
CIPP model, 235
classrooms, concept-based curriculum
    conceptual learning evaluation, 186–187
        evaluation methods, developing,
            187–188
        learning domain considerations, 187
        validity and reliability considerations,
            187
    examinations
        cognitive test anxiety, 188–191
        commercial standardized testing,
            205–206
        evidence of measurement validity,
            196–198
        evidence of test reliability, 202
        general principles of NCLEX®-style test
            writing, 200–202
        NCLEX®-style tests, 189, 192–196
        test item difficulty, 203
        test item discrimination, 203–205
        types of NCLEX® item formats,
            198–200
    papers and projects, 206–207
    quizzes, 206
clinical evaluation tool (CET), 241
clinical imagination, 172
clinical judgment, 169–170
    concept presentation, 251–252
clinical paper assignments, 227–228
clinical reasoning, 169–170

clinical setting, concept-based curriculum
  clinical simulation, 223–224
  direct care activities, 213–222
  evaluation of, 212
  focused learning activities, 224–231
  Objective Structured Clinical Examination
    (OSCE), 224
  standardized patient methodology, 222
  validity and reliability considerations,
    212–213
clinical teaching and learning, CBC and,
  95–122
  activities and assignments, 108–115
    concept mapping, 112
    interprofessional, 109
    organizing, 115–122
    peer-to-peer interaction, 115
    quality improvement, 112
    reflections, 115
    safety-focused, 110
    60-second assignment, 112
    Socratic questioning, 114–115
  classroom, connection with, 106–107
  description of, 97–98
  introduction, 95–96
  laboratory, connection with, 106–107
  preparation for, 98–106
    clinical nurse educator, mentoring,
      100–106
    role of the coordinator, 99–100
    role of the educational resource unit, 100
    selection and management, 107–108
    simulation learning, connection with,
      106–107
  traditional model, 96
cognition, concept of, 194
cognitive domain, 61–63, 68–69, 187
cognitive presence, 132
cognitive test anxiety (CTA), 188–191
collaborative testing, 87
commercial standardized testing, 205–206
Commission on Collegiate Nursing Education
  (CCNE), 235–236
compare and contrast assignments, 231
competencies, 213, 241
competency-based curriculum, 13
completion items, 206
computer-assisted concept mapping
  (CACM), 154
computerized adaptive test (CAT). *See*
  NCLEX®
concept, description of, 26
concept-based classroom, teaching and
  learning in, 73–93

characteristics of today's learners, 74–78
  demographic characteristics, 77–78
  developmental stage, 76–77
  learning preferences, 75
  thinking styles, 75–76
clinical imagination, 80
collaborative learning, role of, 78–79
description of, 73
flipped *versus* scrambled classroom, 79–80
introduction, 73–74
promoting, strategies and activities for,
  81–92
  case studies, 83–84
  collaborative testing, 87
  gaming, 91–92
  graphic organizers, 85–86
  pair discussions, 82–83
  send a problem, 87
  social media, 92
  storytelling, 87–90
  test item checks, 86–87
  video clips and sounds, 90–91
students learning outcomes, relating to, 81
concept-based curriculum (CBC), 13, 234
  case studies, usage of, 167–180
  characteristics of, 26–27
  classroom. *See* classroom, concept-based
    curriculum
  clinical setting. *See* clinical setting,
    concept-based curriculum
  clinical teaching and learning, 95–122.
    See also clinical teaching and
    learning, CBC and
  and concept mapping, 150–153
  model, 244
  nursing, 37–39
    transition from traditional, 39–41
  12-step approach, 37–56
concept-based online learning environment,
  teaching in, 125–145
  cognitive presence, 132
  interactive discussion forums, 137–140
  introduction, 125–126
  management systems, learning, 132–137
    course consistency, ensuring, 136–137
    design and structure, 137
    usage of tools in classroom, 133–136
  methods used in, 126–127
  netiquette and communication, 127–129
  online presence, 129–131
  role of nurse educators, 140–144
  social presence, 131
  teaching presence, 132
  types of, 126

concept-based teaching, 27. *See also*
   conceptual learning
concept mapping, 147–164
   assimilation theory, 148
   in concept-based nursing curriculum,
      150–153
      used in graduate nursing program, 153
      used in prelicensure nursing program,
         151–153
   developing meaningful, 154–156
   faculty and student development,
      161–164
      evaluation, 163
      portfolio and, 163–164
   introduction, 147–150
   step-by-step approach, 156–161
      step 1, 157
      step 2, 157
      step 3, 157–158
      step 4, 158
      step 5, 158–159
      step 6, 159
      step 7, 159
      step 8, 159
      step 9, 161
      step 10, 161
   terminologies, 149–150
concept presentation, 52
conceptual framework, 8
conceptual learning
   benefits of, 28–33
      decreased content saturation, 28–30
      increased focus on nursing practice,
         30–31
      increased thinking and nursing
         judgment, 32–33
      opportunities for collaborative learning,
         31–32
      student engagement, 33
   concept mapping, usage of. *See* concept
      mapping
   description of, 28
   student learning outcomes, developing of,
      59–71
      achievement, measuring, 66–71
      conceptual content, 61–66
      course, 60–61
      introduction, 59–60
   vs. traditional learning, 23–34
constructed response test items, 199
constructivism, 27
content-related evidence, 187
   of measurement validity, 212–213
continuing case study, 179

correction true-false, 206
course decisions, considerations for, 14–15
course development, nursing curriculum and,
      18–20
   course content and evaluation,
      determination of, 19–20
   description, writing of, 18–19
criterion-referenced evaluation, 186–187
critical thinking, defined, 168
curricular drift, 244
curriculum, nursing, 3–21
   approval process, 20
   components of, 6–20
      course development, 18–20
      degree plan, 13–17
      mission, 8
      models, 12–13
      organizing curriculum framework,
         8–10
      philosophy, 8
      plan of study, 13–17
      program outcomes, 10–12
   definition, 3
   essential elements for, 3–21
   faculty role in development and
      revision, 4–6
   introduction, 3–4
   models, 12–13
      competency-based, 13
      concept-based, 13
      traditional model, 12–13
   nursing program accreditation,
      role of, 6

D

data mining assignments, 228–230
debriefing, 80
decision-making trees, 85
deep learning, 25
degree plan, nursing curriculum and, 14, 43
direct care activities (DCAs), 97, 212, 213
   formative evaluation of, 213–216
   summative evaluation of, 216–222
direct measurement of learning, 238
discussion boards, LMS and, 134
Disillusionment with Unprofessional
      Behaviors, 227
distractors, 200
double testing, 87
drag and drop/Rank order/ordered response
      items, 199

E

educational resource units (ERUs), 100
ELLs. *See* English Language Learners (ELLs)
end-of-program student learning outcomes, 238–240
English Language Learners (ELLs), 31, 78
environmental adjustments, 189
evaluation process, definition of, 186
evidence-based assignments, 228
exemplars, description of, 27, 48
exhibit items, 200
expected level achievement (ELA), 236, 239

F

fill-in-the-blank items, 199
flipped classroom, 80
focused learning activities (FLAs), 97, 212, 224–225
    clinical paper assignments, 227–228
    compare and contrast assignments, 231
    data mining assignments, 228–230
    graphic organizers, 231
    reflection papers, 225–227
formative evaluation, 186, 213–216
    quizzes for, 206

G

gaming, 91
gas exchange, lesson plan for concept, 253–254
grading, 70, 135
grading rubrics, 51, 68, 225–226
graphic organizers, 85, 231
group rooms, LMS and, 134

H

Health Promotion and Maintenance, 193–194
high-fidelity simulation (HFS), 223
hot spot test items, 199–200

I

indirect measurement of learning, 238
Integrated Processes (IP), 192–193

internal consistency, 187
interprofessional education (IPE), 32, 109
interrater reliability, 213
IPE. *See* interprofessional education (IPE)
item discrimination ratio (IDR), 204–205

J

Joint Commission's National Patient Safety
    Goals, 251
journaling, 227
journals, LMS and, 135

K

knowledge, skills, and attitudes (KSAs), 13, 23, 27, 212
Kuder-Richardson (KR)-20, 202

L

learning. *See also* clinical teaching and
    learning, CBC and; teaching
    brain functions in, 25
    characteristics of, 25–26
    in concept-based classroom, 73–93
    in concept-based nursing curriculum, 95–122
    conceptual, 28–33
    definition of, 25
    introduction, 23–24
    occurrence, reason for, 25
learning domain, considerations of, 187
learning management system (LMS), 132–137
learning materials, LMS and, 135
lesson plan, 54
let's discuss strategy, 82
linking words, 149
LMS. *See* learning management system (LMS)

M

macroconcepts, 46
matching items, 206
measurement validity, evidence of, 196–198
microconcepts, 46
mission, 8
mobility, concept presentation of, 249–250
multiple-response item, 199

N

narrative pedagogy, 88
National Council of State Boards of Nursing
  (NCSBN), 192
National League for Nursing's (NLN's),
  recommendation, 205–206
NCLEX®, 238
  cognitive levels of, 194–197
  general principles of, 200–202
  item formats, types of, 198–200
  style tests, 189, 192
  test plans, 192–194
NCLEX-PN®, 192
NCLEX-RN®, 192, 243
netiquette, 127
norm-referenced evaluation tools, 187
nullifying, 204
nurse educators, online learning environment
  and, 140–144
nurse generalist programs
  length of, 15–16
  and organizing curriculum framework, 9
nursing concept-based curriculum, 37–39
  12-step approach, 37–56
  transition from traditional, 39–41
nursing concepts, definition, 48
nursing concepts I, 255–256
nursing curriculum. See curriculum, nursing
nursing process, defined, 169, 192–193

O

Objective Structured Clinical Examination
  (OSCE), 224, 239
online course, 126
online learning environment, teaching in.
  See concept-based online learning
  environment, teaching in
online presence, 127–128
organizing curriculum framework, 8–10
  for advanced nursing practice programs,
    9–10
  for nurse generalist programs, 9
outcomes, meaning of, 235
oxygenation, 201
  concept of, 214

P

papers and projects assignment, 206–207
Patient Education, concept of, 216

pedagogies, 81
Performance-Based Development System
  (PBDS©), 239–240
perfusion, 201
philosophy, 8
Physiological Integrity, 194
plan of study, nursing curriculum and, 14, 43
point biserial coefficient (PBS). See point
  biserial index (PBI)
point biserial index (PBI), 204–205
portfolio, 239
prebriefing, 224
process, defined, 235
Professional Nursing concepts, 223
program evaluation, 233
  commonly used models of, 234–235
  evaluating outcomes concept-based
    curriculum, 243–245
  introduction to, 234
  systematic plan for, 235–236
    Course Student Learning Outcomes,
      240–242
    Curricular Outcomes, 238
    End-of-Program Student Learning
      Outcomes, 238–240
    Faculty Outcomes, 242–243
    Program Outcomes, 236–238
program learning outcomes (PLOs). See end-of
  -program student learning outcomes
program of study, 43
propositions, 149
psychomotor domain, 63–65, 69–70, 187
Psychosocial Integrity, 194

Q

Quality and Safety Education for Nurses
  (QSEN) Institute, 213
quizzes, 206
quizzing and testing functions, LMS and, 135

R

reflection, CBC and, 107
reflection papers, 225–227
reliability, evaluation tool, 187
reliability coefficient, factors can affect, 202

S

Safe and Effective Care Environment, 193
scaffolding, 115

Scantron® machine, 203
school of nursing (SON), program evaluation
    plan for, 235
scrambled classroom, 80
Select All That Apply (SATA) question, 199
selected response test items, 199
Send a Problem, learning activity, 87
short-answer items, 206
single-response item, 199
situated learning, 171
SLOs. *See* student learning outcomes (SLOs)
social presence, 131
Socratic questioning, 106
standardized patient (SP) methodology, 222
structure, meaning of, 235
structured controversy, 83
student behavioral modifications, 189
student learning outcomes (SLOs), 10,
    59–71, 137, 238. *See also* learning
    management system (LMS)
  achievement, measuring, 66–71
    affective domain, 70–71
    cognitive domain, 68–69
    psychomotor domain, 69–70
  conceptual content, by domains
    affective domain, 65–66
    cognitive domain, 61–63
    psychomotor domain, 63–65
  course, 60–61
  for Doctor of Nursing Practice (DNP)
    course, 187–188
  introduction, 59–60
summative clinical evaluation tool, 216–222
summative evaluation, 186
superficial learning, 26
synchronous online learning, 126
systematic plan for evaluation
  course student learning outcomes, 240–242
  curricular outcomes, 238
  end-of-program student learning out-
    comes, 238–240
  faculty outcomes, 242–243
  program outcomes, 236–238
systematic plan for evaluation (SPE), 234

T

taxonomy, 61
teaching. *See also* clinical teaching and
    learning, CBC and; learning
  characteristics of, 25–26
  in concept-based classroom, 73–93

  in concept-based nursing curriculum, 95–122.
    See also concept-based curriculum
  in concept-based online learning
    environment. *See* concept-based
    online learning environment
  conceptual, 27
  introduction, 23–24
teaching presence, 132
test blueprint, 196, 198
test item
  difficulty, 203
  discrimination, 203–205
Test Item Checks, 86
test plan. *See* test blueprint
test reliability, evidence of, 202
Therapeutic Communication and Patient-
    Centered Care, concepts of, 222
Think-Pair-Share, 82
traditional learning
  vs. conceptual learning, 23–34
true-false items, 206
12-step approach, concept-based curriculum
    development
  step 1, 42
  step 2, 42
  step 3, 43
  step 4, 43–46
  step 5, 43–48
  step 6, 48–50
  step 7, 50–51
  step 8, 51–52
  step 9, 52–53
  step 10, 54
  step 11, 54–55
  step 12, 55

U

unfolding case study, 175

V

validity, evaluation tool, 187
Venn diagrams, 85

W

What if. . . ? approach, 82
Wikis, LMS and, 134